UNDERSTANDING THE
HUMAN FOOT

An Illustrated Guide to Form and Function for Practitioners

With Introductory Assessments and Corrective Exercises

JAMES EARLS

Author of *Born to Walk* and *Fascial Release for Structural Balance*

Contributor *Lucy Wintle*

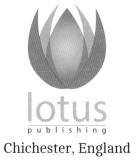

lotus
publishing

Chichester, England

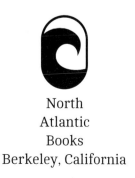

North
Atlantic
Books
Berkeley, California

First published in 2021 by
Lotus Publishing
Apple Tree Cottage, Inlands Road, Nutbourne, Chichester, PO18 8RJ, and
North Atlantic Books
Berkeley, California

Illustrations Amanda Williams
Photographs Rob at Lighttrapper Photography
Cover Design Chris Fulcher
Text Design Medlar Publishing Solutions Pvt Ltd., India
Printed and Bound in the UK by Bell and Bain Limited

Understanding the Human Foot: An Illustrated Guide to Form and Function for Practitioners is sponsored and published by North Atlantic Books, an educational nonprofit based in Berkeley, California, that collaborates with partners to develop cross-cultural perspectives, nurture holistic views of art, science, the humanities, and healing, and seed personal and global transformation by publishing work on the relationship of body, spirit, and nature.

North Atlantic Books' publications are distributed to the US trade and internationally by Penguin Random House Publishers Services. For further information, visit our website at www.northatlanticbooks.com.

Medical Disclaimer
The following information is intended for general information purposes only. Individuals should always consult their health care provider before administering any suggestions made in this book. Any application of the material set forth in the following pages is at the reader's discretion and is his or her sole responsibility.

British Library Cataloguing-in-Publication Data
A CIP record for this book is available from the British Library
ISBN 978 1 913088 26 2 (Lotus Publishing)
ISBN 978 1 62317 657 0 (North Atlantic Books)

Library of Congress Cataloguing-in-Publication Data

Names: Earls, James, author.
Title: Understanding the human foot : an illustrated guide to form and
    function for practitioners / James Earls.
Description: Berkeley : North Atlantic Books, 2021. | Includes
    bibliographical references and index. | Summary: "An essential resource
    for bodyworkers, physical therapists, and sports medicine
    practitioners-a vital guide to understanding the anatomy, form, and
    mechanics of the human foot"-- Provided by publisher.
Identifiers: LCCN 2021023157 (print) | LCCN 2021023158 (ebook) | ISBN
    9781623176570 (trade paperback) | ISBN 9781623176587 (ebook)
Subjects: LCSH: Foot. | Foot--Physiological aspects.
Classification: LCC QM549 .E27 2021 (print) | LCC QM549 (ebook) | DDC
    612.9/8--dc23
LC record available at https://lccn.loc.gov/2021023157
LC ebook record available at https://lccn.loc.gov/2021023158

CONTENTS

CLOSER TO THE HEART

Philosophers and ploughmen
Each must know his part
To sow a new mentality
Closer to the heart

Neil Peart, 1952–2020

THANKS

This book has been a companion to me during the events of 2020. That long, dark year saw much change in the world, with many moments of quiet reflection, of mourning, of loss, and also many moments of hope and new possibilities. There were many stories of the power of community, the power of communication, and connection and I hope that those important lessons are retained as we re-enter the world.

Many of us realised the significance of the people around us and, just as it takes a village to raise a child, so too does it take a village to write a book.

It is with love and appreciation that I acknowledge the support given to me by Owen Lewis (who bravely suffered through early drafts), Mark Parfitt-Jones, Lauri Nemetz, and Holly Clemons, who all gave open and honest feedback.

The wonderful team from Lotus Publishing, especially Jon and Amanda, who patiently receive my constant alterations and edits, thank you!

A special thanks is reserved for Lucy Wintle, author of chapter 9, who wandered into this project halfway through yet still managed to create a fantastic sequence of moves with such little guidance and so few ideas from me.

And of course, my kind, patient, and supportive wife, Liza, who manages to help guide me along the winding paths I somehow find myself on and brings me back to the light— thank you for finding me.

Lastly, a request to every reader of this book—we all have choices to make in this world, let's make good choices, let's make a better world, one that is closer to our hearts.

James Earls
London, May 2021

FOREWORD

Thank you, dear James, for giving me the honor of adding a foreword to this excellent new publication. But this confronts me with the challenging dilemma of having planned to complete my text within a few hours, as I usually do with other foreword invitations, but now finding myself so captivated by the many brilliant chapters of this book, that I want to continue reading every single page of it, just for my own personal enjoyment and education.

Even without your invitation—and beyond my high personal respect for your past contributions in our shared field of exploring the human body from a functional perspective—I would have put this book on my personal "*have-to*" list. I certainly recommend doing so too for everyone interested in learning about the miracle of our living body. Chances are high that several times during one's lifetime one will be confronted with health conditions in the human foot, whether it is one's own feet or those of other people of importance, such as family members or patients.

If I had a few years in my future life to devote myself to studying one part of the human body, I would so far have been torn between different personal options up to recently. But after starting to delve into the exciting journey of this book, I have no doubts: there is no more fascinating part of our body than the human foot, at least when exploring it through James Earls' curiosity-oriented and functional perspective!

Dear reader, please be prepared to face a similar dilemma when picking up this outstanding book. You will certainly profit thoroughly from skipping through the book, like we all do, by sporadically looking at the beautiful images and their well-written legends, as well as reading the subtitles and helpful summaries at the end of each chapter. But I promise that after doing so, this book will captivate your deeper attention, to seduce you into following the author's journey into a deeper understanding of how your body works, as seen from the most fundamental part of it.

One of the many highlights of this book, not found elsewhere in such a captivating manner, is the evolutionary perspective, how the human foot is intimately linked to the specific adaptation of our *Homo sapiens* ancestors to their gatherer and hunter lifestyle. Drawing on the author's extensive background as an internationally renowned bodywork and movement instructor this approach is followed up with a functional review of the musculoskeletal anatomy, in which the foot is not seen in isolation, but rather as part of several myofascial chains connecting it with the rest of the living body.

The author of *Born to Walk* 2020—a previous milestone contribution—takes you into an inspiring exploration of the art of walking as well as running. To me this felt as rejuvenating as being a fish who is re-learning to swim or a bird to fly, yet with improved elegance, refinement, and joy. If not enough, this central part of the book is finally followed up with practical recommendations for how to improve the wellbeing of your feet with specific therapeutic or movement interventions. These are excellently instructed in an easy to follow and clearly understandable manner.

And now I am torn between wanting to continue reading—rather than skipping through—the detailed explorations of this exciting book, or to taking my shoes off and playing with some of the novel exercises described in the last chapters outside in my garden. Dear James, thank you so much, for deeply enriching my intellectual curiosity as well as my sensuous experience with this wonderful choice.

Robert Schleip
Munich, Germany
June 2021

James Earls is a scholar and a gentleman; and it is precisely this quality of scholarship that makes this book an absolute necessity for the library of every serious therapist, regardless of their type or affiliation. This is a book for everyone who wants to build a more comprehensive vision of how the body really moves.

Anatomically, what is the foot? What makes our feet different from the feet of our ancestors? Why are human feet unique in the animal kingdom? Did we develop the shape of our feet, so to speak, as hunter-gatherers in order to migrate to the next food area while expending as few calories as possible? Is walking just controlled falling, or is it more elegant than that? Are my feet genetic destiny, or can I have some mechanical input into their shaping? Does my running form make this better or worse? Should I toe run or heel strike? And, oh my god, shoes! Why are shoes so difficult?

James answers all of these questions and more with uniquely ecumenical spirit. In doing so, he gives all of us the information required to find our own footing with these issues.

He does this by weaving together comparative and evolutionary anatomy, functional anatomy, fascial anatomy, "anatomy" anatomy, muscular forces and actions, morphology, and cellular dynamics, showing how all of these elements combine to impact, and be impacted by, the part of body most designed for impact.

Yet for all his exhaustive research he never exhausts the reader. James is a better author than that. The very necessary exacting level of scientific detail combined with his genial good humor, clear examples, revealing and excellent illustrations make this a joy to read.

And read it with joy I have, and read it with joy again I shall, because it's so full of important, real-life movement and anatomy gems that I want to ensure that I have a thorough working knowledge of all of them. Both to improve my own biomechanical life, and the biomechanical lives of my patients.

So let's turn the page and perambulate with gentleman, scholar, and my friend James Earls. You'll be thinking on your feet in no time.

David Lesondak
University of Pittsburgh Medical Center
Center for Integrative Medicine
Pittsburgh, PA, USA
June 2021

INTRODUCTION

According to Dudley J Morton, a guiding light for this book, "the story of how man became a biped is written in the language of biomechanics." Now that might be because evolutionary texts focus on fossil finds and their analyses of various tendon tunnels and bony bumps, or perhaps it truly is because "anatomy is our destiny." Morton believed it was the development of a modern foot that allowed our first step toward our destiny — toward becoming *Homo sapiens*.

There are many anatomical elements that define our species — the shape and size of the skull, the curvature of our spine, the alignment of the pelvis — but there is only one truly unique feature, our chin. No-one really knows why *Homo sapiens* alone have mental protuberances (the rather odd anatomical name for chins), although theories abound as to why the body wastes some of its finite resources to build bone with no special function or benefit.

This book is not about chins, instead it focuses on the opposite end of the body to explore our feet — those often-ignored extensions on the ends of our legs. Our feet are not unique in the same manner as the mental protuberance, many animals share similar numbers and shapes of bone, ligament, and muscles. But during our evolutionary history, the collection of tissues that constitute the human foot altered in a way that perhaps, single-footedly, set us on a course toward energy efficiency movement. The calories we saved by developing an upright and long stride provided enough surplus energy to produce an expensive bony feature that has no particular purpose other than giving us something to stroke in mental contemplation.

If you are concerned that you might end up scratching or playing with your own chin in frustration as you work your way through yet another dry textbook of anatomy and biomechanics then, please, breathe deeply and relax those jaw muscles. It is my aim and, perhaps, my duty to make this journey as pain-free as possible. I know the frustrations of trying to learn anatomy — the words are obscure and long, the same structures are referred to by different names in different texts, and there are long, complicated descriptors used for just one bone with only hints of its context, purpose, or function.

I aim to deal with each of these frustrations as we progress through the text. There is a beauty to much of the language of anatomy (admittedly, many annoyances too, but we'll concentrate on the positives for now) and we will explore some of the meanings behind the names and the rationale for them. Where numerous terms are used for an individual structure, I will try to list them all and, when possible, explain the reasons for, or advantages of, the different terms. But, most of all, I hope this book will **explain** anatomy—not just repeat the usual dry descriptions but actually put it into context for you.

My experience of anatomy classes and texts has been pretty frustrating—I assume many of yours have been too. Many times, they are designed to hammer in the same facts and figures to get you through an exam and, fingers crossed, through repetition, maybe get you to see how the it all fits together in real-life.

Understanding the Human Foot is my attempt to teach anatomy the way I wish I had been taught 30 years ago. We will start with the big picture— what is a foot and what is it used for? Then, how does it work? How does it work, and what role do all those frustrating little bits with long names play in the foot's many functions?

We will go from the big picture to the small and back out again. I find that if I understand something about a whole system, the features within the parts become much easier to comprehend. As with a jigsaw puzzle, it is so much easier if I know what the final picture should look like. I can slot the pieces in where they belong rather than having to study the grooves, contours, and colors of each piece to try to find where they might fit.

Many facts and figures are bandied about when discussing the foot—26 bones, one quarter of the bones of the body are foot bones, 33 joints controlled by hundreds of muscles, tendons, and ligaments.

I don't care.

Well, I do a little. If I didn't, I would not be writing this text. But being able to list the figures, even name the structures, is not the same as understanding the implications of each feature, and that is where true knowledge and its associated power comes from.

This book cannot be totally comprehensive, to do so would put it beyond the financial and concentration range of most readers.

I have a particular reader in mind for this book—me. Me of 25 years ago, when I was struggling to progress my bodywork practice and straining to decipher my clients' bodies. I tried to read the advanced anatomy textbooks, I attended numerous trainings, but there were few resources that could translate the dense literature and language I encountered.

The language created a barrier and there seemed to be no single book that could give me a helping hand. Searching for something—I didn't know what—I bought a multitude of books, DVDs, and videos (internet was not so advanced in those days), but they were either too advanced or too simple. Eventually, once I had collected a library's worth of texts, I saw there was something missing. I had the introductions and the arcane tomes, but nothing in between. I hope this book will sit in the middle, a step up from basic anatomy that acts as a guide to seeing the full picture with greater clarity and confidence.

Rather than list the numbers of tissues contained in the foot, Morton was much more eloquent when describing its complexities—a *"Multiplicity of mobile parts, the simultaneous actions of many joints, also the constantly changing magnitude and direction of forces in each segment, and the various contributing rules of accessory factors (mechanical and otherwise), give it the complexity of infinite detail that defies direct mechanical analysis."*

Although celebrating its complexity, Morton was also forewarning us. There is much to learn and many of the actions, functions, and interactions of the foot occur at the same time, making them difficult to describe in a linear text. We will have to loop back and forth in our explorations and, although that may feel frustrating at times, the final view is worth it in the end.

I hope this book will provide many tools to help you appreciate the foot's wonder and provide the visual and verbal vocabularies to comprehend its function.

1

THE HUMAN FOOT

▥ INTRODUCTION

There are two heroes in this story: the human foot and Dr. Dudley Joy Morton (1884–1960). Dr. Morton, born in Baltimore, Maryland, completed his medical training at Hahnemann College, Pennsylvania, and became one of the most famous medical authorities in the U.S. during the first half of the twentieth century. A major reason for that fame was his encyclopedic knowledge of the human foot, built on his appreciation of comparative anatomy. Born 25 years after the publication of Darwin's *Origin of Species* (1859), Dr. Morton was quick to use insights gleaned from the developing science of evolution.

Although not often referenced as such, feet are a defining element of the human anatomy. According to Morton, our feet have been *"remodelled so specifically for the pattern of gravitational stresses imposed by our upright carriage that the detailed features call for the same thoughtful regard as is given to the specialized tissues of the eyeball in a comprehensive study of sight."*[1]

As we embark on that thoughtful regard this book will repeat Morton's belief when he quoted Wood Jones—*"If missing links are to be tracked with complete success, the foot, far more than the skull, or the teeth or the shins; will mark them as monkey or man. It is in the grades of evolution of the foot that the stages of the missing link will be most plainly presented to the future palaeontologist."*[2]

Evolutionary changes in the foot coincide with our first adaptations to terrestrial, upright gait, which created a new relationship with gravity. Our new form of locomotion with its vertical alignment to gravity provided numerous efficiencies—efficiencies recouped by savings in calories at a time when the calorie was the only currency that mattered. The math is simple: spending fewer calories in the pursuit of more digestible calories allows reallocation of the savings. Those calorie savings helped fuel the many migrations our ancestors made, spreading far and wide over the African continent and, eventually, further afield.

Of course, our upright gait afforded other benefits as well—reduced exposure to the midday sun as our backs were no longer

---

[1]Morton D.J., *Human Locomotion and Body Form*, 1963, page viii.

[2]Morton D.J., *The Human Foot*, 1935, page 52.

facing directly skyward, hands that were free for tool manufacture and usage, and a new view of the world as we brought our eyes above the level of tall grasses. Each of these benefits, among many others, has been touted as the driving force behind the evolution of bipedalism, but I believe each benefit forms one strand in a complex weave of interrelated factors that set us on the path toward our current anatomical shape. Each listed benefit has some positive effect on calorie expenditure—better heat management reduces metabolic cost, use of tools allows the more efficient capture and processing of food sources, and a better view of the world assists with the hunting of prey and, importantly, early warning of the approach of predators (it should be said that prevention of turning oneself into someone or something else's calories is possibly the most important factor when measuring the success of a species!). The cumulative calorie savings could then be put to good use in the form of expensive tissues, such as the larger brain our ancestors ultimately developed.

However, our evolution is a much more complex story. It is a story that seems to be rewritten almost every week with new paleontological and genetic discoveries, and it deserves more investigation than the simple paragraphs above. But we have limited space and doubtless whatever is written this week will be out of date next. Our research into the role of the foot must be put into context if we are to truly understand the numerous interactions made by its "multiplicity of parts" in response to "the constantly changing magnitude and direction of forces"[3] dealt with in each step.

For Morton, and for this book, the human foot is an essential physical and metaphorical indicator of where we have come from, where we can get to, and how we navigate

our present. Feet have entered our lexicon as symbols of movement, expression, enslavement, or clumsiness—think of how one starts a journey with the best foot forward and we expedite ("free the feet") our deliveries when there are possible impediments in their way. We may get cold feet at a wedding before our clumsy uncle with two left feet asks for a dance. One may also land on her feet after they have been held to the fire while hoping they are not made of clay. After a life lived at pace (from passus, Latin: step), our coffin is carried from the church feet first lest we wish to return. The coffins of Christian priests, however, are removed from the church head-first as it is hoped that they will return in spirit to manage over their flock.

Prior to reaching the coffin, we have probably abused and ignored our feet more than any other part of the body. We have invented myriad encasements of abuse that we call shoes, while using our feet to assist us through dance, sports, and many miles of walking. Feet truly are the Cinderellas of the human form. We squeeze our feet into slippers (glass or otherwise) and, sometimes even train them en pointe. But while feet have been bound, confined, and abused by various means throughout history, so too have they been worshipped.

From Degas' dancers, Botticelli's Venus and the sculptures of Michelangelo, the elegant curve of the foot has been displayed for our admiration. Despite its 250,000 sweat glands, or perhaps because of the associated pheromones, the foot is considered the most common of all sexual fetishes, capable of working its charm more than any other variation of body shape or size.

In contrast to the elegance and attraction of the natural curve, the flat foot has, quite unfairly, become a symbol of the distasteful, inelegant, dangerous, weak, even the "other". At various times, a flat foot was considered the mark of Pan, patron of witches; used by the Nazis as a

---

[3]See introduction for reference to the quotes – you didn't skip the intro, did you???

defining feature of the Jews along with their supposedly short, curved legs; and, during the eighteenth and nineteenth centuries, flat feet were considered a defining feature of the "primitive" cultures of Africa and Asia. Having a flat foot marked you as a bad omen for "first footing" on New Year's Day in Scotland. In fact, the only apparent benefit of having flat feet was that it probably ruled you out of serving in almost any national army (but then one ran the risk of being labeled a flat-footed coward for not enrolling).

Sadly, many of these prejudices are still in our language and cultures, even our medicine. We still tend to see flat footedness as a weakness rather than a possible normal variation along the distribution curve. Like so many things in life, it is not what you have that matters, it is how you use it that really counts. A foot that appears particularly flat, or one that has an overly high arch, may still be able to perform all the functions required of a foot. We just need to know what those functions are.

To truly grasp the complexity of the human foot, we must understand the environment in which it operates. One's choice of footwear is one aspect of that environment, but the foot also operates in the context of the constantly changing focus of gravity, ground reaction force, and momentum. Rather than replicating the non-contextual, force-free world presented in most anatomy texts, we will examine the foot—with Morton's occasional guidance along the way—considering its form, function, and environment.

KNOWING, NOT NAMING

The great physicist Robert Feynman talks of the difference between knowing the name of something and actually knowing something— "You can know the name of a bird, but when you're finished, you'll know absolutely nothing whatever about the bird...So let's look at the bird and see what it is doing – that's what counts."

Have you considered why a bone has a particular shape, why muscle fibers are arranged in different patterns, or why tendons vary in length and thickness? As is often the case, these apparently simple questions require quite long answers, ones I explore in the following chapters. Knowing—or, better still, understanding—a system requires appreciation of both the micro and the macro. Without knowing where a part lies and what function it plays; we can only know its name. Conversely, seeing only the grand picture misses out on the intricacies of the working parts.

Coming to know the system of the human foot will require each chapter to zoom our focus in to the detail and out again to the broader context in which the foot operates. This chapter and the next, aim to give the overall context of the big picture.

FEET, GRAVITY, AND ALIGNMENT

It has long been my belief that anatomy is generally taught in the wrong direction—from the smaller details to the larger form. Then, only once we have the minutiae in place, do we try to understand function. My experience is that any complex system is better understood if we first have an overview of its context. We will start our journey by looking at the overall functions of the foot—what does it do, why does it do those things, and what are the forces involved?

The learning process will not be exactly linear, as to understand the functions we must explore the forces, and to appreciate how the foot deals with those forces we will need a little bit of anatomy. Sadly, functional anatomy cannot be rote learned like the alphabet. A few sections, especially parts of the chapters on bone and soft tissue (3 to 5), may at first appear to be diversions into areas beyond the foot but, rest assured, they are there to assist appreciation of the whole form and its complexity. Spending some time with the less familiar background to tissue development will help build the picture upward beyond the foot to the rest of our anatomy and develop an appreciation of our wonderful shape.

The foot is possibly the most challenging area to begin any study of biomechanics due to the large number of different tissues, each with varying densities and stiffnesses. Thankfully, there is a logic behind both the arrangement of the tissues and the descriptive language used to describe anatomy and function. For many of us that language is foreign, confusing, and frustrating—I hope it becomes less so once we build the picture of the interactions and see how form and function are intertwined. When function and anatomy are seen together, the whole Gestalt is more easily understood.

One of the first questions to answer is "why all the fuss about upright gait"? The short answer is easily provided by mimicking the gait of a chimp, with bent hip and bent knee—the experiment quickly provides us with an immediate sense of the benefit of vertically stacked bones. A few lumbering steps reveal the extra energy required to maintain bent limbs as the increased muscular load rapidly fatigues one's thighs and low back. To measure the effects of bent limbs, Abitbol (1988) compared changes in the metabolic rates between dogs, children, and adults when supine, standing bipedally, walking bipedally, standing quadrupedally, and walking quadrupedally. Abitbol found moving from supine to standing caused a significant increase in energy use for the dog but not so for humans. Our gravity-aligned stance does not require much increase of energy when compared with lying down. The most significant jump in human metabolic rate occurred when adopting quadrupedal strategies as they require bending the limbs and pitching the center of gravity forward.

Numerous experiments, such as Abitbol's, have demonstrated the metabolic efficiencies created by moving away from quadrupedal standing and locomotion. Our characteristic straight knees and extended hips allow an S-shaped spine to enter the skull under its center of gravity and for the overall center of gravity to land between both feet. This contrasts with the costly features inherent in quadrupedalism— bent joints in the supporting limbs, and the forward position of the heavy head and jaws (see fig. 1.1).

This transition to upright stance required evolutionary changes in our feet. Walking with bent limbs may be metabolically costly, but it offers quadrupeds varying degrees of shock absorption. Everything in nature is about finding the best cost-benefit balance between varying demands, in this case, between shock absorption and calorie cost. Our limbs must support and propel us, but they must also manage impact forces created with every step. Angles at each joint between the ground and the hips or shoulders in quadrupeds allow the soft tissue to absorb and manage those forces (figs. 1.1 & 1.2)—beneficial in some ways (which we will explore in chapter 5) but also metabolically costly. The straight-legged gait of *Homo sapiens* has removed most of the bend in the ankle and knee and, by bringing the calcaneus onto the ground, localized much of the shock management role into the feet.

Our straight-legged gait pattern reduces the number of angled joints between the ground and our center of gravity. Any increase in joint angle, or the number of angles between our contact with the ground and our center of gravity, increases the workload on the muscles controlling those joints. Using a stacked-bones strategy for human heel strike reallocates some force management demands away from the soft tissues and into the skeletal system. Allowing the denser and stiffer bones to deal with a greater portion of the reaction forces is one of the factors that helps us walk twice as far as our bent-knee, bent-hip chimpanzee

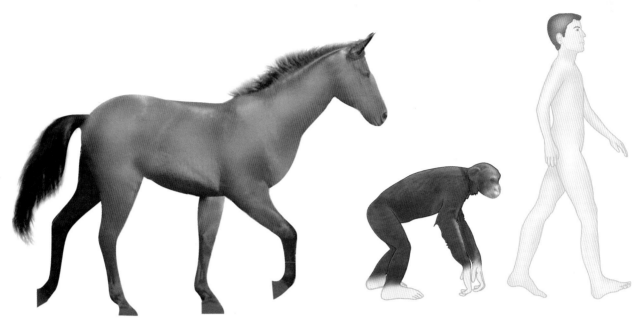

Figure 1.1.   Our upright bipedal stance requires numerous anatomical features including changes in the feet, pelvis, spine, and head. The roles performed by the feet for each species relates to their locomotor strategies and to the abilities of the rest of their anatomy. Our feet have some unique abilities but we have also lost some—most of which have been adopted by other parts of the body, especially the hips.

cousins, using the same number of calories. This disparity in efficiency is reduced when we begin to run, a movement style that tends to use bent-limb strategies and causes metabolic

costs to rise to similar levels as the knuckle-walking chimpanzee (Foster et al. 2013; Pontzer 2017).

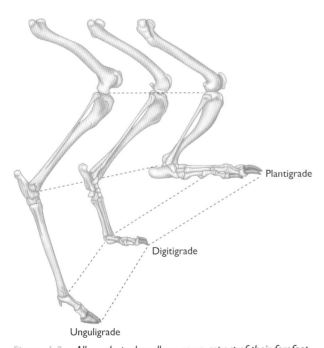

Figure 1.2.   All quadrupeds walk on some aspect of their forefoot. Ungulates have extended their toes and developed hooves, and digitigrades use various aspects of their toes. Plantigrade animals, including Homo sapiens, walk on their full foot and often strike the ground with their calcaneus.

■ SHOCK ABSORPTION, POWER PRODUCTION, AND SUPPORT

Quadrupeds appear to use each limb in a similar fashion when walking but quite differently when jumping and landing. Hind legs are used when extra power is required, and the front legs are used to absorb forces at landing (see fig. 1.3). There are a few reasons for this, the obvious one being that it is easier to push forward from the back than pull from the front, but it is also inherent within the anatomy. The hind limbs are connected to the axial skeleton via the relatively deep and secure hip joints. This contrasts with the muscular sling for the forelimbs, which provides a soft tissue suspension to deal with landing forces.

While horse anatomy may not seem like an obvious place to start our human investigation, it does emphasize the "design" genius of the

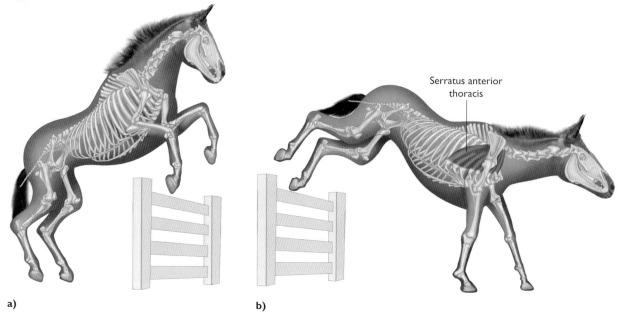

Serratus anterior
thoracis

a)   b)

Figure 1.3.   a) The hind legs of quadrupeds are strongly connected to the axial skeleton and provide efficient force transfer from the limbs to the trunk. b) The equine equivalent of the serratus anterior provides a soft tissue harness for the front legs, which allows the myofascial system to absorb most of the forces on landing.

human foot, which must perform the roles of both hind and forelegs in quadrupeds—providing a stable platform for propulsion as well as shock absorption on landing. A major aim of this text is to appreciate how the aggregation of tissues in the foot combine to create a so-called "rigid lever" and a "mobile adaptor" at the appropriate times.

Our feet are the Swiss Army knife of the body—beautifully designed, compact, and multifunctional. Human feet have developed anatomical features that allow shock absorption and stability, both functions and anatomy that differentiate our feet from those of other primates. The most obvious of these differences are enlarged heels, adducted great toes, and an arched arrangement to the structure of the whole foot. Each feature provides benefits that we will explore through the rest of the text, but it is crucial to keep in mind the complete picture of the foot in context of the rest of the body.

No piece of anatomy works in isolation, whether it be a tissue, organ, or limb. There are always interactions with other body parts,

organs, systems, and the environment. The latter element being particularly true of our feet—they are probably the most frequent points of interaction between our body and the environment, making them an essential source of proprioceptive information for coordination, balance, support, and locomotion.

Structures with conflicting multiple requirements call for complex engineering solutions. It is, therefore, no surprise that feet come supplied with so many sensory endings, bones, joints, ligaments, and muscles. The mechanical requirements for each function do not always complement one another, but thankfully, biology has found ways to work around conflicting demands to find working compromises. For example, our support and balance would be easier with a wider foot and a more flexible big toe but walking straight ahead is more efficient with an alignment of joints from toes, to ankle, knees, and hip.

Balancing on two feet when standing, and on one foot during gait, benefits from an adaptable, mobile foot, but dealing with the forces at heel strike and toe-off is best done with a more robust, compacted structure—we are back to the mobile shock absorber and the stable platform dichotomy. The demand for mobility in the feet is related to our need for support, balance, and overall stability. Humans must support our relatively tall, straight structure over two narrow points of contact. In common with many animals, we gain support from the front of the foot as it projects forward, but we have no tail at the back to counterbalance our body weight. To compensate for the loss of a tail, we have developed a slightly longer heel that projects posteriorly (fig. 1.4). The increased body of the calcaneus also assists with shock absorption at heel strike; its rounded form helps roll us forward through to the ankle and toe joints before toe-off (more below as we investigate the role of momentum).

Most animals are assisted in their balance by supporting themselves with feet placed directly below the hip and shoulder joints. Our other primate cousins also have generally broader feet compared with ours, so we must compensate for lack of width of stance as well as narrow feet. To help us, the human foot is arranged in a way that let its bones spread slightly as our weight comes onto the forward foot during gait. The spreading of the foot is part of the shock absorption response mentioned above

and it gives more freedom to the joints. Letting the bones adjust to the terrain and distributing force into the soft tissues is part of the "mobile adaptor" function of our feet.

Some of the functions performed by feet seen in other species (see fig. 1.2) are offset to other areas of the human body. The wide chimpanzee foot with its abducted strong great toe provides much greater support and control than our narrow alternative. However, our lateral stability during gait has been pushed upward to the hip (see fig. 1.5). By turning the ilia and therefore the gluteal muscles to face outward, we can bring the hip into adduction to swing the center of gravity toward the foot's point of support on the ground. This is supported by the inward angle of the femurs as they come down to the tibial plateaux from the hip joints. During the early stance phase of gait, our feet, especially toward the forefoot, also spread to add support.

BONE VERSUS SOFT TISSUE SHOCK ABSORPTION

To understand the implications of our alignment with gravity, we must appreciate the roles and properties of the body's different tissues. As we saw above, any bend in the

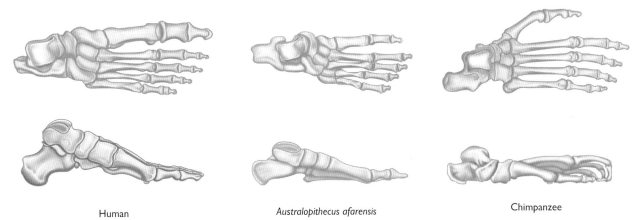

Human   Australopithecus afarensis   Chimpanzee

Figure 1.4.   Numerous adaptations have occurred in the human foot to facilitate our style of gait. These include the adducted big toe, which brings the toe, ankle, knee, and hip joints into closer alignment during a stride; and a posteriorly projecting calcaneus for greater stability and support during stance, and for shock absorption during gait. The feet of Australopithecus afarensis and a chimpanzee are shown for comparison and will be further investigated in later chapters.

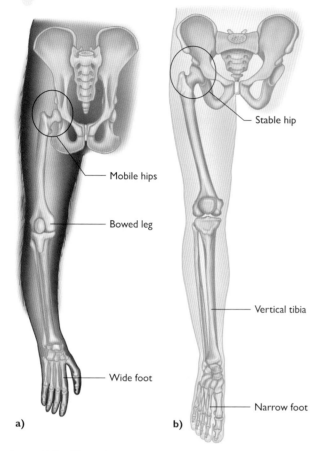

a)

b)

Mobile hips

Bowed leg

Wide foot

Stable hip

Vertical tibia

Narrow foot

Figure 1.5.   The wide platform of the chimpanzee's foot provides a greater range of support, but the anatomy of the hip offers less. The situation is reversed in the human condition, a narrow foot but a laterally stable hip.

joints causes an increase in muscle use, and our reasonably vertical arrangement allows our bones to be "stacked" for some natural, architectural support. However, unlike the building blocks of our childhood, bones are not stable. Our bones have smooth surfaces that curve in many directions, are covered in slick cartilage, and are separated from one another by joint spaces filled with synovial fluid. The skeletal system requires contractile, tensile support from muscles—hence the calorie savings when each bone is kept more closely in line with its neighbor during weight-bearing.

As with most other tissues in the body, bone is a dynamic tissue continually remodeling itself in response to forces passing through it—an idea expressed in Wolff's law, first proposed in 1892 (see chapter 3). The mechanism driving

bone remodeling is complex and not fully understood, but in chapter 3 we will explore how bone balances its mineral and organic composition for apparent weight efficiency in the context of its ability to provide stability, and still bend and compress in response to stress.

Bone is often considered a stable element, but as part of its shock absorption role it can bend (Lieberman 1997; van Wingerden et al. 1993). Bone plays numerous roles within the context of functional anatomy but we must see it as only a part (although a significant one) of the body's stability and force management system. As the function of bones varies according to their shape and position, we cannot analyze or make sense of any bone in isolation.

We can get some sense of the skeleton's significant role in shock absorption by comparing strike patterns during running. The foot's initial contact with the ground during running has had a lot of attention over the last decade in response to the rise in popularity of "barefoot" running. Forefoot or mid-foot landing strategies while running have been suggested by many to improve efficiency and reduce running-related injuries. However, critics of this approach suggest that it simply moves the shock absorption role from the skeleton during a heel strike to the soft tissues. Landing on some portion of the foot in front of the heel bone puts extra demand into the soft tissues that have to control the "bends" created at the ankle joint—essentially, when running "barefoot", we are running like digitigrades (see fig. 1.2) on a series of bent joints.

Relatively stacked bones decrease the stresses placed on soft tissue. The benefits and costs of forefoot versus heel striking when running have been investigated with varying results. Many review papers are inconclusive as to the best strategy, and many suggest it is best to leave the choice to the runner's own sense of comfort and efficiency. The main point to remember is that changing foot strike strategy alters how the body receives and deals with stressors and each of us varies in our functional abilities to adapt. Factors that may limit our adaptation may include skeletal form and soft tissue strength and stiffness—we all differ slightly in our anatomy.

As with running, advocacy for forefoot striking in walking has also been a recurrent theme in some quarters. Forefoot walking seems to raise its head every so often and instructive videos are available via YouTube, but it is not a recent phenomenon. Morton dismissed forefoot walking summarily in *Human Locomotion and Body Form* by clearly stating that, unlike running, forefoot striking is not observed in "primitive cultures" as they walk. Heel striking when walking is not an "invention" allowed by modern shoes. Habitual use of cushioned fashionable shoes is likely to have simply decreased the natural protection of calluses which develop in response to shock.

I mention both strategies, "barefoot" running and forefoot walking, to reassure the reader that this text is not borne from "believerism" in any one system. It is my belief that we need to understand functional anatomy from a complex systems approach and there will be no "one size fits all" recommendations. My hope is that, through appreciation of the anatomy of each tissue and their function, novel assessment and treatment strategies may be developed, and those already learned will have greater context and application.

EFFICIENCY AND ENDURANCE

There are two critical aspects to locomotor strategies—efficiency (the cost of transport) and endurance (the distance one can travel). Morton and many other researchers focused on the idea of increased efficiency helping to drive evolution. It was not until relatively recently that the work of Prof. Daniel Lieberman and

colleagues brought forward the associated dynamic of endurance, particularly with a view to running and its creation of a new hunting strategy to increase sources of calories.

Endurance is related to efficiency—the more efficient one's movement strategy, the further you can go—but endurance is also related to metabolic measures such as oxygen consumption, lactate threshold, temperature, and breath control. From an anatomical point of view, there are certain markers to show the role of the foot in different locomotor strategies, and Lieberman argues that the foot acts as a rigid lever in walking but more as a spring during running, and it is not until quite recently in our evolution that we see the changes in the foot that allow it to act as a spring—to use elastic properties.

While we might not use the foot to its full elastic ability when walking, our stride certainly benefits from the foot's ability to pronate. As the foot opens it can adapt to the surface for grip, and the slight separation between the bones strains the soft tissues with their associated mechanoreceptors. Changing tissue tension is an important element in receiving proprioceptive information about the mechanical environment, and although Lieberman emphasizes the lack of spring in walking, pronation is still a vital functional element to our stride and thereby adds to overall endurance.

The line-up shown in fig. 1.6 overleaf gives us an impression of how each anatomical change helped produce a longer and straighter-legged stride. Increasing the length of the lower limbs produces a longer stride, which means fewer steps can be taken to cover the same distance. But that longer stride can only happen with the ability to heel strike on the forward foot and with decreased angles at each joint.

Stride length is also related to events of the rear limb as well. The longer stride requires the back heel to lift which forces the toes, knee,

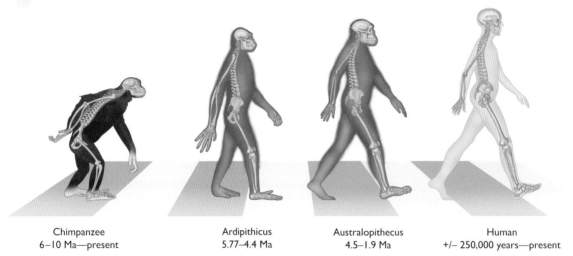

Chimpanzee	Ardipithicus	Australopithecus	Human
6–10 Ma—present	5.77–4.4 Ma	4.5–1.9 Ma	+/– 250,000 years—present

Figure 1.6.   *The black and white bars of the zebra crossing (crosswalk) represent one meter to illustrate the relative stride length for each species. The Beatles-like line-up shows us the changes to the overall form and how they relate to stride length. Those changes include:*

1. The development of the S-shape spine and its central entry into the cranium.

2. The reduction in length of the upper limbs and increased length of the lower limbs.

3. The laterally facing ilia and subsequent repurposing of the gluteal muscles from purely hip extensors to also abductors of the hip.

4. Notice how the ischial tuberosities begin to project backward in Australopithecus *and* Human—*the angle helps improve hamstring leverage for hip extension when upright. Imagine the chimpanzee in quadrupedal stance; the ischial tuberosity projects posteriorly and the trunk angles forward against gravity.*

Many descriptions of the anatomical changes necessary for bipedalism are available in the literature but few focus on what Morton considered the most important—the changes in the feet. With an upright stance, straight-legged walk, and a penchant for running down prey over long distances, Homo sapiens *needed to develop a foot capable of responding to various demands. (Adapted from Pontzer 2017.)*

hip, and spine into extension. While each of the other species shown above can walk bipedally, their strides are shortened by either an anatomical or structural limitation of at least one of those ranges of motions. It is the full suite of joint alignment and range of motion that gives us our long step.

■ GROUND REACTION FORCE AND MOMENTUM

Long strides require a heel strike, and adaptations to the local bone, skin, and fat further support the heel strike as the most natural and normal walking strategy and one that is almost uniquely human. The calcaneus deals with more than just the force of gravity; it also manages forces coming from the impact with the ground and from the body's momentum as it passes over the foot. Being able to visualize the continuous interaction of each force (gravity, ground reaction, and momentum) will be part of the challenge to understand the foot's response but it is also a challenge to present those interactions in this limited two-dimensional space.

Our heel has several shock-absorbing mechanisms that assist efficiency of movement. Some impact force is first absorbed by a firm and thick fat pad on the heel before it makes its way through to the bone. That fat pad is further protected by skin layers that quickly thicken in response to increased change. One only needs to think of the transition from winter to summer habits in temperate climates when one moves from warm, enclosed, and relatively protected footwear to light summer sandals or even walking barefoot in the garden and on the beach. The first few days of summer may leave one's feet a little tender, but the skin quickly adapts, developing calluses designed to protect the area from any increase in the three forces of gravity, ground reaction force (GRF) and momentum.

Gravity is perhaps the most straightforward of the three as it is constant in both magnitude and direction while the other two (GRF and momentum) continuously vary in both these measures. The foot's reactions during side-to-side or backward momentum could both be considered within this text, but to simplify our story we will consider momentum mostly from the view of forward progression (however, understanding forward progression should help your own analysis of side-to-side or backward progression).

The second of the three forces, GRF is perhaps the most challenging to appreciate as it varies according to the force and angle of contact. A reaction force creates the sensation you feel on contacting any surface—your heel hits the ground, and you feel the ground push back to you—with varying degrees of force depending on the characteristics of the surface. The vibration caused by the reaction force is an essential source of information to

the mechanoreceptors in the foot and the rest of the body, which help coordinate the body's response.

GRF is oppositional to the body's contact with the terrain, and as such, it is continually changing as the foot progresses through from heel to toe (fig. 1.7a). The downward forces of gravity and momentum and the upward reaction force negotiate through bones that are not vertically aligned. The offsets between the bones (fig. 1.7b) create a tendency for the bones to move in specific directions in response to the flow of forces acting through them. The relationship between forces, bones and soft tissues is why Morton describes gait as an "interaction". There are many variables to be considered from bone shape to angle of contact, direction of movement, and muscle contraction.

Pressure plate analysis (fig. 1.7c) is often used to help visualize how the foot interacts with the

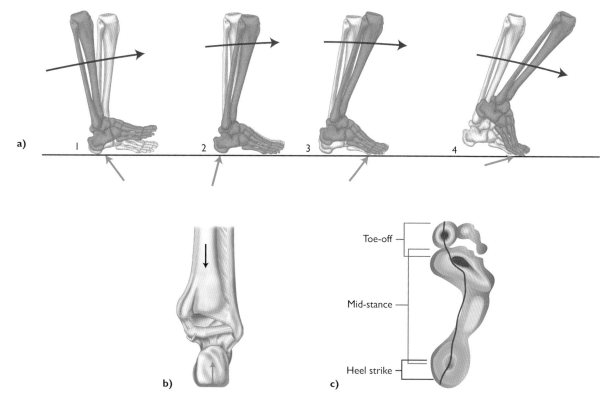

Figure 1.7.   a) GRF, indicated by the green arrow, changes in reaction to the foot's progression. b) The slight offset in the calcaneus and talus bones cause an offset between the opposing forces of gravity, GRF, and momentum to create a relatively predictable response through the rest of the foot and ankle complex. c) Force plate reading—three points marked, heel strike, mid-stance, and toe-off.

ground. Pressure plate readings are useful tools for gait analysis but are not always correctly interpreted unless you understand what is happening with the foot and the pressure through the step. The diagram looks like a footprint, but it is a print left after a step that has involved a heel strike, mid-stance, and toe-off.[4] We see two areas of high pressure at heel strike, and a spread of load during the mid-stance phase. Heel strike is easily understood as an impact and some of the shock is absorbed by the various tissues discussed above. The force reading is high prior to toe-off because less of the foot is in contact with the ground as the heel lifts as the toes extend.

The multi-purpose shock absorption mechanism, known as pronation, occurs as we adapt to the terrain and progress over the foot into weight-bearing. But the opening of the pronated foot must be reversed to create a stable platform able to deal with the many forces associated with toe-off and the foot's relative push back into the ground.

The force reading through the stance phase also indicates changes in foot stability through gait. As mentioned above, the foot can be a stable rigid lever while supinated, or a mobile adaptor while pronated. Handling the associated forces at the two peaks of force (heel strike and toe-off) is easier when the foot is supinated and providing a stable platform and a rigid lever. As weight is accepted onto the stance foot during gait, the other foot is swinging forward, so we only have one point of contact with the ground. Opening the foot into pronation to maximize its adaptability and widening it (albeit slightly) improves stability as the other limb swings forward.

The swinging leg provides the momentum for our forward progression over our specially adapted foot. Each of the phases, from heel

strike to toe-off, is facilitated by a series of rounded surfaces on the foot. The back of heel, the ankle joint, the ball of the foot, and the toe joints form so-called rockers (see fig. 1.9 and chapter 2) to keep us moving onward. The smooth joint surfaces and their alignment then allow the soft tissues to respond appropriately and, preferably, with minimal active input from the muscles. In an ideal foot, with an ideal environment, with an ideal momentum, the foot can be almost a self-working mechanism.

▥ SOFT TISSUES AND BONY ROCKERS

A common mistake is to assume the high force measure at toe-off (see fig. 1.7c) is created by the plantar flexor and toe flexor muscles pushing into the ground to propel us forward. That can be true, but the increase in force also represents the decreased contact surface area (therefore less distribution of bodyweight) coupled with the tensioning of many elastic elements, as the toes extend and plantar tissues stretch. Through this book, I prefer to use "toe-off" rather than the more common "push-off", as I believe pushing-off is an active action. Pushing-off with deliberate muscular contraction is not necessarily our default action, it is just one option available to us in response to movement variables, such as walking faster or uphill. To understand the complexity of the foot, we must appreciate it within the ecosystem of tissues and its response to forces.

Any ecosystem must work toward balancing the varied forces it is exposed to—in the plant world, rock type, ground soil conditions, altitude, aspect, latitude, and longitude, for example, will all affect biosystems. The foot must work within the context of its bones, soft tissues, and environmental forces and, like an active ecosystem, it can adapt in the short-and-long terms to environmental changes by

---

[4]A further breakdown of phases could be made but these three phases serve our purpose to see the foot change from supination to pronation to supination again.

remodeling soft tissues (which includes the skin) as well as bone.

Subsequent chapters will add insight into many of these complex interactions, but we must first see the whole landscape to appreciate the roles of its many parts. By the end of the book, we can zoom out again to view the larger picture to see the richness and beauty of how all the factors interplay and interact.

The impression commonly provided by anatomy texts is that forward propulsion from heel strike to toe-off is created by concentrically driven muscle contraction. To help expand our understanding of muscle action, Morton provides us with the image of muscles acting like someone controlling a wheelchair: at times it will be necessary to push actively, but if you push too hard or if the gradient changes to downhill, you might have to pull back. Sometimes, when the gradient is just right, and the wheelchair is moving, the person steering can relax and simply guide with a light hand. Morton's image provides an analogy of muscles working concentrically to push forward actively, like the actions contained in every anatomy text. But sometimes, the muscles must pull back, to reduce momentum and work eccentrically, and they can often work with minimal effort to lend a guiding hand if everything is moving well.

Just as one would assume control of a wheelchair by instinctively switching between pushing, pulling, and guiding, our muscles will do the same as we move. It is rare, if not impossible, for anyone to take conscious control of each muscle during locomotion. We naturally switch between pushing ourselves uphill and decelerating ourselves as we come down the other side. The positive momentum-creating work (concentric) and negative momentum-decelerating (often eccentric) work both require active muscular contraction to fight against the effects of gravity and gradient.

When walking at an average pace along a flat, even terrain, we recruit momentum to provide efficient progression and our forward momentum is enhanced by a series of joints that are predominately aligned to the sagittal plane. By adducting the human big toe relative to the rest of the foot, its associated joints have been brought into a similar, sagittal alignment. When we compare the track of body weight over the human foot with that of the other primates (fig. 1.8), we see the human foot progress more evenly, and we move with relatively straight limbs to reduce muscle load. Other primates land and lift the feet with greater degrees of hip and knee flexion, and with a shorter stride, thus increasing the metabolic cost of their locomotion.

Streamlining the foot was achieved by adducting the great toe, and this new alignment allows our foot, pelvis, and torso

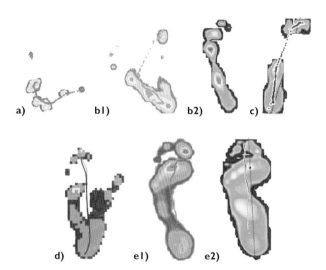

Figure 1.8. *Peak plantar pressure maps (high pressures: red, low pressures: blue) for gibbon (a), bonobo (b), orangutan (c), gorilla (d), human (e1), and human with a "flat foot" (e2). The path of weight transfer (shown by the red line) for the gibbon indicates the abducted big toe makes first contact rather than the heel. Bonobos tend to have quite everted feet (b1) but can be sometimes inverted (b2). The path of transfer for the orangutan (c) and gorilla (d) indicate a relatively sagittal progression but do not show increased peaks of force of heel strike or toe-off. The pressure map for the arched human foot (e1) shows a medial-lateral-medial transfer of pressure in contrast to the more sagittal progression of the flat foot (e2). It should be noted that the reading is a result of contact between the plate and is indicative of the raised medial aspect of the foot. (Adapted from Crompton, Vereecke, and Thorpe 2008.)*

to progress straight ahead over the so-called foot rockers (fig. 1.9). Each of these relatively rounded surfaces helps maintain momentum and the forward direction of our gait. It starts with the roll of the heel immediately following heel strike, and we quickly pass from having only the heel in contact to almost the whole foot. The contact of the forefoot then shifts the momentum to the ankle and we "roll" over the head of the talus, then onto the forefoot rocker as the heel begins to lift to drive us into toe extension.

The effect of speed on efficiency has been investigated many times over the years, and research has told us exactly what we already feel to be true—walking more slowly or more quickly is more tiring than walking at our own preferred pace (fig. 1.10, for further review see Pontzer 2017). Without enough speed in our gait, we use more muscle action to keep moving. Similarly, if we need to speed up, muscles must do the work. To return to Morton's wheelchair image, when the speed is "just right" and we are rolling over our rockers with ease, the muscles can just guide us along. There seems to be a sweet spot for each of us where we can optimize the use of smooth joint surfaces and recycle the energy of our momentum through our many elastic tissues—an analysis treat we will save for later.

It is important to remember that momentum is not just forward during gait; there will also be some up/down force created by the rise and fall of the body as it progresses over the heel rockers. Where one might think that vertical

oscillation—displacing one's weight up and down with each step—would appear to be a waste of energy, it was found that reducing or removing vertical oscillation increased the metabolic cost of moving straight ahead. However, like the speed of gait, there was a "Goldilocks" level of oscillation. If we remove vertical displacement altogether, costs of locomotion increase, and if we create more displacement, we also increase costs.

We mentioned one of the roles of the foot was to help create a rigid lever to manage the forces at toe-off, but the foot is not only negotiating forward propulsion, it is also lifting the weight of the body against gravity as it does so. This is another part of the dynamic we see in the foot pressure readings (see fig. 1.8). A stable foot at toe-off helps contain some of the energy provided by the body's rise and fall as the soft tissue repurposes that movement to optimize efficiency.

It is the momentum of the other leg swinging forward that pulls us through the last two rockers of the back foot. Look at the timing of events during the gait cycle in fig. 1.11. As the left leg comes forward, the right foot responds by lifting the heel and coming into toe extension. From an outside view, that could be interpreted as plantar flexor contractions of the right foot, but it does not have to be. As the other limb swings forward, the planted foot must respond, and that response should help create the stable, supinated foot that we need to lift the body slightly and create the platform to manage the forces at toe-off.

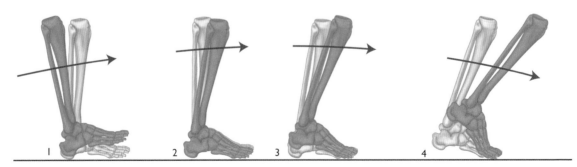

Figure 1.9.   The body's sagittal progression is facilitated by the architecture of the bones and joints of the foot. From heel strike to toe-off there are four so-called rockers—heel, ankle, forefoot, and toe.

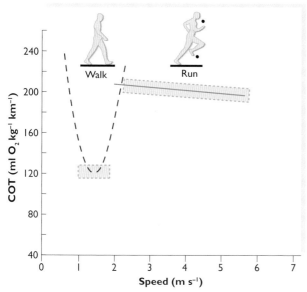

Figure 1.10.   The cost of transport (COT) is calculated according to the amount of oxygen (O_2) used per kilogram per kilometer traversed. Efficiency of walking is very speed sensitive – walking more slowly or more quickly increases oxygen use. As shown by the straighter line, running efficiency is less sensitive to speed in terms of the calorie cost per kilometer traveled. (Adapted from Bramble and Lieberman 2004.)

Although reference is made to our gravity-aligned skeleton and ability to produce an efficient straight-legged walking strategy, bones are often offset from one another, and they have practically frictionless surfaces that provide no inherent stability. The vertically oriented forces thereby need to be stabilized to prevent each joint from moving too much. The amount of offset is yet another 'Goldilocks-type' feature—we need some movement at each joint to deflect impact forces but not so much offset that it diverts a lot of work into the soft tissues. As we saw above, the increased joint angles of the quadrupeds and knuckle-walkers increase the metabolic costs of locomotion. Too much movement at the joints increases muscle work for recovery but conversely, too little joint movement can also reduce efficiencies in the soft tissues.

Getting the joint angles just right allows much of the force to be managed through the bones while some of the force is deflected into the soft tissues. Soft tissues provide responsive shock absorption as they lengthen in reaction to the changes at each joint. The arrangement of slightly offset bones at heel strike creates a series of demands on the associated muscles and their associated collagenous tissues—the tendons and the various levels of fascial wrappings (endomysium, perimysium, and epimysium, see fig. 1.13). The lengthening of the elastic collagenous tissues and the tensioning of the muscles enhances shock

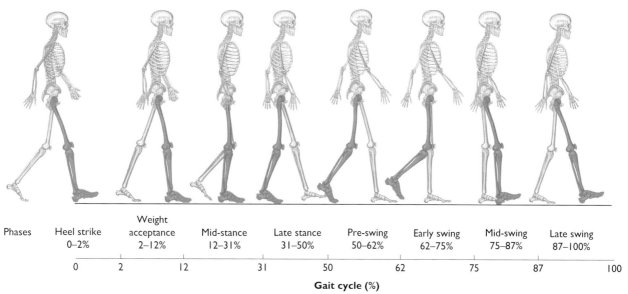

Phases	Heel strike 0–2%	Weight acceptance 2–12%	Mid-stance 12–31%	Late stance 31–50%	Pre-swing 50–62%	Early swing 62–75%	Mid-swing 75–87%	Late swing 87–100%

| 0 | 2 | 12 | 31 | 50 | 62 | 75 | 87 | 100 |

Gait cycle (%)

Figure 1.11.   Gait is traditionally broken into two main sections—stance and swing. Stance phase takes us through each of the four rockers from heel strike (0%) to toe-off (62%). Following toe-off, the limb swings forward and prepares for the next heel strike (62%–100%) and the sequence repeats itself.

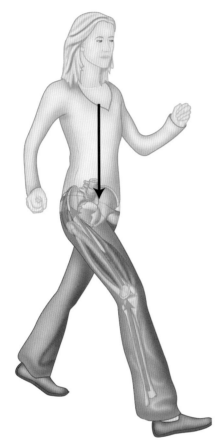

Figure 1.12.   The slight angles at each joint allows some of the forces of momentum, GRF, and gravity to deflect into the soft tissues. Associated muscle tension to prevent the joints from further flexion and the collagenous tissues are stiffened to assist overall efficiency. If the joints are held straight, most of the force would be managed through the bones; if the joints are too flexed, more load is placed on the soft tissues. Achieving the "Goldilocks" degree of offset allows each tissue to do an appropriate amount of force management.

absorption, can load elastic energy to aid recoil, and facilitates efficiency mechanisms to further reduce metabolic costs (these dynamics will be explored later in chapter 5).

A quick walking experiment can reveal how the slightly flexed position of the knee and hip at heel strike causes both joints to flex slightly more in response to impact forces at heel strike (fig. 1.12). We see the same reaction in figure 1.11—as the body weight is received onto the forward foot there is a slight increase in flexion of its joints. The flexed, or slightly offset, position initiates the joint's response to the forces, which then must be controlled by the soft tissues. The kind of unlocking

mechanism we described in the hip and knee joints is very similar to the action of the foot— the offset between the calcaneus and talus (see fig. 1.7b) is the key to opening the supinated, rigid foot of heel strike to let it become the mobile adaptor required for accepting the body's weight. Unlocking the foot allows it to adapt to the terrain's surface and absorb the shock associated with the impact, but then we must create a compact, rigid foot again to help power us forward at toe-off.

■ THE STORY SO FAR

The structure and function of the human foot are essential to the incredibly efficient mode of transport we call walking—we will keep returning to the analysis of gait as it helps to contextualize the anatomy. So far, we have explored a few of the general larger themes—our relationship with gravity, created by numerous skeletal changes, facilitates a straight-legged heel strike on a foot that "rocks" us straight ahead to create and maintain momentum, and our ability to use that momentum (from different directions) and reduce active muscle work.

There is a tissue hierarchy in terms of energy use during movement. As we know from our basic anatomy, one of the main properties of bone is the support it provides. Bone is a relatively stable structure, capable of bending a little under stress but essentially providing the body with an internal scaffolding. This internal scaffolding is held together by ligaments. Ligaments maintain the relationships between the bones, as bony interfaces are notoriously slippery. Like the bones, once they are built, the ligaments provide energy efficient structural support and this contrasts with muscle contractions.

One aspect we will add to this story in future chapters is our ability to recycle energy. Locomotor costs are mostly spent through

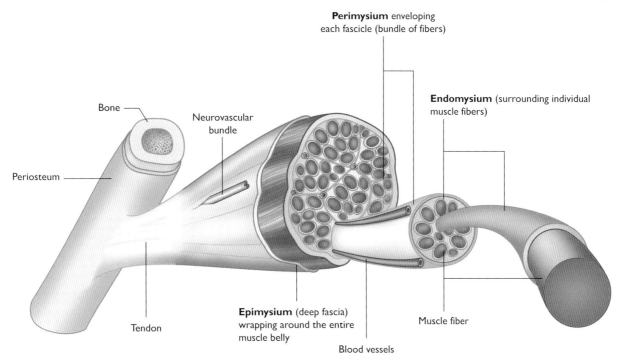

Bone

Neurovascular bundle

Periosteum

Perimysium enveloping each fascicle (bundle of fibers)

Endomysium (surrounding individual muscle fibers)

Epimysium (deep fascia) wrapping around the entire muscle belly

Tendon

Blood vessels

Muscle fiber

Figure 1.13.   *The musculoskeletal system is comprised of tissues with a range of density and stiffness. Stiff, dense bone provides a relatively stable framework, which the other tissues use as an anchor for their management of forces.*

muscle activity (as shown by the effect of slow and fast walking, see fig. 1.10), but the other tissue levels of bone and ligament minimize the outgoings and are joined in their efforts by the collagenous tissues that surround and support the muscle (fig. 1.13). The series of "mysiums" can be considered as wrapping bags for the muscle tissue; they help contain the muscle, give it form, direct and transfer the force of its contractions, and capture some energy from the body's interactions with gravity, GRF, and momentum, to then re-use it to assist our movement.

The degree of support given by any tissue is partly determined by its stiffness—its ability to resist bending. Bone is the stiffest of the tissues mentioned and therefore provides most of the inherent stability of our form and acts to absorb much of the force at impact. The impact force passes through the body in relation to several factors—the angle of GRF, the angle of joints, the center of gravity, and the natural ability of the joints (for a fuller description of these sequences, see *Born to Walk* 2020).

As mentioned above, we do not want to lock out each of our joints at heel strike, nor do we want them to collapse. There is a natural "folding" pattern to each joint based on the factors above. That pattern is determined by the joint architecture, the bony arrangement of contours, grooves, and joint surfaces. The joint surfaces are held together and their integrity maintained by the ligaments, and these determine the angles at which each bone moves relative to its neighbors. The movement of the bones is then controlled via muscle reaction, and this is where energy costs can increase.

An inefficient gait pattern can be created by slow or fast walking, increasing, or decreasing speed, or by creating misalignments between bones and soft tissue that require extra energy to recover. If we look at the toe-off position from the front, we can see how the toes, ankle, knee, and hip are all aligned to deal with forward momentum (see fig. 1.14). There is a reciprocal arrangement between each of these joints and misalignment at one can affect the flow of energy to the others.

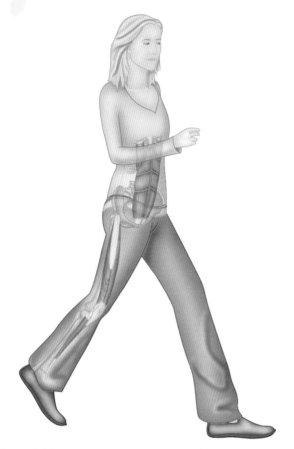

Figure 1.14.   The rigid lever position of the foot at toe-off brings the joints and their associated tissues into alignment. The toes, ankle, hip, and spine are all extended and their associated soft tissues tensioned in preparation for the limb's forward swing.

■ BRINGING IT BACK TO THE FOOT AS A WHOLE, INTEGRATED STRUCTURE

Anatomy repeatedly returns us to the detail of individual structures and discrete dynamics. It gives the impression of being straightforward when the reality is, of course, much more complicated. Most of us were taught about the three or four arches[5] of the feet—medial and lateral longitudinal, proximal, and distal transverse. These can be useful descriptors but none of them helps to appreciate the full

integrity of the foot, considered by Morton to be a discrete functioning organ.

On its journey, the foot's first line of adaptation is the myofascial system, as these soft tissues respond in reaction to the network of mechanoreceptors. As with Morton's wheelchair analogy, muscles adjust their tension to fine-tune movement through changes in tissue stiffness. By "letting out" or "pulling in" (eccentrically or concentrically contracting), muscles control the strain through the tissue network. Our next line of adaptation are changes to muscle strength, which can increase or decrease depending on an imposed workload. This is then followed by changes in the collagenous tissues and, eventually, bone can also remodel itself to the repeated force environment.

Morton liked to think of the foot as having its own specialized properties that helped improve the function of the "total biotic complex". Morton considered the foot to be an organ specialized for human locomotion designed through our response to gravity, a fact beautifully illustrated by the trabecular patterns revealed under X-ray (fig. 1.15).

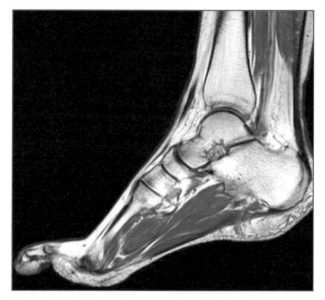

Figure 1.15.   The "total biotic complex" of the foot is highlighted by the continuity of trabeculae direction between each separate bone. Although the bones are considered separate structures, they act together as one functional unit for force management during locomotion.

---

[5]There appears to be considerable inconsistency in the literature with some references claiming three arches and omitting the distal transverse while others count it in. In the end, the matter seems academic when we put the foot into context of the whole.

Trabeculae, explored further in chapter 3, are the internal scaffolding of the bone and they help to reduce weight and increase the bone's overall strength. Built by the osteoblast cells, trabeculae form in response to where strain occurs in the system. The patterns created by these internal structures provide reliable evidence for the direction of force distribution through individual bone. What is most interesting in the X-ray image is the continuity of trabecular direction from one bone to the next.

It is extraordinary how surprising the idea of functional unity can be. Studying discrete anatomy sometimes removes us from the reality of the whole.

Morton's view of the foot as an organ gained support from a contemporary of his, J. McKenzie of the anatomy department at the University of Aberdeen. McKenzie published a paper in 1955 in which he mentions Ellis (1889) and Jones (1944) as all supporting the idea of the foot as a half-dome rather than as a collection of arches. In the *British Medical Journal* article, McKenzie bemoans the fact that *"most students have obviously, and unfortunately, obtained the ridiculous impression that a person uses only the longitudinal arches when walking…"* (page 1069).

With slightly less characterful prose, the concept of the half-dome recently resurfaced in the *British Journal of Sports Medicine* (McKeon et al. 2014). This paper went one step further to show the integration of the soft tissues along with the bony architectural arrangement. McKeon and colleagues present a series of subsystems that go to make up the overall "foot core system", giving an integrated approach to understanding the foot and one that will help guide the overall format for the rest of this text as they break the "organ" of the foot down into three subsystems:

- **Passive subsystem**—bones of the arch (foot half-dome); plantar fascia, ligaments
- **Active subsystem**—intrinsic foot muscles (local stabilizers); extrinsic foot muscles (global mobilizers)
- **Neural subsystem**—musculotendinous receptors, local and global; ligamentous receptors (including plantar fascia); plantar cutaneous receptors

We have already discussed many tissues in terms of energy efficiency and their various other roles in the system. The passive subsystem expends less metabolic energy for support than the active subsystem, and the active subsystem is receiving constant real-time updates on positioning and reactions for proprioception via various receptors. Those receptors are located in and around the joints, and through the collagenous tissues; these are the areas experiencing strain and the proprioceptors are feeding back the body's responses to guide its reaction via the active subsystem.

The three subsystems image may be seen as the body's stiff scaffolding and supporting straps, with the muscles acting as fine-tuning adjusters to draw the bones together or let them out in response to the sensations received through the mechanoreceptors as the forces act through the body. Although we describe them separately, the levels work together simultaneously as a heterarchy—no one system is more important or independent of the other. Each system has its place, and its features must be examined in isolation, but to truly understand it, we must see all of them interact.

SUMMARY

Adaptations to the shape of our feet have provided numerous important benefits, particularly in reducing the metabolic costs of locomotion. One major contributor to that efficiency was an increased stride length due to one foot heel striking while the other foot achieves a sagittally aligned toe-off. Evolutionary forces changed the shape, and therefore function of other bones and joints, especially the pelvis and spine, to provide vertical alignment and stability while much of the shock absorption role was transferred to the foot.

The ability to supinate (lock into a rigid lever) and pronate (unlock and act as a mobile adaptor) is unique to *Homo sapiens* and an essential feature of our efficient gait. Our foot's ability to switch between the two states is illustrated in the ground reaction forces shown in figs. 1.7c and 1.8. The two peaks of force, one following heel strike and one prior to toe-off, relate to the rigid lever position.

Functional anatomy is really the interface between shape, forces, and tissue characteristics. The tissue's response to those forces will depend on its material properties. To appreciate the influence of shape we must see how the structure is loaded with gravity, GRF, and momentum. Understanding forces will help us grasp the influence of shape and tissue make-up; being able to see shape helps us visualize force transfer; and transfer of force will be dependent on tissue properties and its shape.

The following chapters introduce and recap each of those characteristics in a spiraling pattern as we weave and unweave the foot's *"complexity of infinite detail"* for you.

2

EVOLUTION AND THE EVOLVING FOOT

Obviously the underlying reason for
man's adoption of the walking gait....is
its low metabolic demands.

The story of how man became a biped
is history written in the language of
biomechanics.

—Dudley J. Morton, *Human Form &
Locomotion*

▪ INTRODUCTION

Evolutionary theory is both useful and
complicated in equal measures. This
chapter will give an overview of current
understanding and provide a working
knowledge of some tools and terminology used
in paleoanthropology.[1] In keeping with the
idea of understanding our subject, appreciating
basic aspects of evolutionary mechanics
expands our comprehension of the functional
similarities and differences between species.
Seeing the development of the human foot

over time will allow us to contrast the different
shapes of bones and gain a deeper awareness
of what they can or cannot do, as each form
interacts with its neighbors in unique ways.

It is not essential to understand evolution to
understand the foot—I just think it helps. It
is not even necessary to believe in evolution
as my aim is not to evangelize on the science,
but to show a science-based story that assists
the comprehension of anatomical shape and
change. Through that story, we will see the
development of the first feet and some of the
environmental and genetic mechanisms that
allowed them to evolve into modern feet.

The literature describing evolution can be
as frustrating as it is fascinating. It is full of
arcane language, an ever-changing list of
characters with new species being introduced
or re-assigned almost weekly, each dividing
opinion. Where possible, I will point out areas
of confusion or conflict, but the overall aim is
to explore further the implications of shape,
and act as an introduction to comparative
anatomy and ecology.

This chapter challenges our prejudices,
especially in terms of human exceptionalism
and the way we view nature in general.

---

[1]Paleoanthropology is the study of the evolutionary origins of
modern humans and combines evidence from a range of sources
including fossil remains and cultural artifacts.

Many anatomical variations between species are controlled by the interesting Hox genes and we will see how a bone can be repurposed by different species, but the overall vertebrate body plan is recognizable between different families. One hopes that viewing our anatomical relationship to the rest of the animal kingdom can help bring us a deeper connection with the natural world around us.

Mostly, this chapter aims to answer the questions: where did our foot come from; why is it similar to many others; and what is different and unique about it?

True life is lived when tiny changes occur.

—Leo Tolstoy

CHANGE THROUGH TIME

Although we commonly use the word "evolved" in the sense of better, superior, or highly developed, "evolution" only infers change through time and is separate from any sense of hierarchy. Evolution has been commonly perceived as progression toward better and more refined forms, with some form of hierarchical *scala naturae* ("Ladder of Being", fig. 2.1) almost endemic within our thought processes. To better match current thinking, many "trees of life" are now represented within a circle rather than a traditional ladder.

There are also many misconceptions about the speed at which species can change and adapt. Common perceptions range from a glacially slow cumulation of changes to sudden mutations followed by periods of fixation. As usual, the truth is that change can happen at various speeds according to the fluctuations in a complex range of variables. For example, recent work (Grant and Grant 2008) on bird species has shown how population size, group interactions, climatic, and ecological factors all affect which features are emphasized and selected for versus features that are reduced in the population.

Genetic variation occurs naturally within species and the speed at which the positive influence of one trait takes hold in a population depends on many factors. Counter to Darwin's expectation of evolutionary pressures being slow, the work of Rosemary and Peter Grant (Grant and Grant 1993) has shown how normal

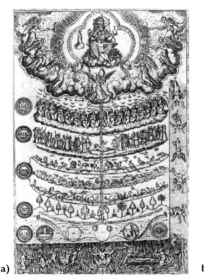 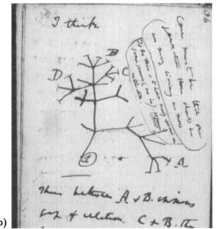 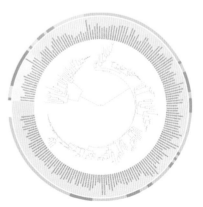

a)   b)

Figure 2.1.   *The natural world has been represented in numerous ways over the millenia. Originally ordered as a "scala naturae" by Aristotle (a), and as a tree by Darwin (b), both presentations give the impression of progression and order in the natural world. More recent representations prefer a circular arrangement (c) that still visualizes evolutionary relationship but with more equivalency between species.*

climatic variation can drive changes in form within a generation.

The Grant's prize-winning work was carried out on Daphne Major island in the famous Galápagos archipelago, on which they camped for six months every year since 1973 to catalog a wide range of data, including a long-term study of the Galápagos finch. The Grants showed significant changes of beak size and shape in the Galápagos finch in response to variations in rainfall from year-to-year. The amount of water available influenced vegetation growth which, in turn, affected food resources for the birds. Variation in the availability of seed-types (large and hard, or small and soft) influenced which finches were able to eat, as some had beaks suitable to either extreme, and therefore, for example, finches with smaller beaks could not manage the larger, tough seeds when there was shortage of the smaller versions. Following years of higher rainfall, when seeds were abundant, smaller beaked birds had an advantage over their larger cousins and could flourish by consuming more calories, more quickly.

Intergenerational shape change among finches contrasts with the conservation of the shark's general body plan, which has barely altered in 420 million years. We often find geological time difficult to appreciate so, to put that time scale into context, mammals only began to appear around 250 million years ago (MYA), the split from monkeys to apes happened about 220 million years later, and chimps and humans shared an ancestor 6 or 7 MYA. In less than 2% of the time sharks have been around, the shape of humans has evolved from something resembling a chimpanzee to our current anatomy. The secret to the shark's success in staying incredibly consistent over time is not due to any regular self-care routine but mostly down to the consistency of their ecology.

The ecology experienced by a species has a huge influence on its shape. Variations in climate, access to food, and competition with other species are among the many factors that will influence the niche within which the species can operate (see fig. 2.2). The introduction of a large predator may drive a species into the trees, the size of branches will affect those that can move from branch to branch—lighter species tend to operate in the higher canopy, heavier ones toward the bottom where the branches are thicker. Body weight determines the amount of food needed to be consumed for survival, which may influence the size of litter and reproduction rates, which also affect the rate at which a species evolves.

The evolutionary history of the human foot is like a review of the progressive stages in the development of an automobile. For in both, each improvement over the crude original model has had a functional significance which is more impressive and better understood as we gain familiarity with the conditions that brought it about.

—Morton, *The Human Foot*, 1935

Although there are many drivers to evolution, as evidenced by the consistency of the shark's features and the rapidity of the finches' changes, fluctuations in climate is probably the most common. It is likely, although we do not know for sure, that climate change set us on the road to upright stance. The standard textbook story is that the human family tree sprouted sometime in the middle-to-late Miocene epoch (16–5.3 MYA), a time period characterized by significant climate alterations that reduced tree coverage in areas populated by apelike primates.

Reduced tree coverage and increased grasslands placed new pressures on arboreal-based species. Trees provide food, protection from the elements, and safety from predators and it is assumed that developing an upright posture helped to mitigate the loss of tree

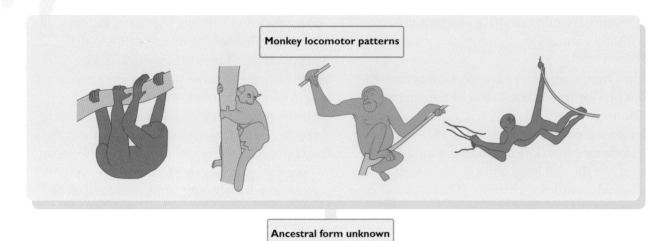

Figure 2.2.   *Monkeys show a range of arboreal strategies (upper portion of the illustration)—walking over or under a branch, climbing, leaping, brachiating, or using suspension. Through a complex interplay between locomotor style, anatomy, and ecosystem, each of the apes (gibbon, orangutan, gorilla, chimpanzee, and human) have evolved their own movement specialisms. Although each has a range of gait and posture options, gibbons specialize in brachiating, orangutans also use their upper limbs to climb hold onto overhead branches as they walk along sturdier lower branches. As they spend less time in the trees, chimpanzees and gorillas have both developed knuckle-walking as a primary form of terrestrial locomotion. Only humans consistently walk upright—although they can stand and walk on two legs, the other apes all do so with effort caused by bent hips and knees. The anatomy of each species has specialized to facilitate their locomotion patterns and the movement patterns can be interpreted from the shape, alignment, and size of their bones.*

coverage. Standing up freed the hands from locomotor duties and allowed our ancestors to carry and manipulate tools and weapons; an upright stance exposes only the top of the head to the midday sun, helping reduce the metabolic costs of thermoregulation (creating the possibility of midday hunting when other animals are resting); bringing our eyes higher also provided a better view for hunting and early sighting of other predators; and, of course, bipedal gait is less metabolically expensive, thereby increasing daily movement range (fig. 2.3). Furthermore, widening our range may have helped us be less susceptible to local changes—if we did not like the local conditions we could just up and move.

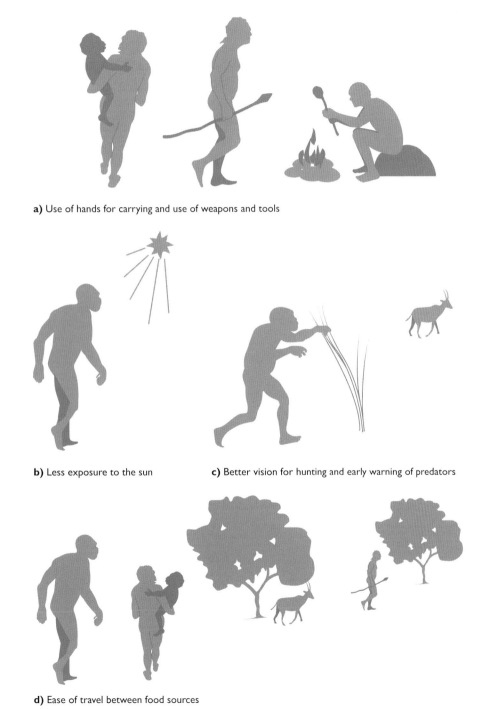

a) Use of hands for carrying and use of weapons and tools

b) Less exposure to the sun   **c)** Better vision for hunting and early warning of predators

d) Ease of travel between food sources

Figure 2.3.   *Many advantages of bipedalism have been proposed as a driving force toward its evolution. It is unlikely that there was any one driver, but rather a mix of each that fed a circular process toward an ever-increasing upright stance. (Adapted from Fleagle 2013.)*

The transition to terrestrial life was probably not immediate or absolute. Trees still offered the same advantages as they had before, it was only their proximity and abundance that had changed. Our hominin line (see figs. 2.2 & 2.11) shows a range of species between the split of our common ancestors from other apes and our current, modern anatomy. The most likely scenario, supported by fossil evidence, is that our anatomy gradually adapted from an arboreal to a terrestrial-based bias as we became less reliant on trees and more able to stand on our own two feet.

■ FORM AND FUNCTION

Although we can use other measures to define species, for our functional purposes we are interested in the change of form that coincides with adaptation to new environments. Form can be defined as a composite of the two characteristics of *size* and *shape*. As we saw above, size plays an important role in determining which ecosystem one can fit into— slender upper branches will not hold a heavier weight and smaller beaks limits the seeds that

can be eaten. The other aspect of form is shape, which plays an essential role in determining our functional ability within the environmental niche we find ourselves.

Shape plays an essential role in biology and it is changes in shape that inform us about movement patterns and ability, however, shape is more difficult to define in a way that allows us to measure differences between species. Shape varies within species according to environment, age, or stage of development, and variations in form can be used to define species. The problem of comparing variation was partially solved through a mathematical analysis of shape using a process first developed by Scottish polymath D'Arcy Wentworth Thompson (1860–1948).

In his classic text *On Growth and Form*, Thompson proposed that shape comparisons could be analyzed by mapping comparable fixed landmarks on Cartesian grids and the various deformations could then be quantified (fig. 2.4). Thankfully, there have been significant improvements in computing

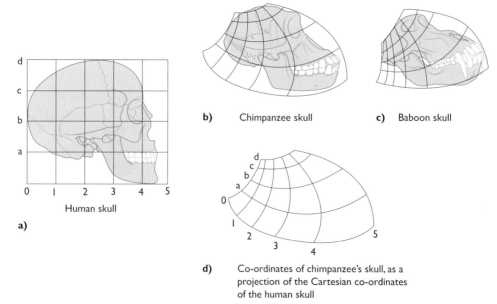

b)   Chimpanzee skull   **c)**   Baboon skull

Human skull

a)

d)   Co-ordinates of chimpanzee's skull, as a projection of the Cartesian co-ordinates of the human skull

Figure 2.4.   *By removing the variables of size and direction, the variable that is left is "shape". To compare and contrast shape between samples, base landmarks are marked on a Cartesian grid, in this case using an adult human skull (a) and then compared with the landmark positions on other species—chimpanzee (b), and baboon (c). The resulting figures, such as (d), provide visual and mathematical comparisons, illustrating, for example, the smaller brain cases and enlarged jaw of the chimp. (Adapted from Thompson 1968.)*

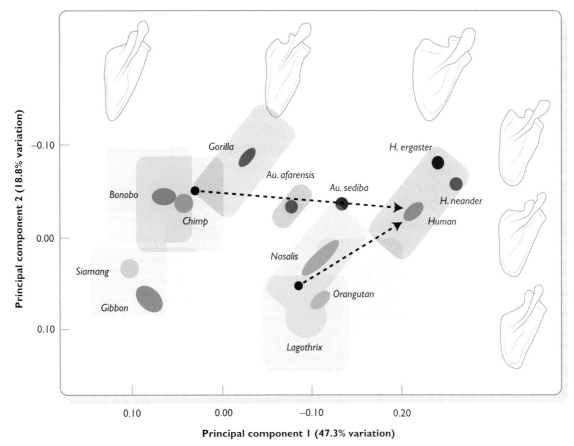

Figure 2.5. To allow mathematically-based comparison, individual scapulae were landmarked and subjected to geometric morphometric analyses. Results showed most of the shape variation occurred along two axes of change—angle of spine of scapula (principal component 1, explained 47.3% of variation) and borders of the supraspinatus fossa (principal component 2, 18.8% of variation). The plot shows a strong trend for species to group together according to species and locomotor patterns. More arboreal species tend toward the bottom left of the graph and terrestrial species toward the upper right. Colored points indicate individual samples; dark ellipses, 90% confidence interval of the mean; light ellipses, 90% confidence interval of the sample. (Adapted from Young et al. 2015.)

power since Thompson first developed his ideas in the early twentieth century. Powerful computer analysis is now able to process large amounts of three-dimensional data and provide in-depth statistical analysis of shape variation. Known as geometric morphometrics, this mathematical type of "form and function" measurement allows researchers to better identify bones of unknown species and provides new insight to species and functional variations.

Although the image in fig. 2.5 illustrates the scapula rather than the foot, it provides a clear example of how one bone varies between species and locomotor styles. The analysis of the scapula was carried out in a similar method proposed by Thompson, and the mathematical

comparison showed that most of the variation between the species occurred along the two directions of shape change shown in fig. 2.5. The directions of change are plotted along each axis of the graph and are known as the "principal components".[2] The *x* axis[3] measures variation in angle of the spine of the scapula—notice how the glenoid fossa faces superiorly on the top left scapula and more laterally in the top right. Differences in the borders of the supraspinatus fossa are plotted along the *y* axis[4]—the scapula on the bottom right has

[2]Principal component analysis is complex and burdened with obtuse terminology—one can think of the principal component as simply a direction in which change occurs.
[3]I know, I struggle to remember high school maths as well—the *x* axis is the horizontal one.
[4]And, the *y* axis is vertical.

very little space available for the supraspinatus muscle, but the fossa becomes more developed (indicative of more muscle bulk) toward the upper scapula.

The analysis of scapula shape introduces us to the many benefits of using a math-based approach. In the chart, a number of samples from each species are represented by colored points. The scatter for each species indicates the amount of shape variation within, as well as between, species. We can see some overlap of shape between species—especially between the chimpanzees and gorillas, but we also see that the averaged shapes (shown in darker shading) are quite distinct from one another. This data then becomes useful in identifying bones from unknown species.

One of the many advantages of geometric morphometrics is that it removes preconceptions from the measurement. Landmark data from an unidentified bone can be subjected to analysis and its position plotted on a similar graph. Proximity to the shape of other species can then help identify its species and, because of incremental change in shape over time, in some cases, the shape analysis can help position evolutionary relationships to other species.

As we mentioned at the start of this chapter, we often consider evolution to be a progression toward improvement with us at the pinnacle. Comparison with our ancestors shows that we are neither better nor worse—we are just different. The upper right portion of the graph in fig. 2.5 plots the data from two extinct species, *Homo neanderthalensis* and *Homo ergaster*. The direction of shape change is toward the upper right quadrant, but *Homo sapiens* falls inside the extreme—do we have less evolved scapulae? No, we just have different demands in a different ecology.

Professor Daniel Lieberman argues that one of the many problems with discussion around the evolution of the foot is the focus on walking, but the foot has to perform many more tasks and it is not restricted to gait only. The foot also must support our ability to turn, crouch, creep, push, pull, leap, jump, land, and, importantly for Lieberman, run. Most evolutionary discussion involves the almost binary comparison between tree-climbing and bipedal creatures, but real-world, environmental, and functional pressures are rarely so well categorized.

There is a current trend to see the human foot as the epitome of evolution—it isn't. The human foot is wonderfully adapted to the many demands placed upon it, but it is not ideal for climbing, it is not specialized for fighting, nor perfect for long-distance running. It can do many of those things. As Leonardo da Vinci famously put it, the human foot is "a masterpiece of engineering and a work of art", but we should not let ourselves succumb to the temptation of human exceptionalism. We are no more or less *evolved* than our other animal neighbors, we all arrived here through the process of change and we are still subject to change.

■ EVOLVING IN GRAVITY

Let's be honest, we are not the only creatures that walk on two legs. Birds do it, kangaroos do it, even hungry chimpanzees do it. There are many important differences though.

The literature tells us we are the only *"obligate plantigrade biped"*—but what does that mean?

Well, for one, *obligate bipedalism* means that walking on two feet is our main mode of locomotion. We can walk and run on all four limbs, but we choose not to do it, mostly for the reasons explained in the previous chapter—it is metabolically expensive and hard work, making it a great form of exercise if required. Other quadrupedal primates use bipedalism occasionally (referred to as *facultative bipedalism*) but it is not their first choice nor are they efficient with it.

Birds hop on two feet, but they are not *plantigrade*, their heels (the calcaneus for us) do not touch the ground, and their locomotion style is bouncing rather than the rolling action discussed in chapter 1. Kangaroos and other macropods (big-footed animals) do walk on the soles of their feet and use the heel during walking gait, but the heel is assisted by their large, muscular tails, which are often recruited as a kind of fifth limb.

Much debate exists on the origins and driving force behind the evolution of human bipedalism and anyone wishing to delve into the intricacies of evolutionary literature should be forewarned. There are many papers that give clear and detailed analysis of a fossil, stating its position and functional interpretation with confidence. However, lurking in competing journals will be a paper or two written with similar precision and giving equal assurance but of an opposing view. As is often the case, the situation is muddied for us by simplified presentations in press and social media. Those reports are driven by our desire to find the most ancient biped, but fail to inform us about the fragile nature of the analyses they describe.

Paleoanthropology is a young science with a very small sample size of fossils (fig. 2.6).

Most fossil finds do not include the small foot bones, and interpretations of those that have been found are restricted by sample size, challenged in their reconstruction (as we will see below), and sometimes based on untested assumptions (DeSilva et al. 2018). Sadly, the debate on the development of bipedalism is sometimes taken as evidence for lack of credibility of the theory of evolution, but that is a naïve understanding of scientific process. Any young science requires time to accumulate evidence, analytic tools, and a body of literature that can be subjected to rigorous debate.

The theory of evolution is often said to be just that—a "theory"—but the all-important aspect of a theory is that it can be tested. One can make predictions based on a theory and then analyze the results of any experiment to support or reject it. Until now, there has not been any significant evidence to challenge the "theory". Of course, we do get improvements as methods are refined or discoveries made, but the underpinning dynamic of change over time has not been improved since first put forward by Darwin and Wallace.

Prof. Neil Shubin applied the predictive ability of the theory of evolution for his discovery of *Tiktaalik roseae* (see fig. 2.7), a transition species between fish and amphibian. Describing the

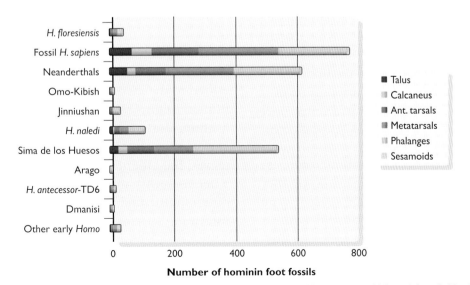

Figure 2.6.   In absolute numbers, there are very few foot fossils attributed to various Homo species. (Adapted from Pablos 2015.)

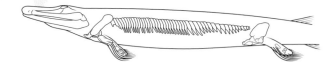

Figure 2.7.   Dated to 375 MYA, Tiktaalik roseae was one of the first amphibians and shows numerous adaptations to life on the land rather than sea. These include a flat head, a cervical spine, and more developed fin apparatus that could support its body on land. (From Shubin et al. 2014.)

search process in his book, *Your Inner Fish*, Shubin describes how he realized few fossils show transitional features between fish and amphibian. He calculated that amphibian features should have appeared in the animal kingdom around 375 MYA and so he started checking geological records. He was looking for sites of rock beds of the correct age that had experienced the appropriate climatic conditions that would have encouraged the evolutionary jump from water to land. A few possible sites were identified and, after several visits to Canada's Ellesmere Island, *Tiktaalik roseae* was discovered.

Commonly known as Tiktaalik, the fossil has features that identified it as a fish (scales and gills), but it also has a flattened head, cervical vertebrae, and developed fin bones that could be used to support its body in gravity—i.e., this was one of the first species to walk out of the water. Subjecting itself to gravity rather than water resistance required a rearranged anatomy, one that allowed it to support its head and to propel its body by pushing against ground rather than water. But Tiktaalik did more than just support itself—the finding of Tiktaalik also supports the application of scientific method to evolution in a simple three step process:

1. **The development of a question.** Analysis of the fossil record showed a gap—a so-called "missing link" or transitional species. Would it be possible to find a transitional fossil?
2. **Forming a hypothesis.** Dating the gap led to the hypothesis that a fossil species with transitional features would be found in geology of that era.

3. **Testing the hypothesis.** The theory was tested by searching in appropriate sites and, in this case, was proven correct.

SHAPE CHANGE

One of the many stepping stones that helped guide Darwin toward his theory of evolution was the organization of the natural world into families, genera, and species. When developing his classification system, the Swedish zoologist, Carl Linnaeus (1707–1778), used physical features to separate animals and plants into groups. Linnaeus refined his system through his lifetime as he gained experience and better access to information, a process that continues as we struggle to find better, more consistent ways to categorize species.

Using shared anatomical features to define a species was mostly replaced in textbooks by the biological species concept introduced by Ernest Mayr in the 1940s. Mayr proposed that a species should be defined by its inability to reproduce outside of its group. However, the idea of reproductively isolated species comes up against many issues, including asexual reproduction, hybridization, and provides no certainty when dealing with extinct species.

The reality of ligers and zonkeys[5] and many other apparently mixed-species hybrids has made it easier to accept fluidity of breeding between related species. Acceptance of reproductive mobility between species has added to the increasingly complex picture of human origins. At one time, there was hope of a straightforward lineage reaching back from *Homo sapiens* to a common ancestor between us and the other apes. The reality seems to be a network with numerous lines, branching off and returning as they interact again with migrating species (see fig. 2.13).

_____

[5]A liger is a cross between a male lion and female tiger, and a zonkey is a cross between a zebra and any other equine.

In contrast to the amount of media attention and the number of scientific articles they attract, hominid fossil finds are rare. This makes functional interpretation and species identification difficult and often hotly debated (hence the number of articles written). Rather than follow the common (and rather tedious) practice of listing and analyzing each find in turn, relevant contrasts are made throughout the text when they serve to highlight important functional differences (and the dedicated investigator can find further texts to explore in the bibliography and through the references, if desired). Nuanced discussion of fossil foot mechanics is unnecessary for our purposes, but some understanding of the mechanisms of anatomical change is useful, as there is a lot of misunderstanding around evolutionary dynamics.

As mentioned above, there is still a common perception of hybrid forms positioned in evolutionary forks between species. There is also the popular idea that we developed from chimpanzees, or something very similar to the current chimpanzee anatomical form. The truth, indicated through genetic and fossil evidence, is that we shared a common ancestor, but both chimpanzee (including their bonobo cousins) and humans have changed since we last shared a meal over 6 MYA.

The fact of common ancestry is evident in our shared anatomy, not just with other apes but with the rest of the vertebrate world. All vertebrates share a similar blueprint, which has altered in each species in the context of its own evolutionary history. This shared blueprint is evident in the skeletal arrangement of the hands and feet (see fig. 2.8), a fact first recognized by the fathers of comparative anatomy, Vicr d'Azyr (1748–94) and Sir Richard Owen (1804–92, founder of London's Natural History Museum).

In his recent text, *Some Assembly Required* (2020), Neil Shubin (the researcher who discovered Tiktaalik) provides an excellent summary of the current understanding of evolutionary change. Shubin explains that soon after the publication of Darwin's *The Origin of Species* (1859), many people objected to Darwin's idea of gradual change over time as they could not conceive how an animal could survive with half a wing or part of a beak. According to Shubin, Darwin added five important words to the sixth edition of *The Origin of Species* (1876) when he answered critics of his idea and suggested "that natural selection is incompetent to account for the incipient[6] stages of useful structure. This subject is intimately connected with that of the graduation of the characters, often accompanied *by a change in function.*"

Darwin correctly saw that organisms rarely developed new structures, they repurposed old ones—swim bladders of fish became lungs of amphibians and fish gill arches eventually formed the human jaw, middle ear, throat, and larynx. This kind of anatomical repurposing can happen because each species has evolved from that original vertebrate blueprint. We can still see evidence of the shared blueprint reflected in the embryos across species (see fig. 2.9) but its alteration in different species occurs through genetic mechanisms that were only discovered during the second half of the twentieth century.

It was well after Darwin's death that the hidden forces responsible for anatomical change were revealed. The discovery and swift application of genetic theory to inheritance enhanced and expanded our understanding of evolution. Although, as with paleoanthropology, DNA analysis is still a young science, it has provided many essential insights. One particularly important element for the analysis of shape has been the discovery of the homeobox genes.

Where the overall genome provides the recipe from which a body is built, genes supply the

---

[6]Incipient—"to come into being". Not to be confused with "insipid"—Darwin's approach to his science was anything but insipid.

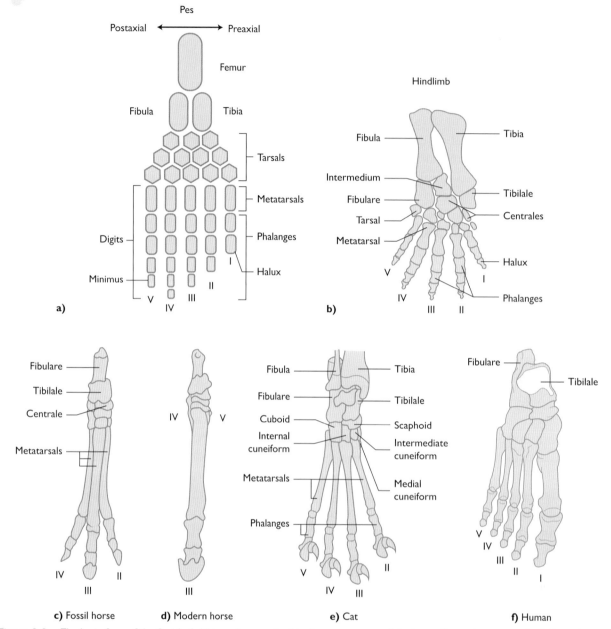

Figure 2.8.   *The basic form of the foot (a & b) is easily recognized in the arrangement of the bones from other species (c–f). Specialization can be seen in the reduction of the metatarsals IV and II between the fossil and modern horse condition (c & d), the long, separate metatarsals of the predatory cat (e), and the modern human form explored through this text (f).*

code for the ingredients and inform cells which proteins to produce. Homeobox genes guide the timing of protein production—they are responsible for the body's overall structure, such as limb placement. One type of homeobox gene, the Hox gene, manages the development of body structures in their correct place. When we look at the basic arrangement of limb bones, we see the arrangement barely changes from one species to another. The overall pattern remains the same, but the relative shape and size vary according to species type (fig. 2.8).

Sequencing of limb development occurs in three zones—upper (arm/thigh), mid-portion (forearm/leg), and distal (hand/foot)—with Hox genes allocated to the control of each section. The twisted structure of DNA strands makes them susceptible to twisting further on themselves causing changes to the positioning of the genetic switches for protein expression. Moving the position of protein switches changes the timing of its signal, and altering the timing will have consequences for bone placement, shape, and size. For example, *Sonic*

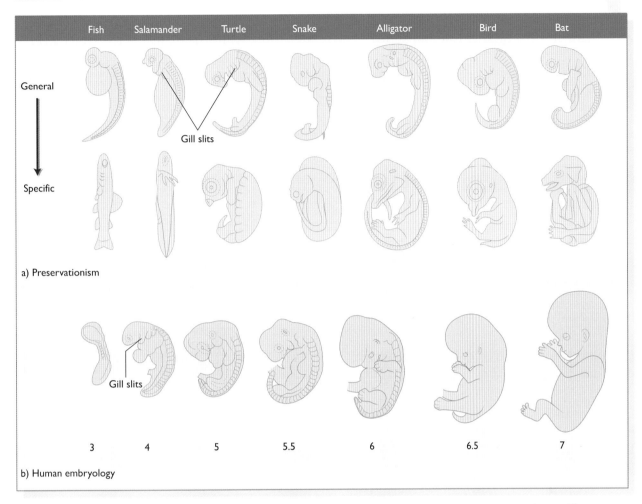

Figure 2.9. *Embryos across numerous species share a common layout in early stages of development prior to specialization. This is especially clear in the three gill slits, which are repurposed during growth* in utero *according to the adult shape, becoming the jaw, middle ear, throat, and larynx in the human form.*

hedgehog, a well-known example of a Hox gene, is responsible for the number of digits and is involved in cases of polydactyly.[7] When investigators looked at the *Sonic hedgehog* gene, no mutation was found on the gene itself but rather in a genetic switch determining when *Sonic hedgehog* would be active and for how long.

Although the *Sonic hedgehog* gene is involved with development of many organs, including the heart and spinal cord, any mutation in the limb control portion only affects the limbs. Likening the arrangement to a central heating system, Shubin suggests that we consider the *Sonic* gene like the furnace that could affect the

heating within the whole house. Switching the whole gene off, as has happened with snakes, stops the development of limbs altogether. In most cases, the gene remains active but the settings are tweaked by genetic switches positioned further along the DNA sequence, and these switches alter certain protein production, acting like the thermostats within each room.

Using on/off and finely tuned genetic switches to affect the growth of each bone has a number of benefits. The arrangement allows the inheritance of the generalized body plan (seen with embryonic generality, fig. 2.9), which is then given species-specific adaptations through fine-control of protein switches. And, importantly, any mutations are more likely to be restricted to one area (such as the case with polydactyly).

[7] The condition of having more than the usual number of fingers or toes.

Although unknown to Darwin, the Hox gene arrangement is the mechanism that allows modification of existing structures and partly explains why we might share significant proportions of genetic material with apes (96% with chimpanzees), cats (90%), and even bananas (60%), but have quite different shapes. Shape is not only determined by the genetic code but also the timing of codes being switched on and off to guide protein production.

FOSSIL FINDS AND THEIR EVIDENCE

The first steps taken by Tiktaalik (or another similar amphibian) exposed the animal kingdom to gravity for the first time. Morton considered gravity a major factor in the evolutionary modeling of our foot, and he made a bold prediction of what the transitional arboreal-to-terrestrial foot might look like (fig. 2.10a). Very few fossils were available to Morton in 1935, so he was speculating on the anatomy of a transition species unknown to him.

Morton assumed the transition foot would show *mosaic* features, i.e., a grasping foot alongside new features adapted for bipedalism. The grasping, prehensile ape foot provided hints of what the transition might look like as the alignment changed when the big toe became less used for grasping and parallel to the other toes, encouraging a long straight stride. It was some time after his death that Morton appeared to be proven correct, when a fossil was unearthed from a cave in Sterkfontein, South Africa. The talus, navicular, medial cuneiform, and first metatarsal of the so-called "Little Foot" fossil skeleton, were first found in 1980, but the fragments had been left in a mislabeled museum storage box until 1994, when they were correctly identified by paleoanthropologist Ronald Clarke. Clarke recognized the fossils to be

hominin and revisited the original site of the fossil find, where he managed to extract a very complete skeleton generally recognized as belonging the species *Australopithecus africanus* (figs. 2.10b & 2.11).

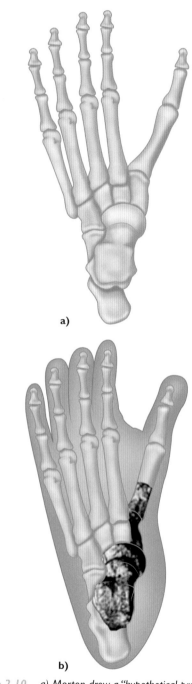

a)

b)

Figure 2.10. *a) Morton drew a "hypothetical prehuman foot" in 1935, which shows a range of arboreal and bipedal features. b) The reconstruction of "Little Foot" appears to match Morton's prediction. The fossil has been allocated to the species* Australopithecus africanus *and is dated to 3.6 MYA.*

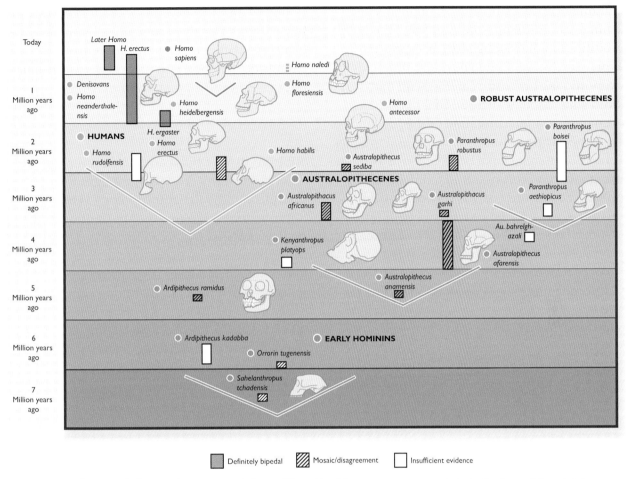

Today

1 Million years ago

2 Million years ago

3 Million years ago

4 Million years ago

5 Million years ago

6 Million years ago

7 Million years ago

Later Homo
H. erectus
Homo sapiens
Homo naledi
Homo floresiensis
Denisovans
Homo neanderthalensis
Homo heidelbergensis
Homo antecessor
● ROBUST AUSTRALOPITHECENES
Paranthropus boisei
● HUMANS
H. ergaster
Homo erectus
Homo rudolfensis
Homo habilis
Australopithecus sediba
Paranthropus robustus
● AUSTRALOPITHECENES
Australopithacus africanus
Australopithacus garhi
Paranthropus aethiopicus
Kenyanthropus platyops
Au. bahrelghazali
Australopithecus afarensis
Ardipithecus ramidus
Australopithecus anamensis
Ardipithecus kadabba
● EARLY HOMININS
Orrorin tugenensis
Sahelanthropus tchadensis

█ Definitely bipedal   ▨ Mosaic/disagreement   ☐ Insufficient evidence

Figure 2.11.   Species with features that appear to indicate obligate bipedality appear more recently in the fossil record. As a defining characteristic of the Homo *family, bipedality correlates with increased size of the cranium and reduced size of the jaw.*

Although "Little Foot" and other specimens are sometimes touted as such, there are no hybrid "missing links"—and, sadly, no "crocoducks",[8] the imaginary chimera of a shared crocodile/duck ancestor. There are however plenty of fossils that indicate the adaptive ability of change through time. The "Little Foot" fossil possesses both *primitive* (inherited from its ancestor) as well as *derived* (new adaptations) features. It has inherited an opposable hallux, but both the hallux and the calcaneus are more robust than those of its predecessors. The mosaic arrangement of features marks "Little Foot" as one of many transition fossils.[9]

As mentioned earlier, one can easily get the impression that evolution follows a linear progression, but this is far from the case. It is tempting to create a narrative that shows a step-by-step change from an ancestral to a modern foot, but this is not possible for numerous reasons. A major reason is the paucity of the fossil record (see fig. 2.6). Fossils are not easily formed as, contrary to popular thinking, they are not bone remains but minerals that have replaced the tissue. The conditions must be right for minerals to replace the bones tissue and the bones have to remain intact, free from scavengers, erosion, and movement. Finding and identifying fossils is also difficult, one has to know where to look and how to recognize them among various other types of fragments—as in the case of "Little Foot".

[8] For an amusing few minutes try searching for "crocoducks" on the internet. Further exploration of the arguments surrounding evolution is given in Jerry Coyne's excellent text, *Why Evolution is True* (2014).

[9] Although each species is, to some extent, a transition species, as all species inherit features from their predecessors while possessing novel characteristics that differentiate them from others.

Discovery of fossil remains triggers another sequence of difficulties, as they must be dated, classified, reconstructed, and interpreted. Thankfully, several reliable dating methods exist, and the literature can focus on the interesting debates surrounding species allocation and interpretation of the functions of the bone's various lumps, bumps, and grooves. Each characteristic on a bone can provide some information on soft tissue attachments and direction of strains (see also chapter 3), but this is an inexact science with many untested assumptions (DeSilva et al. 2018). For example, even the generally accepted idea of the robust calcaneus mentioned in chapter 1 as a development for shock absorption during heel strike is yet to be properly validated (Holowka and Lieberman 2018).

Although the timeline in fig. 2.11 is constantly updated in response to new and better information, we can see that *Australopithecus africanus* ("Little Foot's" species) and *Australopithecus afarensis* are both placed in the fork of a "Y". Coming up from the early possible bipeds, *Sahelanthropus tchadensis, Ardipithecus kadabba,* and *Ardipithecus ramidus,* there seems to be a divide from the *Australopithecine* species. The left arm of the chart follows the changes to the *Homo* family, while the right arm goes off into the *Paranthropus,* the robust *Australopithecines* that all seem to disappear around 15–2 MYA.

Sitting in the crux of the "Y", the *Australopithecines* represent another turning point in our evolutionary story. The two main species, *afarensis* and *africanus,* differ in foot and overall body shape. Being the slightly more recent of the two species, *Australopithecus africanus,*[10] the species reconstructed by Clarke and Tobias (1995), is often put forward as the more direct link to the *Homo* family, a claim Morton would surely have supported.

Perhaps Clarke and Tobias were influenced by Morton's sketch or some unconscious bias, but more recent reconstructions have shown "Little Foot"[11] to have had a more adducted first metatarsal and may have been an even more efficient biped than first thought (DeSilva et al. 2018).

Subjectivity and bias can cause confusion among the many schools of thought in any discipline and paleoanthropology is not immune to its own forms of in-fighting and rivalry. Some of the emotion can be removed from the debate by exposing the data to mathematical analyses such as the geometric morphometric analysis mentioned above. This has been done for samples of the calcaneus and talus (fig. 2.12), both of which show the bone-shape of *Australopithecus afarensis* are closer to that of modern humans (DeSilva et al. 2018; Sorrentino et al. 2020).

Most fossils attributed to *Australopithecus afarensis* have been found in East Africa, particularly in the eponymous Afar region. "Lucy",[12] possibly the most famous of all fossil finds, belongs to this species. Having been found in 1974 by Donald Johanson and named after a Beatles song, Lucy's 40% intact skeletal remains supplied many insights to the potential locomotor patterns of earlier hominins.[13] Like Tiktaalik, Lucy is a transition species that shows a mix of primitive (inherited) anatomy associated with life in the trees and derived (newly adapted) features showing significant modification to terrestrial locomotion (fig. 2.12).

---

[10]*A. africanus* is dated as being around between *3.7 and 2 MYA* while *A. afarensis* appears to disappear from the fossil record almost 1 million years earlier (3.9–2.9 MYA).

[11]Officially recognized by its reference StW 573 (StW refers to Sterkfontein in South Africa, the original site of the fossil find.).
[12]Lucy is given the reference A.L. 288-1 and features in the graph of fig. 2.13b. The reference in this case identifies Lucy as found in the Afar region of Ethiopia.
[13]Should you ever wish to bore people at dinner parties—hominin refers to humans and chimpanzees and their shared ancestors; hominae includes gorillas, hominids include orangutan, and only hominoidea includes all the apes by bringing gibbons into the group. However, frustratingly, other conventions do exist so it's not worth arguing over.

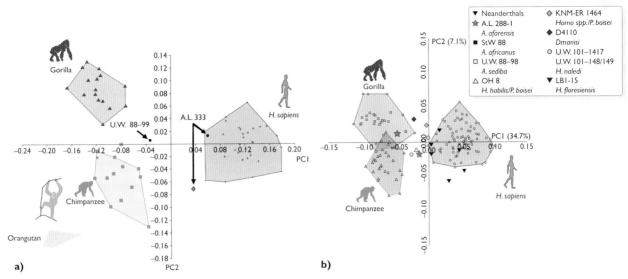

Figure 2.12. *Geometric morphometric analyses were performed on the calcaneus (a, adapted from DeSilva et al. 2018) and talus (b, adapted from Sorrentino et al. 2020). Both plots show the difference in shape between modern human and other apes, but the proximity in shape between modern human and samples from Australopithecus afarensis (A.L. 333 and A.L. 288-1).*

■ WE WALKED AND THEN WE RAN

Early hominins began to show adaptations to being upright 5–7 MYA. These changes included a central foramen magnum, modified lower limbs, and the development of a lumbar curve—all of which improved the ability to take calorie-efficient longer strides. At that time, terrestrial-focused locomotion did not replace tree-climbing. Retaining the ability to climb trees for safety, food, or rest was still an option; it was not until *Homo erectus* (approximately 2 MYA) that we begin to see the specialized derived features of a committed obligate biped—the rounded robust heel, the locking domed foot, and the adducted big toe.

It should be no surprise that locomotor efficiency provided by the anatomical changes enabled long-distance migrations and allowed at least one group of early *Homo* to reach Europe around 500,000 years ago. This group(s) developed into the species we now recognize as *Neanderthal* and the lesser known *Denisovans*. Meanwhile the species remaining in Africa continued to evolve into

anatomically modern humans that co-existed in at least three sites within Africa. The sites, which have all produced fossil remains, are at extreme distances from one another (Morocco, South Africa, and East Africa, see fig. 2.13), and therefore point toward the development of *Homo sapiens* within Africa around 300,000 years ago, after the outward migration of earlier species (Galway-Witham and Stringer 2018). As we now know from many genetic analyses, once *Homo sapiens* came out of Africa into the Middle East and Europe they interbred with the *Neanderthal* and *Denisovan* populations that had already settled there.

Lieberman has posited that running, more than walking, provided the final touches to modern anatomy, as detailed in an influential paper published in 2004 with Dennis Bramble. Bramble and Lieberman argue that many skeletal changes show adaptations to endurance running that are unnecessary for efficient walking. Those changes include a longer waist, a more developed occipital protuberance, and, most significant for our area of interest, some significant adaptations in the feet: shortened toes, lengthened heel, and increased arch height.

Recent African Origin Model (With Modifications)

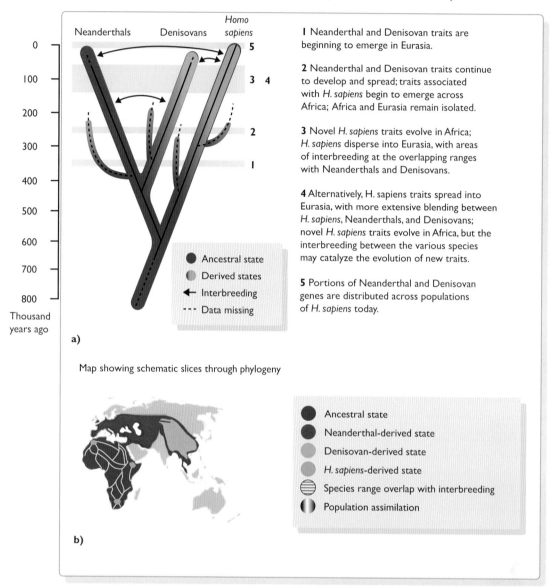

1 Neanderthal and Denisovan traits are beginning to emerge in Eurasia.

2 Neanderthal and Denisovan traits continue to develop and spread; traits associated with *H. sapiens* begin to emerge across Africa; Africa and Eurasia remain isolated.

3 Novel *H. sapiens* traits evolve in Africa; *H. sapiens* disperse into Eurasia, with areas of interbreeding at the overlapping ranges with Neanderthals and Denisovans.

4 Alternatively, H. sapiens traits spread into Eurasia, with more extensive blending between *H. sapiens*, Neanderthals, and Denisovans; novel *H. sapiens* traits evolve in Africa, but the interbreeding between the various species may catalyze the evolution of new traits.

5 Portions of Neanderthal and Denisovan genes are distributed across populations of *H. sapiens* today.

Figure 2.13.   a) Recent finds suggest that ancestral humans left Africa in at least two waves. An earlier wave into Europe, Middle East, and parts of Asia led to two groups known as the Neanderthals and Denisovans. These then interbred with the anatomically modern humans that had developed in various parts of Africa around 300,000 years ago. b) A suggested snapshot of distribution approximately 250,000 years ago shows three sites of modern humans in Africa, Neanderthals throughout Europe, and Denisovans in Asia. (Adapted from Galway-Witham and Stringer 2018.)

Lieberman 2014 and Holowka et al. 2018 argue that these are adaptations that assist running and are unnecessary for economical walking. Efficient endurance running is believed to have opened new hunting possibilities that provide extra calorie input with minimal calorie expenditure. Lieberman's work was popularized by Chris McDougall's book, *Born to Run*, and has been immensely influential among distance runners and fans of a "barefoot" approach to movement and health. Coinciding with the popularity of "barefoot" running has been a growth in "functional training" that uses variable loads, directions, and tasks, and is often performed barefoot.

Many advocates of "functional movement" like to point out how their approach to exercise is reflective of the evolutionary legacy in our anatomy. Although our skeleton has evolved—a comparison of the features of the chimpanzee, *Australopithecine,* and modern human in fig. 2.14, shows the many differences as well as similarities—and modern humans have developed features that facilitate efficient running and walking, those features do not prevent us climbing or swinging through the trees. Our mobility options are reflected in our anatomy; the evolutionary changes that occur are not absolute and therefore, as Lieberman points out, skeletal adaptations can be difficult to place into binary categories of terrestrial or arboreal. The truth, as illustrated by the scapulae in fig. 2.5, is along a sliding and variable scale. We have specialized our anatomy toward terrestrial locomotion while retaining some anatomical elements of our arboreal past.

Homo erectus fossils are indicative of a long-waisted species with larger semi-circular canals in the ears for improved balance and coordination and with a pronounced nuchal ligament for stabilization of the head—all features of a long striding, habitual, and efficient terrestrial biped. Movement had to be efficient as higher metabolic demands were being placed on the evolving species. Body size and brain size had increased and both gestation length and time to maturity had become longer for their young (Aiello and Wells 2002). Any anatomical adaptation that could save a few

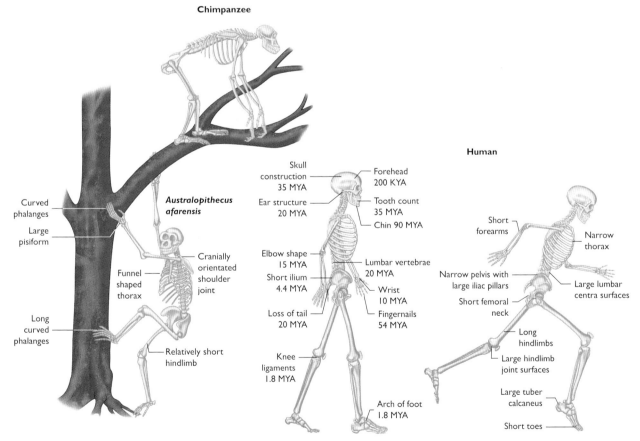

Figure 2.14.   *Although the last common ancestor (LCA) is unknown, its body plan is thought to be a close resemblance to that of the chimpanzee.* Australopithecus afarensis *is one of a number of hominin species that appear to be transitional between the LCA and modern humans. Skeletal changes occurred at various stages that allowed more efficient walking and, eventually, running. Major changes toward modern human are estimated to have evolved approximately 2 MYA, with the emergence of* Homo ergaster *and* Homo erectus, *coinciding with the final adaptations that enabled endurance running. Anatomically, modern humans are considered to have evolved around 2–300,000 years ago. (Adapted from Fleagle 2013.)*

calories to offset these demands would have been selected, and, of course, there is no real order to those changes. It was not a case of first developing efficient movement to facilitate increased metabolic demands, nor was it the metabolic demands that created the need for locomotor adaptations, they are likely to have co-developed gradually, generation by generation.

A suite of shape changes had to occur before *Homo erectus* could take long, straight-legged strides, and these had to include changes in the feet. Increased toe extension for toe-off and increased robusticity and roundedness of the calcaneus for heel strike contribute to a long stride (Holowka and Lieberman 2018; Webber and Raichlen 2016). The extension achieved at toe-off lets the free leg swing further forward and straighten to land on its heel. Look again at the line-up in fig. 1.6 to compare joint angles for each illustrated species. The earlier species all have a shorter stride and only *Australopithecus* (4.5–1.9 MYA) demonstrates any degree of toe extension, but the anatomically modern human shows increased joint extension through the whole system from toe, to knee, hip, and spine.

Heel strike and toe-off correlate with the two peaks of force we saw in fig. 1.8 with very little pressure evident though the mid-foot. The other ape species all show some degree of high pressure in their mid-foot, indicating the flexibility of the mid-foot and their inability to heel strike or toe extend. When watching chimpanzees, bonobos, and gorillas walking we see the foot being planted down almost flat. As we shall see in chapter 4, the limited toe extension in tree-climbing species is due to the downward curve of the bones. The downward curve facilitates grasping but inhibits extension when walking on flat surfaces—a perfect example of form determining functional ability.

Our modern human foot bones have arranged themselves into a dome-like arch but it is still uncertain exactly when this occurred.

The famous footprints in Laetoli,[14] most probably left by Lucy's species, *Australopithecus afarensis,* show an ability to heel strike and toe-off in an almost modern fashion and might be indicative of an early arch. However, some researchers have argued that the lack of mid-foot pressure only indicates that the foot stiffens as the heel rises and the foot progresses to toe-off, and that the requisite stiffening of the foot could be created by at least two mechanisms independent of the presence of a high arch (Sorrentino et al. 2020). Once again, the lack of fossil remains limits our ability for certainty.

The stabilizing mechanisms for the foot's "rigid lever" will be explored in detail in the following chapters, but can be summarized as using a combination of form and force closure dynamics. Form closure results from close-packing of the bones in response to the natural movement through the foot, an architectural arrangement that requires the vaulted doming of the bones. This contrasts with force closure, which refers to the tightening of the soft tissues that span the foot and support the bones by drawing them together. The soft tissues involved with this are located both within the foot itself, the so-called intrinsic muscles, as well as the better-known muscles of the leg, the extrinsics.

Both mechanisms of form and force closure are assisted by having a long stride. As we will see, supination of the foot is driven by rotation of the lower leg and a longer stride provides the rotation that turns the bones—form closure. The ability to heel strike also requires the toe joints of the back foot to extend. Toe extension stiffens the soft tissues on the plantar surface and initiates the windlass mechanism to increase the overall stiffness of the foot and prevent the midtarsal break seen in chapter 1—force closure.

---

[14] A series of bipedal footprints found in Tanzania, they are preserved in solidified volcanic ash dated to 3.7 MYA.

To support his endurance running model of human evolution, Lieberman points out that the two more recently derived features, short toes and high arches, are unnecessary for efficient walking. The arched foot, with its associated soft tissues, only acts as a spring during running, as running distorts the foot's arch much more than walking and creates higher strains within the soft tissues. The soft tissues are then better able to return that energy to assist with forward propulsion—this mechanism is almost entirely absent when walking because of the lower forces involved.

The higher ground reaction forces passing through the foot in running are partially controlled by the toe flexors as the body moves over the foot and the toe joints extend.

Shorter toes reduce the amount of work necessary to control the forces involved (Rolian et al. 2009). Both of these changes—toe length and arch height—make no difference to the work load incurred by walking but do contribute to running by reducing energy costs.

Appreciating the role of the shape of the foot in different locomotor patterns has allowed Holowka and Lieberman (2018) to put forward a three-stage summary of the foot's evolutionary path (fig. 2.15). The model takes us from the abducted hallux and long-toed *Ardipithecus,* through the adducted hallux but still long-toed condition of *Australopithecines,* to the eventual short-toed and high-arched characteristics of the *Homo* lineage.

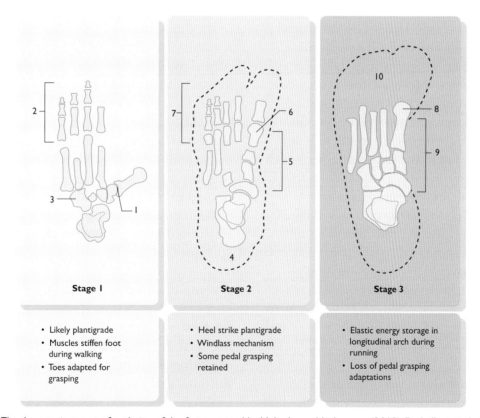

Figure 2.15.   *The three main stages of evolution of the foot proposed by Holowka and Lieberman (2018). Each illustrated species is placed as an example, other species may also fit the criteria.*

Stage 1—Ardipithecus ramidus shows an abducted hallux capable of opposition (1), long toes (2), but elongation of the mid-foot (3).

Stage 2—Australopithecus afarensis has the ability to heel strike (4), a low medial longitudinal arch (5), slightly abducted hallux (6), and long toes (7). The dashed line indicates the footprint from Laetoli.

Stage 3—Homo habilis and erectus shows a fully adducted hallux (8), a human-like medial longitudinal arch (9) and, based on footprints from Ileret, Kenya (dashed line), short toes.

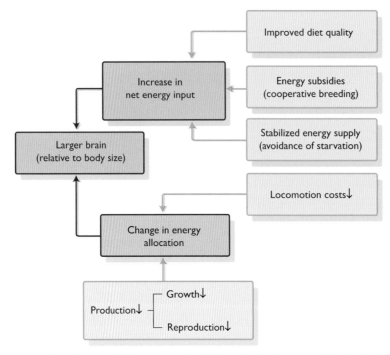

Figure 2.16.   Numerous anatomical and perceptual changes went hand in hand to feed increases in brain size. (From Navarette et al. 2011.)

Developing an elastic arch brought reduced locomotion costs and opened new hunting possibilities. The structural and thereby functional changes of early *Homo* is only one of several factors that allowed reallocation of energy to feed our larger brain. Slowing the pace of life (in terms of growth rate and reproduction, not in the sense of kicking back on the sofa!), improving the quality and regular supply of food, and forming cooperative groups all helped with the virtuous cycle of improving our ratio of brain size to body[15] (fig. 2.16, Navarrete et al. 2011). The realloction of resources toward brain size initiated a relatively rapid succession of body shapes, each given its own species assignment—*Homo habilis, Homo erectus, Homo heidelbergensis,* and *Homo naledi,* to name a few.

There is still debate on the order of shape change that was necessary for the development of the domed elastic foot. Morton emphasized metatarsal torsion (1935), (see also chapter 4), others considered it was an elongation of the lateral forefoot that brought the metatarsals toward the big toe (Kidd, O'Higgins and Oxnard 1996), or that the subtalar axis was altered to adduct the big toe toward the rest of the foot. Regardless of which change came first, the whole structure of the foot became domed to produce an adducted big toe, a line of relatively aligned metatarsal heads, and an elasticated arch—as well as one of the suites of changes that also occurred in the leg bones.

A comparison of primate malleoli, which encase the talus bone, shows human legs are torsioned laterally compared with their ape relatives (fig. 2.17). We shall be further exploring the functional relationship between the talus and the tibia and fibula in further chapters, as the two malleolar extensions from the leg bones encompass and can control the talus of the foot. The intimate relationship of these three bones means that if one changes direction or alignment, the others are likely to follow. If the tibia torsions laterally it will require the above changes to occur

[15]Absolute brain size is not so important; elephants and whales have larger brains. Humans have a high encephalization quotient meaning a large brain relative to their body size, that ratio is smaller for whales and elephants. Shape and proportions of brain areas are also important factors for cognitive procession. Size is not the only important factor.

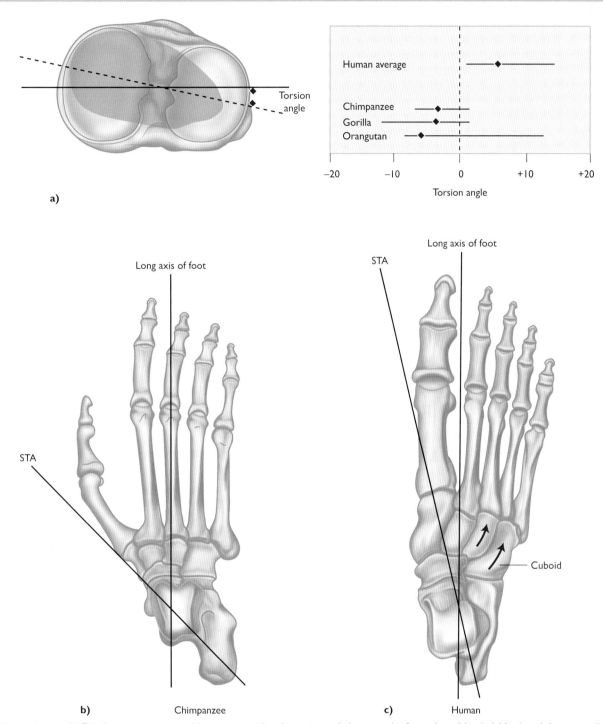

a)

b)   Chimpanzee

c)   Human

Figure 2.17.   *(a) Tibial torsion is measured by comparing the change in angle between the femoral condyles (solid line) and the two malleoli (dotted lines). The chart shows chimpanzee, gorillas, and orangutan are all internally torsioned in contrast to the lateral torsion of the human tibia. (b & c). A direct comparison of the human and generalized ape foot shows the adduction of the big toe, elongation of the lateral tarsals, and the realignment of the subtalar joint in the human foot. This view also shows how the human great toe has torsioned from facing toward the foot in the ape condition to toward the ground in the modern human foot.*

(adducted big toe, torsion of the metatarsals, and elongation of the lateral foot) to let the toes contact the ground. Although it is tempting to try to find the *first* bone to change, it is just as likely that the whole foot complex was adapting, as any change in one area would alter the forces received through the rest of the structure.

Which leaves us with the question of where would we be if we had not developed the spring in our step?

SUMMARY

Cumulatively, the evidence does seem to align with Morton's prediction as discussed at the start of this chapter—walking upright reduces metabolic costs of locomotion, and changes in movement strategies are reflected in changes in the skeletal and fossil records. Those changes in form are intertwined with ecology, in that any change in the environment influences the niches that open to us and form a never-ending feedback loop that drives evolution. But not evolution in the sense of progress, only in the sense of change and adaptation to find a best fit to the niche we find ourselves in.

We started this chapter with three major questions regarding where the foot came from, why is it similar to so many others and what makes it uniquely human? We have seen how the first feet arrived on land and explored the mechanisms through which the body accumulates change over time. Built from the same vertebrate Bauplan, the human foot has adapted in its unique way to manage environmental forces, first with upright walking and then specializing further into running while still maintaining the ability to stand, climb, fight, pull and push.

While Morton said that *"The story of how man became a biped is history written in the language of biomechanics"*, we could rewrite that to the *"..language of 'shape'"*. New tools for the analysis of shape have allowed the extraction of bias from analyses. And to understand biomechanics, to enable a vision of what a form can or cannot do, we are really talking about understanding the language of shape.

Any student of anatomy is a student of shape, therefore we will not leave our comparative anatomy in this chapter but carry it with us along our journey. Seeing the implications of shape during movement, with its associated forces, is an important goal of this book and leads us directly to the next chapter.

3

THE SHAPE OF BONE

◼ INTRODUCTION

As we have seen so far, to understand the foot, we must appreciate the many roles of its bones and how their shape affects our movement. Moving bodies require some element of stiffness as a base for movement. While a variety of stiffening strategies can be found among invertebrates, vertebrates solved the problem of a stiffness requirement with the development of bone. Bone plays an essential role in the ebb and flow of the body's tensegral balance and it is a complex role that requires constant monitoring and updating of bone morphology.

Bone is shaped at two different levels of development, firstly through evolutionary inheritance (or *phylogeny*)—a general pattern of the number and position of bones is determined through genetic heritage, and through Hox gene sequencing. The overall bony scaffolding blueprint of vertebrates has been relatively consistent for 500 million years (Gould 1989, cited in Carter and Beaupré 2001). As we saw in fig. 2.9, each portion of the highly conservative skeletal framework has been adapted, altered, and repurposed to allow novel movement strategies for each species within their environment.[1] Following birth, the inherited bone shape will influence overall movement possibilities, but a fine-tuning system is in place to let individual bones shape themselves to the movement demands of the local environment. This second mechanism allows the evolutionary blueprint to be updated and refined during development (or *ontogeny*).

In this chapter, we will explore the ontological development of bone. Functional and mechanical requirements imposed on the body throughout its lifespan lead to complex interactions within each tissue type. In the case of bony tissue, a feedback loop exists to allow specialized cells to sense the stress experienced by a bone and for the cells to then direct construction and maintenance of the bone.

---

[1] A solid introduction to the relationship between form, function, skeletal, and genetic adaptation is contained within Neil Shubin's *Some Assembly Required* (One World 2020).

This real-time mechanism allows bone to constantly, albeit slowly, update its form in response to the force environment. It is a bit like setting your computer to automatic downloads and updates for new operating systems—provided you have the power switched on, and the computer has the available processing capacity—everything takes care of itself. However, for our bones to do a similar job, the correct nutritional and movement environment must be in place.

Bony tissue is laid down in response to the overall mechanical environment, and the communication of force from bone to bone is beautifully illustrated in the X-ray image of the foot (see fig. 1.15). The trabecular pattern illustrates the reality of force transfer through a system rather than a collection of bones that somehow make up a series of arches. Understanding how the body manifests and organizes itself is rarely explored in texts of this type and so we will take a little time to appreciate the complexities of bone building and design in general before we dive into the specifics of the foot bones in chapter 4.

Tension and compression, the defining forces of tensegrity systems, are the major designing forces for the bone, as the bone can sense the mechanical environment and remodel itself to optimize its shape. Bone's mechanoreceptive ability allows tissue strain patterns to guide cellular action and provide a self-organizing system, one that manages the competing needs for lightness, flexibility, and strength.

In this chapter, we explore the body's ability to sense, distribute, and respond to strain, a dynamic that has been explored in the context of tensegrity (see Solórzano 2020 for a comprehensive overview). Throughout this text, we will become aware of the complex interplay between the stiffer tissue of the bone and how the body uses contractile soft tissues to adjust the tension and support for the skeleton. The skeleton, in turn, provides the stiffness required to anchor muscle and tendon in the continual balancing act between tension and compression, an underpinning dynamic in determining bone shape.

BONE'S ABILITY TO SELF-MODIFY

Although bone is mostly thought of as a stabilizing element, we should not view it only from such a restricted perspective. For full appreciation, we must examine the relationship between bone's structure, its properties, and its, often contrary, needs. Those needs include bone's ability to create more stable conditions that facilitate movement, provide protection (for itself and the various other soft tissues), and adapt to the varied strains the moving body is exposed to—tension, compression, shear, bending, and torsion (fig. 3.1). Bone must also be compliant enough, not only to absorb some of those forces but also to experience the organizational dynamic of movement.

Bone's compliance in response to movement forces allows it to self-modify, as cells contained within the structure of the bone sense and respond to repeated changes in the force environment. This dynamic feature helps bone self-organize its structure in context of the overall force environment, as strains passing through the bone create a constant feedback loop—movement—strain—response—build/remodel—movement—strain—response—, etc.

Pure compression and tension are difficult to recreate, and bones will most commonly experience bending forces. Bending creates tension on one side and compression on the other, and the experience of these forces guides the cells within the bone to adjust its shape (fig. 3.1). However, bending of long bones is potentially dangerous, allowing tension and compression on either side of the bone, which can create a point of weakness—once a structure starts to bend, applying more force will bend it further. The counter to the weakness of bending would be to build bones

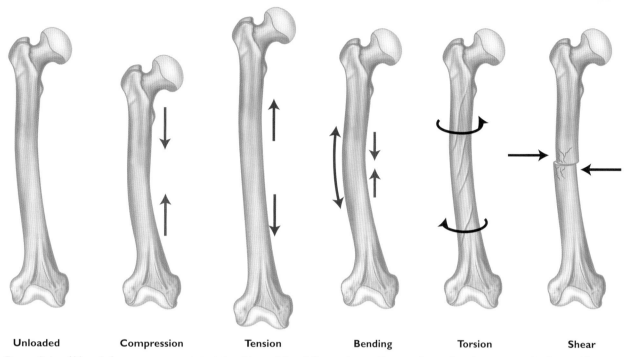

| Unloaded | Compression | Tension | Bending | Torsion | Shear |

Figure 3.1. Although forces never occur in isolation, it is useful to define each type. Compression and tension are opposite forces, either directly approximating tissues or pulling them apart. Most structures will experience some degree of bending, which creates tension on one side and compression on the other. Torsion is a result of a twisting action or torque. Shearing occurs when there are two opposing forces acting through the tissue.

that do not bend, but that would make them fragile: any bending force will cause them to snap, and a little bit of pliability is a good thing in some cases.

Bone is a truly fascinating dense material worthy of the metabolic cost required to build and carry it around in our bodies. During development, our body works to find the optimal balance between the potentially opposing demands of using enough of the correct materials to provide support with a margin of error, without creating too great a metabolic requirement. Thankfully, as we will see below, nature has provided a range of best-fit solutions to this conundrum.

▤ DIFFERENT MATERIALS FOR DIFFERENT JOBS—CORTICAL AND CANCELLOUS BONE

Bone has two major forms—a strong and dense outer lining and a woven, mesh-like inner scaffolding (fig. 3.2). Known as either cortical or compact bone, this outer layer of bone is

densely packed, relatively rigid, and strong (see also fig. 3.4). But being dense, it is also heavy and makes up approximately 80% of the bone mass. To lighten itself, bone constructs an inner scaffold system known as cancellous, spongy, or trabecular bone. This inner construction is relatively weaker but allows the bone to bend under stress and therefore makes the bone less fragile.

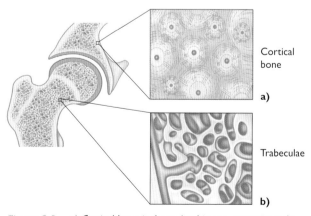

Cortical bone

a)

Trabeculae

b)

Figure 3.2. a) Cortical bone is dense (making up approximately 80% of bone mass) and smooth. Its periosteal covering provides attachment for various soft tissues. b) Trabeculae (Latin: "small beam", also known as cancellous bone) form in long bones to provide a scaffolding that both strengthens and, as it is less densely packed, lightens the overall structure.

Terminology

Through the text we will discuss stress and strain. If this is new terminology for you, don't panic. It will make sense eventually as we approach the topic from different directions in different chapters, and each chapter will help build the picture for you. While below is an official definition, it may be easier to remember that stress is applied, and strain is felt.

Stress is a measure of the force acting on a tissue.

Strain is how the tissue responds.

Stress = force divided by surface area—or, the amount of force that is applied to a measured area.

Strain = the structure's response and is measured in changes to length or volume.

Generally, if the strain creates tension there will be a lengthening response and, if the strain causes compression, there will be a density response.

To give a real-world example:

Consider the difference between someone walking on a wooden floor in flat shoes and in stiletto heels.

The floor would show no evidence of the first walk but is likely to indent with every strike of the stiletto. The bodyweight is the same in each shoe, but it is focused on a smaller area when wearing the stiletto. This is the reason why stress is measured as force (bodyweight multiplied by gravity) divided by the area (flat shoe versus pointed heel).

Because the same force (bodyweight and gravity) is focused on a smaller area (the stiletto heel), there is more stress on the floor. The wooden floor then deforms, or strains, as a result.

To use a simple comparison of a stiletto heel with a surface area of $1cm^2$ versus a loafer type heel with a $35cm^2$ surface area, the stiletto has around 35 times less surface area to distribute the force.

Or, to put it another way, the floor under the stiletto will receive 35 times more stress.

There are, of course, many calculations that can be done that involve new and relatively complex mathematics, but they are available in most biomechanics texts. What is important for us at the moment is not the mathematics but the principles of stress and strain.

Each bone will have a unique ratio and arrangement of bone type according to the stresses and strains it has been exposed to. The ratio of cortical to cancellous bone is one of the ways in which the body adapts itself by placing the right materials in the right place in response to a complex costs and benefit analysis.

As an analogy, consider the expense of building a skyscraper in temperate London only for it to be immediately relocated to Moscow and exposed to the extremes of Russian weather. Would you have used all of the costly materials needed to insulate the skyscraper in Moscow if you thought it was staying in London? Probably not, as it would be an expensive and inefficient use of material. So, our relocated "designed-for-London" skyscraper would now be experiencing temperature fluctuations that are likely to create structural flaws and eventually cause the building to collapse. What if the materials could automatically, though slowly, adjust according to the demands of the environment?

Just as one would balk at the expense of using Moscow levels of insulation for a building in London, the body tries to find the right balance of material appropriate to its mechanical load—a dynamic you might be familiar with as Wolff's law.

Inspired by reading von Meyer's observations on the similarities between trabeculae in femoral heads and the supports of overhead cranes, Julius Wolff published his well-known "law of bone transformation" in 1892 (Barak et al. 2011). However, the idea of a strict mathematical law has come under scrutiny in the last 20–30 years as Wolff's law, with an emphasis on *law*, implies that mechanical force is the primary designing factor, whereas the reality is much more complex. Age, injury, and hormone levels all influence the size and form of bone, and the term "bone functional adaptation" has been suggested to replace Wolff's law as a description of bone formation and modeling (Ruff et al. 2006). However, mechanical strain remains a major influencing factor that can still be used to predict and interpret trabecular patterns according to locomotor strategies (Barak et al. 2011), and even facilitates the kind of interpretation and comparison of fossil remains and related species that we saw in chapter 2.

The ability to design a skyscraper that can adapt to different environments would require communication through the many different levels and materials involved in its construction: the walls, windows, air conditioning pipes, electricity ducts, and all the associated bolts, screws, and nails, etc. would have to coordinate as new layers were added, and service ducts would be required to change paths as the building adapts. The process of change would require a host of instructions to manage it, with many architects, managers, supervisors, and workers able to feed appropriate information backward and forward to make best use of available material and resources.

Bone (and many other tissues in the body) has to self-organize in this way and it does so with

a hierarchical[2] series of tissues similar to the architects, managers, supervisors, and workers in our fantasy skyscraper. Skeletal morphology is argued to be an expression of genetic and mechanobiological "morphogenetic rules" (Carter and Beaupré 2001), a phrase indicative of the interrelationship between mechanics and cellular expression, and the overall genetic blueprint—a blending of the phylogenetic and ontogenetic processes.

This fascinating interface between cells and their mechanical environment was investigated by Chen and Ingber (1999) who proposed that each level of organization, from cell to tissue to organ, is part of an intercommunicating hierarchy arranged to facilitate structural optimization via mechanotransduction—the transformation of mechanical force into electrochemical stimuli for the production, maintenance, and alteration of tissue. Specific cells within the body's tissues sense mechanical strain. These cells can then signal for appropriate responses to correct the amount of strain in a way that will balance the mobility/stability conflict. Even when using minimal material but building with appropriate safety margins, the bone appears to be perfectly formed to deal with the everyday forces it is exposed to. Tension and compression created during movement provide the stimulus element within a feedback loop, as bone uses its mechanoreceptors to instruct and guide the remodeling of individual bones.

■ BONE AND TISSUE RESPONSE TO FORCES

As mentioned above, providing the body's "solid" framework sets up conflicting demands for bone—to be dense enough to create a reliable base for movement and absorption

---

[2]In this case the hierarchy is one of complexity of tissue levels, from simple to complex, but no level is actually more "important" than the others, and in that sense, it is really another heterarchy.

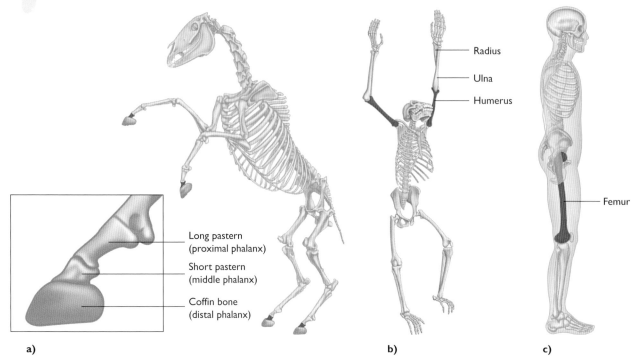

Long pastern
(proximal phalanx)

Short pastern
(middle phalanx)

Coffin bone
(distal phalanx)

Radius

Ulna

Humerus

Femur

a)   b)   c)

Figure 3.3.   Bones' shape and size have adapted to their function. a) The horse phalanx has become cube-like and sturdier to resist compressive forces. b) The gibbon's upper limb bones have elongated to assist brachiation and manage tensional forces. c) The long human femur deals with compressive forces which can cause the bone to bend.

of forces, but to be as light as possible to ease calorie demands and facilitate faster acceleration for the local body part and the body in general.

The position, size, and shape of the bone, coupled with style of locomotion, will determine angles, amplitude, and rate of force interactions. Square foot bones of a quadruped are exposed to heavy compression, a brachiator's upper limb will be under significant tension, while a biped's femur will experience compression leading to bending forces (fig. 3.3). The shape and size (especially the length) of a bone affects the forces that act on it and influences the animal's overall biomechanics.

Square bones give solid platforms for areas of high force, and long bones provide efficient movement. Our longer lower limbs, for example, are one reason for our economical walking as they allow a longer stride. Placing just the two long bones of the femur and tibia between our pelvis and feet significantly increases the length of a step. The long bones

also provide a mechanical advantage as they increase the distance between the joints and improve leverage.

We have already mentioned the idea of the foot becoming a "rigid lever" at the point of toe-off. Creating a "solid" foot between the toe and ankle joints improves our ability to create the force to propel us forward. The advantage of a longer bone might be easiest visualized by the increased popularity of the throwing sticks used by dog walkers worldwide. The long plastic arm of the stick will significantly increase the distance a ball will travel with little added effort.

Having longer leg and foot "levers" provides us with similar benefits, but the downside of long bones is that they are prone to bending and require extra monitoring to prevent them bending too far. The human body has placed small square bones around the rearfoot where there are higher forces and "long" bones for the metatarsals.[3] In later chapters, we will see that

_____

[3]The metatarsals are not very long but anatomically they are classified as such.

the foot uses an ingenious range of strategies to satisfy the competing functions of shock absorption and force production and it does so partly through the shape of its bones.

Bone must cope with impact compressions, pulling tensions, shearing, and bending forces, and each individual bone has adapted over time to manage the forces it is exposed to in its environment. However, creating a totally robust bony system that managed all the forces on its own would be metabolically costly in the production and maintenance of the bony material, as well as heavy and costly to move. The vertebrate body has developed several solutions to this issue, through variation in bone shape and size as well as through the development of tissue variety—bone, ligament, tendon, and muscle. Each tissue has different material properties and plays a role in the management of forces.

Of the tissues illustrated in fig. 3.4, bone has the greatest degree of stiffness, which is a measurement of its resistance to stress (both terms are defined above[4]). The shallow gradient to the curves of ligament and tendon contrasts to that of bone, showing them to be less stiff. However, although bone is stronger, in that it can withstand greater forces before breaking, it does not strain (lengthen) much in response to stress (applied force). Ligament and tendon can lengthen much more than bone under low loads before reaching their plastic and failure phases—they are therefore less strong, but more elastic and resilient than bone. The bone, ligaments, muscles, and tendons work together to manage forces, with the ligaments and tendons providing elastic support and pliability in contrast to the stiffness of bone.

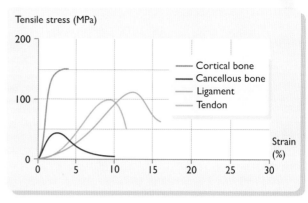

Figure 3.4.   *Each tissue has a unique response to stress depending on its material properties and overall shape. The lines shown here illustrate an average response for each tissue type—cortical and cancellous bone, ligament, and tendon. Their ability to lengthen is measured as strain along the bottom of the graph and the force applied (stress) is measured along the vertical axis. Both types of bone material do not lengthen much before reaching their plastic and failure lengths, but cortical bone requires the application of a lot of force to break. Ligament and tendon will both lengthen more than bone, reaching strains of up to 10–13% before they lose their integrity. The drop in the ligament and tendon curves indicates that they have lost some of their integrity and will lengthen with less force applied. After the peak of the curve, they are said to have entered the plastic phase. The plastic phase is when the material deforms and is unable to return to its original length; it has been permanently deformed. If force is increased further, the tissue will eventually reach failure and break entirely. Before any material enters its plastic phase, it has the possibility of returning to its original length and is therefore elastic—it has the ability to spring back to the start position. (Stress and strain is explored further in chapter 5.)*

Factors that influence bone response to load are numerous and complex, and they include composition (the balance between minerals, organic material, and water content), type (cortical bone or trabeculae), density and orientation of trabeculae, bone length, cross-section, and joint position. For example, the femur and the tibia, both long bones, illustrate how different requirements correlate with different features. The femur has the ability to bend in response to load but the tibia less so. The femur has a relatively circular cross-section along the shaft compared with the more triangular tibia—the thicker bone and its triangular shape make the tibia sturdier and less prone to bending (see figs. 3.5 & 4.8).

---

[4]Hans Selye, who developed the famous General Adaptation System analysis of the human response to stress was quoted as saying that he regretted his lack of understanding of English as he would have used a better word than "stress" to describe our response to stressors. Stress is the measurement of an applied force, "strain" is the correct term for the response to a stressor. https://www.stress.org/what-is-stress. Stress and strain are explored further in chapter 5.

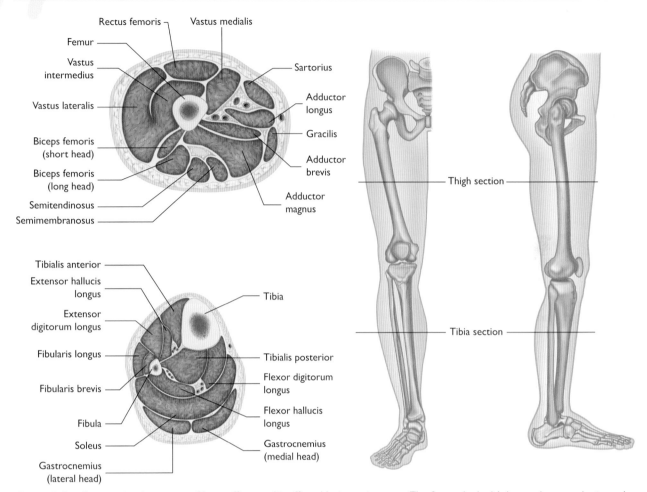

Figure 3.5.   Cross-sectional geometry of bone affects, and is affected by, its environment. The femur, the body's longest bone, angles inward from the hip to the knee and is slightly curved anterior/posterior. It is surrounded by large strong muscles with an adaptable joint at the top. In contrast, the tibia lies vertically between the ankle and knee joints, neither of which have many degrees of freedom. The cross-section also demonstrates the thick, dense cortical layer of bone within the tibia, a further indication of its less compliant nature.

Morton talked of locomotion as an interaction and the same is true within anatomy. It is not only the material properties of the bone that affect its response but also its immediate environment. The femur is surrounded by strong contractile tissue and a number of studies demonstrate muscle's ability to preserve the bone's integrity by decreasing the amount of bending in a long bone and, potentially, putting the long bone under compression (Duda et al. 1998; Lutz et al. 2016), see fig. 3.6.

As mentioned above, bending a bone increases its potential to bend more and eventually break—bending long bones under high loads is dangerous. A simple experiment with a pencil will show how easy it is to break if you bend it, not so easy if you try compressing it by pushing directly inward from either end. However, we cannot analyse bone shape and material properties as if they are separate from the rest of their environment. Using complex analyses, Lutz and colleagues (2016) showed the contraction of muscle around the femur reduced significantly the bending forces it experienced when under high load (fig. 3.6). We cannot analyze bone shape and material properties as if they are separate from the rest of their environment. The surrounding muscles affect a bone's response and are recruited to minimize its bending under high loads.

It therefore appears that long bones are able to bend under normal loads, but are compressed

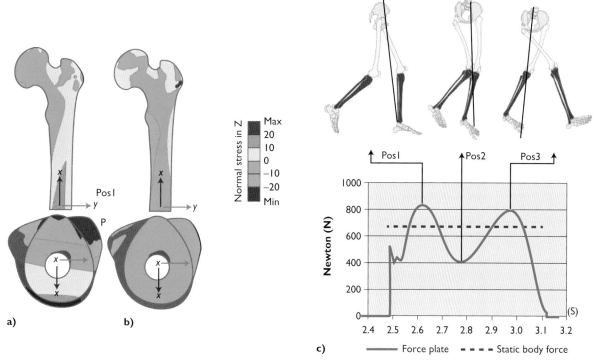

Figure 3.6.   *Using complex computer modeling, known as finite element analysis, several experiments indicate that long bones may experience almost pure compression during peak loading. Stress distribution shown in (a) and (b) represent the bone's reaction at heel strike (position 1, (c)). The image is adapted from a paper by Lutz et al. (2017) where they used a new calculation method using real-life data. The solid color-scheme on the cross-section, (b), indicates the bone is not bending, unlike bone (a), which has a range of stress measurements indicative of tension and compression.*

(i.e., no bending) under high loads, which is a safer balance of the characteristics. But some bones, as we saw in fig. 3.3, are designed for compression—they are short and square, therefore unlikely to bend and experience tension.

Demands in a system with limited resources and a reasonable level of predictability are best met using materials that support and reinforce the structure in specific directions. To return to the skyscraper analogy, it would be a waste of materials to build the structure to resist high winds from every angle if storms only blew in from the west. To save on construction materials, biological tissues show various degrees of anisotropy—i.e., their ability to withstand forces is direction dependent, (fig. 3.7)—another indication of active and localized modeling of bone in response to its recurrent stress environment (Chen and Ingber 1999).

Creating consistent layers of densely packed, solid bone would be metabolically expensive. The compromise is to create a hard, outer layer and a scaffold, which is sometimes hollow inside. The outer layer of dense, compact bone provides strength to the overall structure.

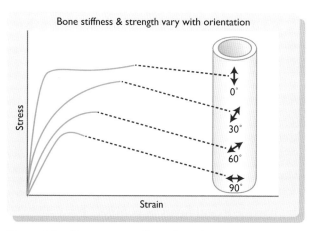

Figure 3.7.   *The anisotropy of bone. Bone does not have a single stress/strain curve, due to variations in shape and trabecular orientation, it reacts differently according to direction of stress and may show weakness in uncommon vectors.*

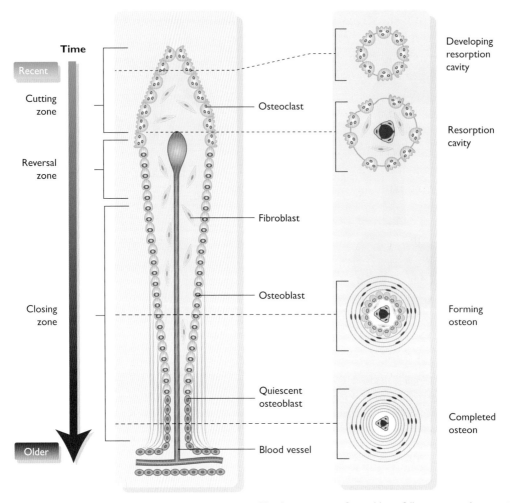

Figure 3.8. *A cutting cone showing the concentric ring pattern created by the sequence of osteoblasts following osteoclast erosion. Note the trapped osteoblasts, now osteocytes, within the completed osteon. (Illustration from Standring 2008.)*

As we have seen with the differences between the femur and tibia, the body modifies cortical thickness and cross-sectional dimensions to accommodate the forces experienced through the bone (Main et al. 2010). Compact bone also provides solidity for periosteal connections to musculotendon contractile tissues and cartilaginous interactions at joint surfaces, and reinforces areas of compression, as shown in fig. 3.4. The body modifies cortical thickness and cross-sectional dimensions to accommodate the forces within the bone (Main et al. 2010; Chen and Ingber 1999).

The hard, cortical layer of compact bone also protects the inner sections of the bones, the honeycombed trabecular bone (see fig. 3.2), (Standring 2008). The benefits of a solid outer and a trabecular core are to lower the overall density and therefore the metabolic costs of bone production, maintenance, and movement (Chen and Ingber 1999), and to provide space for marrow or gas (Currey 2002). The struts of trabecular bone, like the Volkmann's canals (fig. 3.9), are aligned to maximize strength by triangulating their connections (Chen and Ingber 1999). The triangulation of the struts, as we saw in figure 1.15, helps to distribute load, just as von Meyer recognized in the arms of cranes back in the 1890s.

■ CELLULAR ACTION AND MATERIALS

Bone is developed and maintained through the actions and interactions of its cells: osteoblasts, osteoclasts, and osteocytes, illustrated in fig. 3.8. These cells form a construction system based on the role played by each cell type— the builders (osteoblasts) and demolition crews (osteoclasts) respond to signals from the managers (osteocytes), who can sense how their local area is responding to the strain environment and instruct accordingly. Osteocytes are sensitive to changes in pressure and strain, and act as mechanoreceptors for bone in a system that is not yet fully understood.

While much more detail is available in other sources, the outline below is designed to give an appreciation of the interplay between mechanics and cellular behavior. However, the message is easily summarized: given the correct nutritional environment, bone should be able to self-optimize its shape in response to the mechanical environment around it. So, you can skip this section if you want to, but you will miss out on a lot of cool stuff and a little bit of revision of basic bone anatomy if you do.

The physical properties of bone are created by a balance between the compliancy of collagen and the stability of crystalline elements. These materials are exuded from the osteoblasts located on the surface of bone, under the periosteum (the fibrous lining of bone; its interface with contractile tissues) is shown in fig. 3.9. The osteoblasts often lie dormant as "bone-lining cells" until called upon by changes in strain (Currey 2002). Once stimulated into action, the osteoblasts produce materials including tropocollagen—single-strand collagen—and osteoid— the initial fibrous network protein for the bone. Once outside the osteoblast, tropocollagen fibers bond together and form type I and some type V collagen fibers (Standring 2008). These fibers create the scaffolding for hydroxyapatite crystals (the calcium that gives bone much of its rigidity) that lie between the collagen strands (Currey 2013).

The collagen fibrils, especially type I, provide the bone with elasticity and pliability, while the calcium sulfate and hydroxyapatite crystals provide solidity and rigidity to the bone. The interplay in positioning and ratio between these two primary materials, collagen and crystals, can give bone a variable and complex arrangement of properties along the elastic to rigid axis.

This building process is kept in check by balancing the actions of osteoclasts and osteocytes. Osteoclasts remove unnecessary or redundant bone material under the guidance of the "sensing" osteocytes. Osteoclasts are polymorphic cells (i.e., they take on many forms and roles depending on need) that dissolve bony minerals with acid and break down the fiber network with collagenase (Standring 2008). Osteoclastic activity appears to be moderated via signals processed through osteocytes (highly dendritic cells embedded within lamellar bone). This process is managed according to local and systemic demands in a circular feedback loop—the force experienced by the bone determines much of its shape and the shape of the bone determines how it receives force.

BONE REMODELING

Numerous theories exist to explain the adaptive modeling of bone by the osteoblasts and osteoclasts and they all center on the characteristics of the third type of bone cell, the osteocyte (see figs. 3.8 & 3.9). Osteocytes are repurposed osteoblasts that have been embedded within mature bone during the modeling and remodeling processes.

During the remodeling process (see fig. 3.8), osteoblasts are left behind within the "closing zone" and remain in the lacunae—the spaces in intermediate layers between the growth rings of the Haversian canals (see fig. 3.9). These stranded osteoblasts cease to produce bone and develop a complex dendritic network through the canaliculi (small canals) of the bone matrix and change their function to become

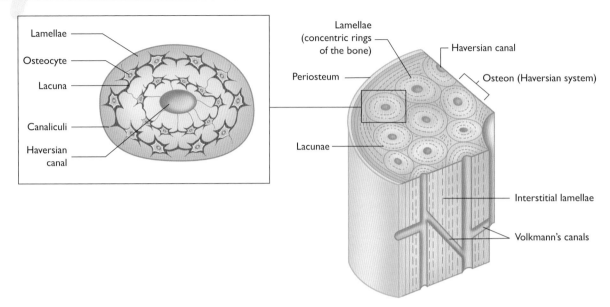

Figure 3.9.   A schematic illustration showing major features of bone. (Illustration from Standring 2008.)

osteocytes. Osteocytes communicate chemically and electrically with each other via their dendritic branches and fulfill their new role of monitoring nutritional and mechanical levels through the bone (Currey 2002).

Local variations in tension or electrical flow initiated by the strains of compression and tension are sensed by the osteocytes and they, in turn, organize bone remodeling to balance out the strains acting through the bone. It seems reasonable to say the osteocytes act as bone-centered mechanoreceptors. The interconnected, mesh-like placement of osteocytes within a relatively pliable series of concentric layers gives them access to numerous sources of information on the forces acting on the bone. Information reaches osteocytes from chemical and electrical flows, as well as through changes in the fluid mechanics that alter and affect mechanical tension along their dendrites.

Via the canaliculi, osteocytes have access routes for "diffusion of nutrients, gases and waste products" (Standring 2002, page 88), and so it stands to reason that osteocytes both give and receive information in numerous forms between themselves and their environment. That exchange includes degrees of mechanical

force interchange (including amount, rate, and amplitude) that allow cellular regulation through mechanochemical transduction—a system proposed by Chen and Ingber (1999).

The ability of bone to self-regulate in response to mechanical demand is well documented (Currey 2013) and often observed by clinicians. One has to assume, however, that the optimization will only be for the more common loading patterns that have driven the remodeling. The body must construct some degree of resilience—too much saving on building materials would create fragility. Likewise, constructing for every eventuality would be overly costly and heavy to move. Remodeling involves its own feedback system to find a balance between too much and too little support in response to loads.

Support for the idea of systemic optimization comes from experiments into the remodeling of the cranial and caudal portions of the radius of horses (Batson et al. 2000). The remodeling aligned the collagen fibers of the lamellar layers in such a way as to better resist compression during loading of the caudal cortex. While the remodeling appeared to come at the expense of decreased strength under tension, it is much less likely for that area to experience such stress in normal usage. The bone showed adaptation to resist and support the most common strains and ignored the possibility of uncommon ones.

Bone appears to have its own design team, but it requires information to operate smoothly. Part of this communication system is provided by the natural architecture of the bone's Haversian systems, which create areas of potential stress concentration. The canaliculi, the Volkmann's canals, and the lacunae, can all generate points of weakness (see fig. 3.9). Perhaps counter to expectation, the presence of the canals is necessary for the many other benefits they bring to the system—by being placed in the canals, osteocytes provide the mechanical feedback and they need to receive nutrition and disperse their waste and signaling materials. Further, the angle of the various channels and the orientation of the lacunae are all found to minimize mechanical deformation but only from the common directions of load to save on expense and weight (Currey 2013, see also fig. 3.7).

▨ STRAIN DISTRIBUTION AND TENSEGRITY

As we saw in fig. 3.7, bone prepares itself for strains in certain directions, so changes in force direction will alter how it is able to respond. Soft tissues are also aligned according to the arrangement of the bones and joints, and the tension network created by the contractile tissue helps support and reduce strain levels within bone. Any change to one system affects the response of the other, with the potential for the response of both systems to be sub-optimal and create tissue disruption in the event of unexpected and unusual forces.

However, evolution seems to have provided our musculoskeletal system with a certain degree of "anti-fragility"—the ability to adapt to demands and be strengthened by them (Taleb 2013). According to Taleb, anti-fragility differs from resiliency as resiliency implies

returning back to the same position. Due to cellular feedback loops that are constantly alert to changes in strain, the system can adapt to novel strains acting through the body.

The body's ability to make fine adjustments to shape and material properties in response to strain distribution illustrates the power of its innate tensegrity (fig. 3.10). Tensegrity, the balance between tension and compression elements that communicate strain

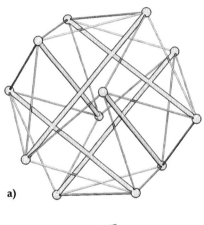

a)

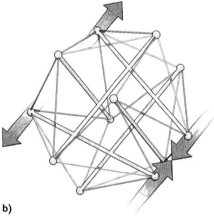

b)

Figure 3.10.   Tensegrity. a) This simplified model provides an image of the stiffer compression elements suspended by the tensional elements. In real-life, however, the body's "compression elements" experience degrees of tension within their normal tolerance levels and are self-designed to be under compression when the surrounding contractile tissues are optimally tensioned (see fig. 3.6). b) The body's whole tensegrity system responds to stress by distributing strain, causing tension and compression to be present simultaneously. Strain to the bone is perceived by the osteocytes, the mechanoreceptive osteocytes then guide osteoblasts and osteoclasts to remodel the bone in a way that balances forces so that only compression of the bone is felt under repeated high loads. (Image from 'Movement Integration: The Systemic Approach to Human Movement', Lundgren & Johansson, Lotus Publishing, 2019.)

throughout the system, has been proposed as an organizational principle of the body. It underlies much of the work on cellular response by Inger and Chen and explains why the long femur bone experiences compression under optimal load rather than bending.

As the body's stiffest element, bone gives support and provides leverage to the soft tissue, but there is a need for inherent safety factors to be built in. If long bones could not bend, they would be brittle and subject to breaking when minimally strained (see fig. 3.4). But if they bend too much, they would be likely to create a weakness when experiencing high loads. A safe zone has developed, wherein the bone is able to strain a little but, rather than always supporting the soft tissues, the tensioning and stiffening of soft tissues also helps support and compress the bone.

The tensioning of surrounding soft tissue prevents the femur from bending and turns it into a "rigid lever", as shown in fig. 3.6, a solid strut between the pelvis and the tibia. Importantly for our current area of interest, the foot, a series of soft tissues will have to do the same for its collection of bones by drawing all of them together to provide stability between the toe joint and the ankle. Thankfully, we have a tensegrity-based musculoskeletal system that adapts to the requirements of our movement patterns.

▪ SUMMARY

This chapter has introduced a lot of possibly unfamiliar and complicated terminology. But the general message is simple—overall bone shape and position are determined by genetic inheritance, and then its construction and

upkeep is fine-tuned by a feedback loop that is sensitive to changes in strain.

Or, if you want a jargon-laden sentence, the morphogenetic model of bone adaptation blends both phylogenetic and ontogenetic dynamics to describe how the shape of bone adapts to fulfill its function.

We have a self-organizing dynamic for bone modeling and remodeling; there is an interdependent relationship between shape and movement. Bone shape will influence movement possibilities, and the experience of strain created by movement will influence bone shape. We saw that square bones are designed to receive high forces, and long bones can help produce greater force but also create the fragility of bending, which is then reduced by the muscle tension around it.

The adaptation of our bones to the mechanical environment allows us to make the kind of interpretations from fossil remains we saw in chapter 2. The shape, size, and orientation of bone and its trabeculae all create fossil artifacts that can be read to understand what use the bones were put to and allow us to interpret usage patterns of long-dead species.

And so we return to the constant feedback loop mentioned at the start of the chapter: movement—strain—response—build/remodel—movement—strain—response … repeat.

The body's tensegrity creates a self-organizing system that adapts itself to repeated strains and allows tissue to constantly remodel itself, using mechanoreceptive cells that signal and guide bone shape. We will explore how this mechanism works in the foot in chapter 4.

4

THE BONES OF THE FOOT

The ease of our walking step makes it
seem a simple action. But since
it includes some degree of motion
in all parts of our physical structure,
the action in its entirety is a highly
complex one.

—Morton, *Human Locomotion
and Body Form*

▦ INTRODUCTION

Our hero, Morton, regularly discussed the
foot's expertise in dealing with the forces
of locomotion and gravity. As we saw in
chapter 3, bone adapts itself through a constant
feedback loop, with the mechanoreceptive
osteocytes directing the balance of construction
and "destruction" by the osteoblasts and
osteoclasts. By looking at the trabecular pattern
in the bones of the foot in the X-ray image
(see fig. 4.1), we can appreciate the continuity
of force flowing from one bone to the next—a
perfect illustration of strain distribution and
tensegrity in context.

If we look at the overall pattern, we can see two
important features:

1. There is a general anteroposterior pattern
   to the trabecular lines, indicative of the
   strongly parasagittal pattern of use of the
   foot as we roll from heel to toe. Of course,
   there are twists and turns in each direction,
   but the primary vector of strain is from front
   to back.
2. The pattern fans down and out from (or up
   and into) the talus. The talus is the top of
   the half-dome and is the interface between
   the leg and foot. The talus, therefore,
   negotiates the flow of force up from the
   heel, along from the forefoot, as well as
   down from the leg.

By building on the image introduced toward
the end of chapter 1 of the foot as a half-dome,
our goal is to build a detailed picture of how
the foot is a structure that can be mobile to
allow pronation yet also provide a "rigid lever"
for the two points of high stress—heel strike
and toe-off (see fig. 1.7).

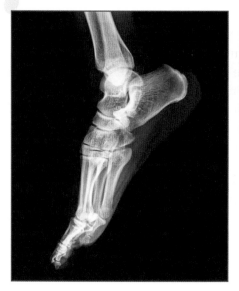 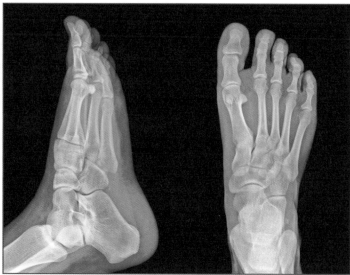

Figure 4.1.   Our previous chapter looked at how force forms and shapes individual bones. This series of X-ray images illustrates the continuity of force communication from one bone to its neighbors to create a functional unit.

There is a strong argument from those involved with tensegrity that "there is no such thing as a lever in the body". This is true. Mechanical levers do not exist in biological structures. However, I believe we can use the principles of leverage to understand many—not all—of the interactions between bones and joints during real-life movement. For example, evolving longer lower limbs boosted locomotor economy because of the way our long femur and tibia allow us to vault over the planted foot to lengthen the stride. Just like trying to prise open a box, having a longer implement to work with can provide a mechanical advantage commonly referred to as "leverage".

Once there is better, more accurate vocabulary, I will happily use it but, for now, this is the best descriptive language that we have, and it mostly works.

It is easy to see that the femur is a rigid bone between two relatively limited joints (knee and hip). It is much more difficult to see the collection of oddly shaped bones with so many tissues and joints that we call a foot in the same way. However, the principles remain the same for the tissues of the foot as for those of the thigh, as positions of high stress will also recruit high levels of tissue strain and tension. As we saw in chapter 3, the femur provides some inherent stiffness, but, in an intricate

play between form and force, it is actually the tension of the surrounding soft tissues that provide rigidity to the bone. To see how and why this happens at the foot first requires an appreciation of bone shape and function.

To get a taste of the foot's adaptability, stand with your feet comfortably below your hip joints and turn your head to the right to look over your right shoulder – turn as far as you can, letting your trunk and pelvis follow your gaze but keep your feet in place. Pause at the end of your comfortable range of movement and feel the reaction of your feet. If you let the movement pass through your pelvis, your left foot will have moved toward pronation and your right foot will have supinated. This ability to unlock (pronate) and lock (supinate) is driven by the bony architecture of the foot and ankle. Understanding the shape and relationships of the bones will help us see how and why the foot reacts in this way and we will return to this exercise at the end of the chapter to reveal why this reaction is so universal.

■ THE FOOT AS A WHOLE AND IN SECTIONS

The 26 bones of the foot come in a confusing variety of shapes and sizes with equally confusing names that are tricky to pronounce and spell. As with much (certainly not all!) anatomy, there is some reasoning behind the names, but only if you have a strong working knowledge of Greek and Latin.

There are a few ways to divide and conquer the foot. One is by **bone group**—*tarsals*, *metatarsals*, and *phalanges*—and they bring us to the Greek and Latin. Like many native English speakers, I struggle with other languages, but once I started to know the meaning of these difficult and strange polysyllabic terms, I realized they had their place and even made life easier. Another way to divide the foot is by **area**—*rearfoot* (calcaneus and talus), *mid-foot* (cuneiforms, navicular, and cuboid), and *forefoot* (metatarsals and phalanges). I recommend, therefore, that you allow yourself some time to let each term become familiar. Many joints are named according to the associated bones, and knowing the names of bone groups as well as individual bones, stands one in good stead to progress from bones and joints to ligaments.

Be sure to spend a little time cracking the logic of the system now as it helps make sense of the rest of the anatomy as we go forward. I have often found that one of the main reasons people get lost with anatomy is because the basic building blocks of the vocabulary were not in place first.

▪ TARSALS, METATARSALS, AND PHALANGES

The tarsals are a group of seven bones: the talus, the calcaneus, the three cuneiforms, the navicular, and the cuboid. *Tarsal* is the Greek word for "wicker basket". Look at the X-ray images and imagine the trabeculae as the intricate weave of a basket. If you turn the book so the sole is facing upward, you can (with a little imagination) see the inside of the half-dome as the inside of the basket.

As we will see, this area can act like a wicker basket that can tighten and loosen its weave depending on load and direction. The basket is therefore a helpful image to use to understand pronation and supination. Imagine the soft tissues and bones are the basket material and that they stretch and strain as the holes in the basket open—pronation. Twist the basket in another direction and the holes close up, close-packing the basket—supination and our rigid lever position. Provided the weave remains flawless, at no point should the basket lose its integrity. Whether the weave is open or closed the basket retains its strength.

The tarsals form the *rearfoot* and *mid-foot* while the metatarsals make up most of the *forefoot*. If you had the advantage of a classical education, you probably already knew the prefix "meta" simply means "beyond" (think of physics and metaphysics—metaphysical means beyond explanation by physics). The forefoot consists of many long straight bones, first the row of five metatarsals and then the 14 phalanges that make up the toes.

In general terms, long bones provide leverage, and short ones give adaptability. Think of the femur and tibia, for example—their length provides significant locomotor efficiency, and the knee joint provides a lot of leverage. But leverage comes at a cost as the longer the lever, the more force required to stabilize and control it. The relative proportions of the human foot provide an effective lever, but that long lever must be stable. The stability is partly provided by the unique, wicker basket-like arrangement of the human tarsals, which twist and lock together to provide a rigid lever, and then untwist to spread, thereby allowing the soft tissues to strain, as they absorb shock.

There are two compound joint lines[1] across the human foot—the *tarsometatarsal* and *transverse*

---

[1] A compound joint is one "joint" made up of numerous joints. I know, it didn't make sense to me either when I read it, but it will make sense shortly.

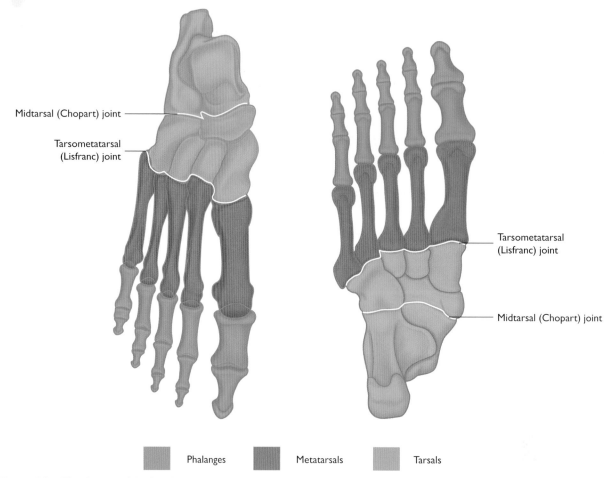

Midtarsal (Chopart) joint

Tarsometatarsal
(Lisfranc) joint

Tarsometatarsal
(Lisfranc) joint

Midtarsal (Chopart) joint

Phalanges   Metatarsals   Tarsals

Figure 4.2.   The divisions of the foot. The tarsals make up the rear- (calcaneus and talus) and mid-foot (cuneiforms, cuboid, and navicular) regions. The forefoot consists of the metatarsals and phalanges. There are two important joints traversing the foot—the midtarsal (or, transverse tarsal, or Chopart) and tarsometatarsal (or Lisfranc) joints. As they include several bones they are referred to as compound joints.

tarsal joints (fig. 4.2)—which facilitate some of the foot's unique range of functions. The distal joint line across the foot is the interface between tarsals and metatarsals, the aptly named tarsometatarsal joint. The tarsometatarsal line looks like a coastal map with a rough outline of inlets and projections. This ragged arrangement of interlocking bones provides some natural stability to the joint line to help prevent shearing.

The more proximal transverse tarsal joint is also commonly known as the midtarsal joint because it occurs roughly in the middle of the tarsal section. Both the superior and inferior views of this line show its elegant curve; however, this curve creates a potential instability that must be stabilized by a locking mechanism between the calcaneus and the cuboid (fig. 4.3). The midtarsal joint is also known as Chopart joint—Chopart was a French surgeon who chose this line for its ease of amputation.

The tarsometatarsal joint, also known as Lisfranc joint (yet another French surgeon), suffers from being at the base of a series of long bones. Just as the knee joint is commonly challenged by trauma due to its placement between long bones, the same is true of the tarsometatarsal/Lisfranc joint. Though less common than the various injuries to the knee, the tarsometatarsal joint can be dislocated by falls and accidents.

Understanding the Greek and Latin anatomical terms is difficult enough, but once surgeons start naming things after themselves, we can really start to lose our place, especially if references cannot make up their mind which naming tradition they wish to use. Until recently, I would find myself looking for the new structures of Chopart or Lisfranc joint (for instance) because the reference did not make it clear that there are alternative names. Where possible in this text, I will adhere to anatomical terminology and avoid any further unnecessary boosting of dead egos. The retired French surgeons are mentioned here purely to help you avoid the moments of confusion I experience myself.

If we look at the groups of bones in the foot—tarsals, metatarsals, and phalanges—and then at the joints so far—midtarsal and

tarsometatarsal—it makes sense that the next interface is the line of the metatarsophalangeal joints. This line of joints forms the "ball of the foot" (one of the rockers). The only potential confusion here is that the **m**e**ta**t**arso**p**halangeal** **j**oints[2] are variously abbreviated to MTPs, MTJs and, sometimes, MTPJs.

Our last line of bones, the phalanges, are so-named because they are relatively long and straight, just like a group of Greek soldiers as they march into battle. There are 14 phalanges on each foot—two for the big toe and three in each of the other toes. The joints between them are therefore the interphalangeal joints, and because there are three bones in the smaller toes, they have a **p**roximal **inter**p**halangeal** and a **d**istal **inter**p**halangeal** joint, cutely abbreviated to the PIPs and DIPs.

▪ FUNCTIONAL DIVISION

In keeping with the tradition of naming the same parts in various ways, we can divide the foot into functional units. We can see the foot as two functional halves: the medial aspect made up of the talus, navicular, cuneiforms, and metatarsals one to three, the lateral aspect comprised of the calcaneus, cuboid, and metatarsals four and five (fig. 4.3).

As we will see later, the medial/lateral split divides the foot according to each part's roles during weight transfer through the foot and the function of each "half" during standing and locomotion. While I dislike dividing the foot in this way, preferring the complete image of the half-dome, the medial/lateral split can be a useful image for gaining functional insights into the foot.

Another common terminology used to reference areas of the feet is *"ray"*—as in the common diagnosis of a hyper- or hypomobility

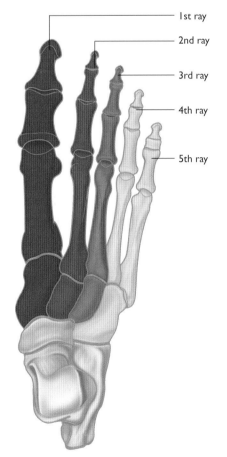

1st ray
2nd ray
3rd ray
4th ray
5th ray

Figure 4.3. *The foot can also be divided up medial to lateral as a series of "rays" or lines, which are numbered according to their associated toe (one to five). Some references also like to differentiate between the medial group, which aligns rays one to three with the talus, and the fourth and fifth ray to the calcaneus.*

_____

[2]Highlighted letters are those used for the various abbreviations of the joints.

of the *first ray*. A ray is simply a line of bones, so the line of each distal phalange to the metatarsal constitutes a single ray. The rays are named from medial to lateral, from the big toe as the first ray, to the little toe as the fifth ray (see fig. 4.3).

RELATIONSHIP TO THE LEG

The foot only makes sense in relation to the rest of our anatomy, particularly when put into the context of our movement strategies, and having an understanding of the gait cycle aids appreciation of the interface between the foot and the leg. It is important to remember that anatomical divisions are almost arbitrary, as the overall structure works as a system to seek and find the essentials of life—water, calories, safety, and sex. As we saw in chapter 2, adaptations of the foot are often emphasized in the story of *Homo sapiens'* rise to bipedalism, but changes to the foot were part and parcel of the alterations to our overall anatomy.

In chapter 2, we saw the relationship between tibial torsion, foot alignment, and adduction of the big toe. The twist within the foot provides the half-dome formation, a mobile shock-absorbing system that communicates force upward to the rest of the body. The foot's "fall" into pronation is corrected by supinating back into a "rigid lever" to control the force involved with toe-off. Much of this correction is provided to the foot by the movement pattern of the rest of the body, which is communicated through the leg bones (tibia and fibula) to the talus (fig. 4.4). Thus, the ankle complex (the relationship between the tibia, fibula, talus, and calcaneus) plays an important role in determining the foot's direction and alignment.

The ankle complex is formed by three joints: the inferior tibiofibular joint, the talocrural joint, and the subtalar joint. There are three bones involved in the first two joints—the tibia and fibula (inferior tibiofibular joint), and then the tibia, fibula, and talus (talocrural joint).

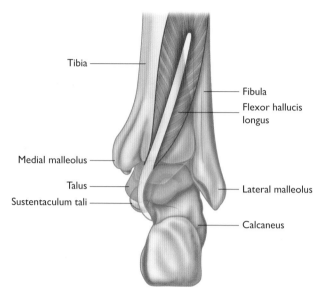

Figure 4.4.   The center of gravity of the talus (in pink) is slightly medial to the center of gravity of the calcaneus. The talus rests on a projecting ledge of the calcaneus called the sustentaculum tali. The bony projection is supported by the tendon of the flexor hallucis longus from below. We should also note how the talus is "captured" between the two malleoli of the leg bones.

The subtalar joint is the interface between the calcaneus and talus.

Although the terminology can be daunting at first, it can be broken down into manageable chunks. As mentioned above, many joints are named by the bones involved, such as the tibiofibular joint. The same thing is true of the talocrural joint—we just need to know that crura refers to the portion of the lower limb between the knee and ankle. Crura is shorthand, in this case, for the tibia and fibula. So, talocrural is just short for talotibiofibular joint. The subtalar joint will be explored later in this chapter as it describes the relationship between the talus and the bones below (*sub*) it.

The *talus* (from Latin: ankle) is placed directly below the sturdy, triangular, and weight-bearing tibia (fig. 4.4). Both bones of the leg, the tibia and fibula, have bony projections known as *malleoli* (Latin: little hammer, mallet) that encase the talus on either side. The top of the talus, also known as the dome or *trochlea* (Greek: pulley) forms the second of the four rockers (see figs. 1.7 and 4.5). The talar dome

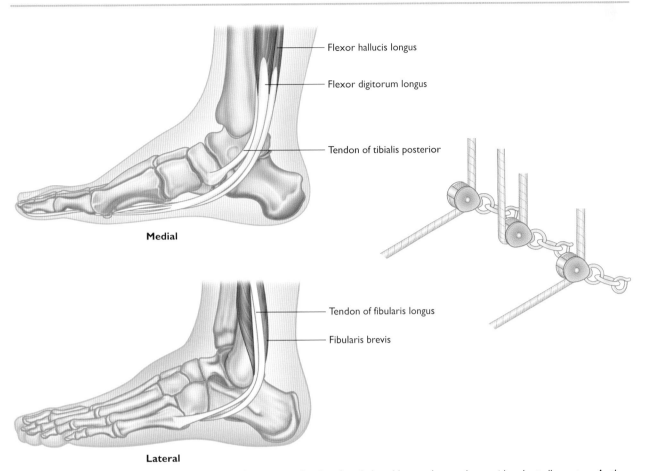

Flexor hallucis longus

Flexor digitorum longus

Tendon of tibialis posterior

Medial

Tendon of fibularis longus

Fibularis brevis

Lateral

Figure 4.5.   The trochlea (dome) of the talus translates as a pulley but the whole ankle complex can be considered a pulley system. As the ankle moves into dorsiflexion, the tendons passing around the bones will tension and help stabilize the foot.

(or, trochlea) receives the weight coming down from the tibia and the bony arrangement between the three bones means that this talocrural joint facilitates dorsiflexion and plantar flexion (see fig. 4.6).

The bony arrangement creates a mortise and tenon joint, a carpentry term where one piece of wood is slotted between two projections without the use of glue. Slotting together two pieces of wood creates a very stable join in every axis except the one plane where the joints are aligned, and stability in this plane is provided by the tightness of the fit—a determining characteristic of the carpenter's skill. We do not wish the same amount of congruence in the talocrural joint as it benefits from a little looseness but, as ever, there is a balance in the body between mobility and stability.

The angle created by the overlapping malleoli allows a predominantly sagittal plane movement. In this axis, the tibia and fibula move together over the talus (see fig. 4.6b) or the talus and the rest of the foot move under the leg bones (see fig. 4.6c). The trochlea of the talus provides the smooth, rounded surface for this action. The trochlea acts like the groove in a pulley easing the movement of the cables passing around it—and this is precisely the translation of trochlea.

The dome of the talus, the trochlea, is wide anteriorly, and narrow posteriorly (see fig. 4.6a). Regardless of whether the movement is open- or closed-chain, when the ankle is in relative dorsiflexion, the interface is on the wider, anterior portion of the talus. The extra width requires the tibia and fibula

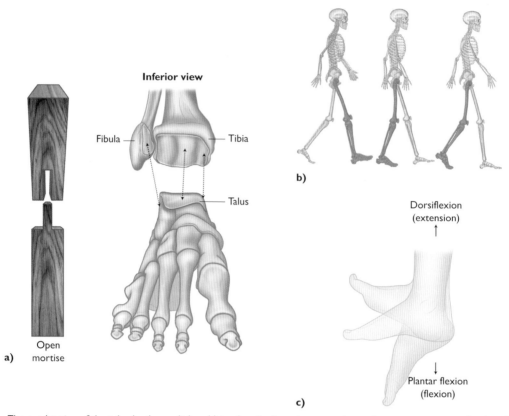

Figure 4.6.   *The overlapping of the talus by the medial and lateral malleoli creates a mortise and tenon arrangement for the talocrural joint (a). The joint alignment facilitates dorsiflexion and plantar flexion but limits rotation. During stance phase of gait, the tibia and fibula move over the foot in a closed-chain reaction (b). In an open-chain movement, the foot moves under the leg (c).*

to move slightly to accept the increased dimension (see fig. 4.11).

The tibia and fibula are held together by a fibrous layer between the two bones (fig. 4.7) and this interosseous membrane arranges its fibers along common lines of strain. The upper portion of the membrane shows cross patterning of fibers as they pass from superior-to-lateral from the tibia and superior-to-medial from the fibula. This contrasts with the lower two-thirds where fibers pass down and out from the tibia to the fibula. The criss-cross pattern helps stabilize the proximal portion from moving too far up or down, tethering the proximal fibula in both directions, and protecting the proximal joint. However, distally, the down and out fiber design allows the fibula to move up and away from the tibia slightly to accept the trochlea of the talus as the joint moves into dorsiflexion.

■ BONE SHAPE AND MUSCLE FUNCTION

To further appreciate the relationship between shape and function, we can compare the position, roles, and form of the body's two longest bones, the tibia and femur (see fig. 4.8). The tear-drop shaped shaft of the femur angles inward from the hip to the knee and has an anteroposterior curve along its length. In contrast, the tibia is relatively vertical, has a triangular form with a thick layer of cortical bone. The long shaft of the femur is surrounded by strong muscles that control forces at the knee and hip. Although the lower leg also deals with high degrees of force, the tibia is not surrounded by muscle; the associated muscles are mostly located posterior to the bone.

Although it has not been fully researched and investigated, the contrast between the

THE BONES OF THE FOOT

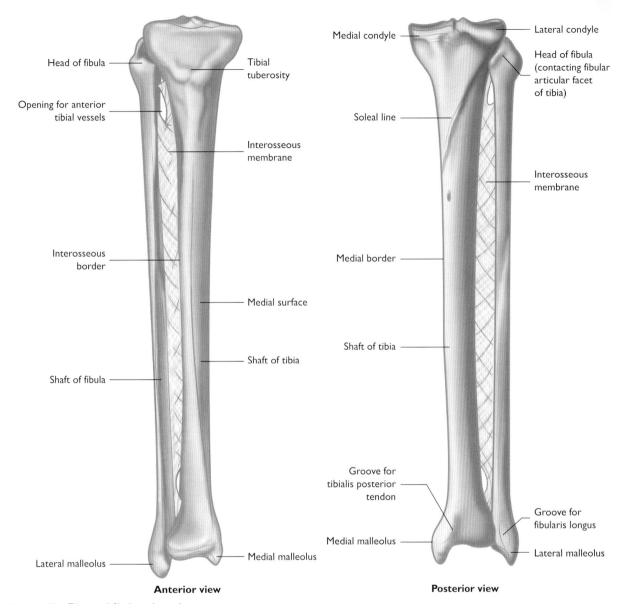

Head of fibula

Tibial
tuberosity

Opening for anterior
tibial vessels

Interosseous
membrane

Interosseous
border

Medial surface

Shaft of tibia

Shaft of fibula

Lateral malleolus

Medial malleolus

Anterior view

Medial condyle

Lateral condyle

Head of fibula
(contacting fibular
articular facet
of tibia)

Soleal line

Interosseous
membrane

Medial border

Shaft of tibia

Groove for
tibialis posterior
tendon

Groove for
fibularis longus

Medial malleolus

Lateral malleolus

Posterior view

Figure 4.7.   Tibia and fibula with syndesmosis arrangement.

position and shape of these two bones appears to emphasize their differing roles. As the femur shaft is fully encased by muscle, the tension created by muscle contraction supports the bone and inhibits the bending under high loads (see fig. 3.6). Because of the lack of muscle on its anterior medial aspect, the tibia does not receive such support and must reinforce itself with extra cortical bone; it also tends to receive force from two relatively flat joint surfaces.

The tibia sits quite firmly on top of the talus and the tibial plateau creates a neat interface for the femoral condyles. Sitting between two relatively flat joint surfaces, the thick, triangular tibia receives a limited range of quite predictable forces during normal movement. The ball-and-socket joint at the hip, however, allows the femur a large and three-dimensional range of motion, most of which is used during our daily routines. As we saw in fig. 3.6, the solution to supporting the long femur while allowing it to be lightweight appears to be surrounding it with contractile, tensional tissue. That solution is unnecessary, or not possible, for the tibia.

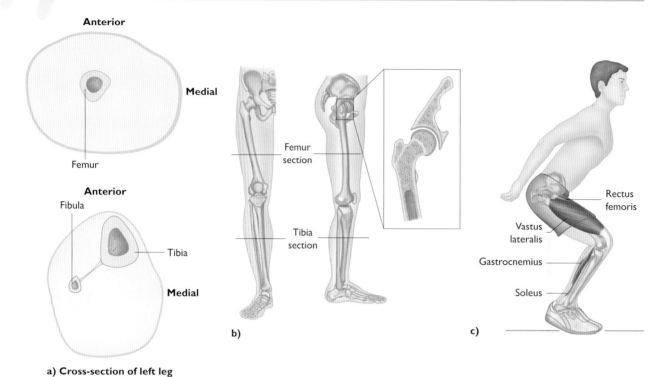

a) Cross-section of left leg

Figure 4.8.   a) The femur has a narrow, tear-drop shaped shape in its mid-shaft in contrast to the more robust tibia, which also has a thick layer of strong cortical bone (see also fig. 4.9). The femur is surrounded by contractile tissue; the soft tissue is predominately posterior to the tibia. b) The tibia has two flat surfaces that interface with relatively limited joints at either end and the femur has a large-range ball-and-socket joint with the pelvis. The vertical tibia therefore receives more predictable forces in contrast to the femur. c) The patella prevents the knee from passing into extension. Because of that limitation, the ankle is driven, most commonly, into dorsiflexion. As a result, the muscle arrangement around the tibia is biased toward the deceleration of dorsiflexion and therefore is predominantly posterior to the triangular bone (see also fig. 3.5).

Tibial movement is limited by the joints at either end. The malleoli and talar dome at the ankle contain the tibia to mostly sagittal plane movement. The patella at the knee joint prevents the knee from moving much beyond neutral into extension. As the knee is limited to almost only flexion (a few degrees of rotation and extension are available, but very little compared with the range of flexion), the tibia is driven forward into ankle dorsiflexion in reaction to knee flexion. The joint arrangements determine the reaction, and the soft tissue develops to decelerate the high and rapid deceleration forces (fig. 4.8c). The combination of these features—bone position and adjacent joint reactions—explains why the tibia changes shape during development from a relatively circular cross-section to a triangular cross-section—indicating it is strengthened along its anterior/posterior axis (fig. 4.9, Gosman et al. 2013).

Unlike the vertical and sturdy tibia, the human fibula does not carry any body weight and is the more mobile of the two bones of the leg (figs. 4.10 & 4.11). The human fibula contrasts with that of the chimpanzee, which does have to carry some body weight and has a joint with the talus bone (figs. 4.10 & 4.15). Chimpanzee legs are bowed, and wider ranges of motion are required to deal with their terrain. Our feet and legs have adapted to minimize locomotor and postural metabolic costs, and this was supported by redesigning the tibia as a relatively vertical strut. To compensate for the inward "Q" angle from hip to knee, the thigh and hip complex has developed a series of soft tissue adaptations, including the iliotibial band and its associated fascia lata to distribute mechanical forces (Cowgill et al. 2010; for more information see, *Born to Walk*, 2020).

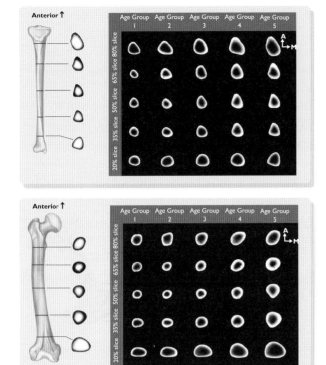

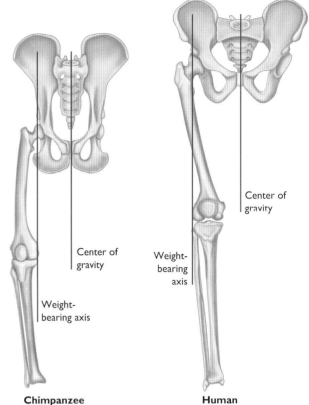

Figure 4.9.   A study by Gosman et al. (2013) compared cross-sectional shape across several areas of the femur and tibia for different age ranges. The cross-sectional slices were taken at 20%, 35%, 50%, 65%, and 80% of the length of each bone. Each section shows an increase in asymmetry during ontogeny (development) in response to the force environment experienced. The age groups used are: 0–1.9 years; 2–4.9 years; 5–8.9 years; 9–13.9 years; and 14–18 years. (Adapted from Gosman et al. 2013.)

Figure 4.10.   Several features of the lower limb of the chimpanzee prevent it from being an efficient biped. These include the bowed legs and laterally tilted tibia relative to the vertical alignment of the human tibia. The inward "Q" angle of the human hip requires increased mobility and stability at the hip complex, which is partly assisted by the positioning of the hip abductor hip muscles.

The distal tibia rests on top of the talus, which is wider from back to front, requiring the joint to open to accept the front of the talus as the ankle dorsiflexes (fig. 4.11). This widening of the joint to receive the wider portion of the talus tensions the soft tissue around the joint (joint capsule, ligaments, and interosseous membrane) and creates a "close-packing" of the joint. A "close-packed" joint provides a stable position from which to launch strong forces, one reason for starting a sprint from a dorsiflexed position. The joint expansion that happens during dorsiflexion should be palpable—both as a self-palpation and as an assessment for clients. Lightly place a finger on each malleolus; the gentle movement of the fibula should be palpable as the ankle passes toward end-range of dorsiflexion.

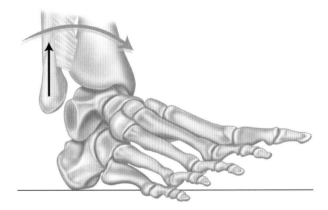

Figure 4.11.   When compared with neutral, as the ankle dorsiflexes, the wider portion of the talus pushes the fibular malleolus upward and laterally. This action provides the extra space for the talus and tensions the supportive tissues. (The relationship and the changes have been exaggerated for visual representation.)

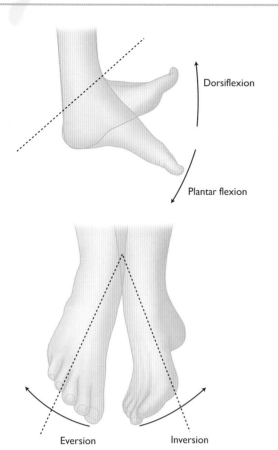

Dorsiflexion

Plantar flexion

Eversion   Inversion

Figure 4.12. *The mortise and tenon joint arrangement of the talar (or, talocrural joint) allows for 20–30° of dorsiflexion and 40–50° of plantar flexion. Inversion and eversion mostly occur in the subtalar joint and range from 20–30° for inversion and 10–20° of eversion.*

While the bony arrangement facilitates dorsiflexion and plantar flexion, rotation at the talocrural joint is restricted by the overhanging malleoli (see fig. 4.8). This "limitation" is not a negative feature as it facilitates the coupling of rotational movements from the leg to the talus and from the talus to the leg. We will explore the implications of rotational coupling as we go through the rest of the text, but this coupling relationship is quickly and easily felt by standing and turning to your right (as we did at the start of this chapter). The rotation causes a predictable reaction as your left foot should pronate and the right foot supinates.

As we saw in chapter 2 when exploring tibial torsion, lateral rotation twists the foot up into the supinated half-dome and medial rotation leads to pronation—the reaction of the foot is

mostly determined by the direction in which the leg bones rotate. Rotation through the lower limb and pronation/supination are "coupled" because of the overlap between the malleoli and the talus—if one bone in this trio (tibia, fibula, and talus) rotates, the others will follow. Movement of the three ankle bones is coupled in transverse plane rotation because of the mortise and tenon arrangement but, because of the joint arrangement, they are uncoupled in the sagittal plane. During dorsiflexion and plantar flexion, the leg bones and the talus can move relatively independently through mid-range. It could be said that the talus is a leg bone in rotation and a foot bone in dorsiflexion and plantar flexion.

As we saw above, the tibia is a sturdy weight-bearing bone, while the non-weight-bearing fibula lies to its side. The strong quadriceps and iliotibial band both attach to the superior portion of the tibia. These and many other muscles around the knee complex help give the area support and stability. In contrast, the only support given to the fibula from above is from the biceps femoris (fig. 4.13). The fibula provides attachment sites for eight of the muscles coming down to the foot, a fact that would result in pulling the fibula inferiorly if not for the fiber angle of the interosseous membrane and the upward pull of the biceps femoris.

Only primates and carnivores (for example, cats and bears) have a separate tibia and fibula with "give" at the ankle. The slight movement between the two bones provides extra mobility and allows better handling of the strains created during complex combinations of sagittal and transverse plane movement. Considering the varied terrains and required speed for turns performed by these agile predators, it is clear that they require that ideal combination of mobility and stability. In contrast, deer and giraffe have no fibula and although they excel in graceful, elegant prancing, they struggle a little with turns.

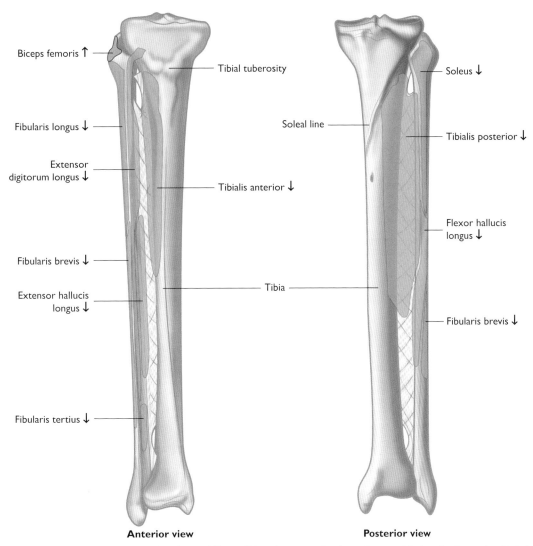

Biceps femoris ↑

Tibial tuberosity

Soleus ↓

Fibularis longus ↓

Soleal line

Tibialis posterior ↓

Extensor
digitorum longus ↓

Tibialis anterior ↓

Flexor hallucis
longus ↓

Fibularis brevis ↓

Tibia

Extensor hallucis
longus ↓

Fibularis brevis ↓

Fibularis tertius ↓

Anterior view

Posterior view

Figure 4.13.   *The muscle attachments on the tibia and fibula. Although a more slender and non-weight-bearing bone, the fibula has nine attachment sites, with only one of them, biceps femoris, pulling the bone upward.*

The syndesmosis arrangement of the human ankle facilitates mobility and stability to assist our varied locomotion. The arrangement of ligaments and the interosseous membrane around the ankle complex allows the fibula some freedom of movement (see fig. 4.14). The fibula's movement provides adaptability, shock absorption, and force distribution, and also allows the bone to move inferiorly at heel strike. The small downward glide of the lateral malleolus helps stabilize the ankle by adding more overlap between the talus and the fibular malleolus, while also stretching the interosseous membrane and tibiofibular ligaments to distribute soft tissue strain (Aiello & Dean 2002).

A *fibula* refers to a "pin" or brooch that was often used to attach robes. The human fibula is obviously too long and blunt for this purpose, but the equivalent chicken bone perfectly matches the shape and length of the metal pins that were used.

The malleolus of the human fibula extends further distally than the tibial malleolus and provides some support to the ankle by creating a bony block to eversion sprains (see also "end feel" in chapter 8).

The posterior surface of tibia provides an essential anchor for the strong soleus muscle (see fig. 4.13). This soleal line should be visible on any skeleton and is indicative of the strength, and therefore importance, of this muscle. As we explore each bone, the significance of each line, groove, bump, indentation, projection, and tuberosity should become more evident, but it will require circling back and forth between function, skeletal, and musculotendinous anatomy. The significance of each feature, such as the soleal line, is revealed through understanding its functional context.

The dome-shaped, pulley arrangement of the trochlea (top of the talus) is complemented by the two rounded ends of the malleoli (see fig. 4.5). The medial malleolus provides a "pulley" for the tendon of the tibialis posterior, and the lateral malleolus performs the same role for the fibularis longus and brevis muscles (previously known as peroneus longus and brevis). The roles of the soft tissues will be examined further in the next chapter, but they require mentioning here to mark the importance of the bony architecture.

The distal joint surface of the tibia is horizontal, which helps the tibia "vault" over the pulley of the trochlea, but the trochlea is angled slightly medially. Coupled with the front-to-back offset between the encasing malleoli, the trochlear angle gives a tendency for dorsiflexion and plantar flexion to also create rotation within the joint. The amount of rotation is variable and is questioned by some researchers (Brockett and Chapman 2016) but it is worth noting in the case of complex clients who may exhibit unusual patterns.

Comparing our ankle complex with that of our chimpanzee cousins illustrates several points made so far (fig. 4.15). Chimpanzee fibulae are more robust, share a joint surface with the talus, and carry a significant portion of body weight. This contrasts to the gracile human fibula which stays truer to its pin-like descriptor. The chimpanzee tibia and fibula form a rounded dome over the talus, producing a rolling gait, but the human tibia remains relatively horizontal, correlating with our straight-ahead glide.

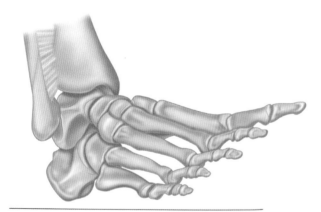

Figure 4.14.   As the ankle is dorsiflexed in preparation for heel strike, the fibula is pulled inferiorly to provide extra protection to the ankle and to tension the syndesmosis and ligaments. The fibular malleolus is more distal than the tibial and blocks eversion—therefore inversion sprains are more common but eversion sprains are more serious as they often injure the bone of the fibula.

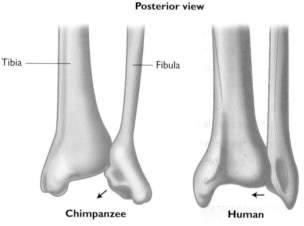

Figure 4.15.   The chimpanzee tibia and fibula have numerous differences to the human condition. Due to the bowing of its lower limb (fig. 4.10), the chimpanzee fibula carries more body weight and articulates with the talus, which reduces some of its potential for mobility. The sturdier human tibia is vertically aligned with a larger articulation to the talus.

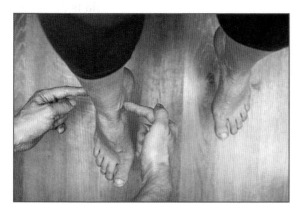

Figure 4.16.

Palpation—Getting to Know the Ankle Complex

As in fig. 4.16, use your fingertips to feel for the two malleoli (L. = Little hammer).

The medial malleolus is a projection from the tibia, and the lateral is from the fibula—notice that the medial is slightly anterior.

If the knee is bent (fig. 4.17), one can compare the angle between the axis of the knee joint (close enough to the frontal plane) and the angle made by the imaginary line passing between the two malleoli. This angle is indicative of the tibial torsion, a natural twist of the tibia that occurs during development. The normal range is a 12–15° lateral rotation. Variations on this will influence ankle tracking and the height of the foot's dome. Just as we explored above in the rotation exercise, medial rotation pronates the foot; lateral rotation supinates it. It would, therefore, be normal for someone to have a tibial torsion less than 12° and be flatter footed than someone with a tibial torsion greater than 15°. *The example shown was measured at 13° and is therefore 'within normal limits'.*

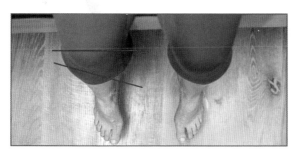

Figure 4.17.

Explore your range of motion at the ankle and watch what happens with the foot as you pass between the extremes of plantar flexion and dorsiflexion (fig. 4.18). The angle of difference between the malleoli leads to offset axis for the movement and couples various degrees of inversion during plantar flexion and eversion of the foot during dorsiflexion.

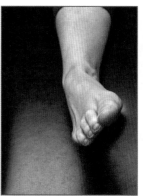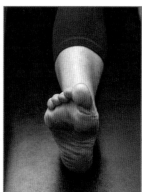

Figure 4.18.

▪ MOBILITY AND STABILITY OF THE FOOT

The human foot has many special powers— along with its ability to change from mobile adaptor to rigid lever, the foot can sense the terrain, provide proprioceptive input to the central nervous system, and absorb and recycle kinetic energy for locomotor efficiency. This combination of abilities is due to the way the foot's collection of tissues combine to allow locking and unlocking of its form. To truly understand Morton's idea of the foot as an organ requires an appreciation of the ecology of the bones—their many interactions with their neighbors, the soft tissue, and the constant changes in their force environment.

We explored some of the compound joints above, but to really appreciate the beauty of this collection of oddly shaped bones, we must investigate each bone in turn. Each bone has its place and its functions, and we will continue to unravel both aspects below.

The bony arrangement provides much of the foot's stability. Earlier, we saw how the trabecular pattern weaves from one bone to the next, and we can also see how the bones weave themselves together with each shape slotting in neatly to allow certain movement and prevent others—just as we saw with the arrangement between the tibia, fibula, and talus. But full stability of the foot requires assistance from the soft tissues, as we will explore in detail in later chapters. The foot's bony form is complemented by force provided by the contractile tissues in the back and forth between mobility and stability.

Dutch physiotherapist Andry Vleeming uses the terminology of form and force closure to describe the mechanics of the complex sacroiliac joints (SIJs). The bones of the SIJs fit together to provide support through their form, but the joints still require extra reinforcement from the muscles crossing the joint lines. The concept of form and force closure fits perfectly for many of the mechanics we see in the feet. The architectural arrangement of the bones almost creates a self-supporting dome, but it requires a ligamentous tethering and a forceful regathering to draw the bones tightly together.

The interactions between the bony and soft tissues allow the foot to fulfill its three major functions listed by biomechanist Bruno Nigg (Nigg 2010):

1. Provide support;
2. Provide protection; and
3. Act as a lever system.

As mentioned above, we can argue over the usage and what is meant by his use of "lever" but I doubt if anyone questions the necessity of the bones providing stiffness to our locomotor system. That is quite straightforward in the case of the two major bones of the lower limb—the femur and the tibia. Both bones are long and interface at the knee joint, a relatively straightforward arrangement compared with the foot.

If we consider the major bones and joints of the lower limb—the hip joint supported by the deep acetabulum, the long femur, the strongly ligamented knee joint, the sturdy, vertical tibia on top of the talus contained within its malleolar box—each segment seems to have some degree of inherent stability and support. The stability and support available to the foot are far less obvious. Consider the foot's position at toe-off, with the toes extended, the heel lifted and a LOT of force acting along its length between ankle joint and toes. This is an impressive feat of engineering for a collection 26 oddly shaped bones with 33 joints.

The foot can unlock into pronation to absorb shock and adapt to the terrain's surface and then regather itself to create a stable structure strong enough to deal with the high force load at toe-off. The foot can do this because of its complex interaction between form and force.

In the last chapter we saw the femur's stiffness increase due to the tension of its surrounding soft tissue. The tibia, as it is not surrounded by soft tissue and has a more limited range of force requirements, has evolved through a change in bony architecture to provide a rigid lever. Each of these areas, the thigh and the leg, consist of one major load-bearing bone. It is mechanically easy to produce a rigid lever if you only have one element lying between each joint. Somehow, the foot manages to produce its rigid lever from ankle to toe—creating a compound bone.

Each joint of the body has some combination of form and force closure—architectural support from the bones and tensional assistance from the muscles. The femoral shaft is stabilized by the force of its encasing muscles while the tibia's form is its main source of stability. The compound bone—the foot as a rigid lever—has combined these two strategies to let the loose arrangement of tissues be held together as a functional unit.

While we explore each bone individually and in small functional groups, we need to keep in mind the bones' greater context—their role in the compound bone that is the foot.

▦ REARFOOT—TALUS AND CALCANEUS

The talus and calcaneus make up the rearfoot, and their major roles are to negotiate the forces involved at heel strike and to pass forces up to, and down from, the leg.

The dynamics of the talar joint previously discussed, highlighted important concepts in the coupling and uncoupling of movement across joints. The talar joint is quite free in sagittal plane flexion but its form-limited rotation "couples" the rotation of one bone to its neighbors. How the forces of gravity, momentum, and GRF pass through joints is directly affected by the degrees of freedom available at each joint.

There are a few oft-quoted facts about the talus: it is the only bone with no muscle attachments; 70% of its surface is synovial cartilage; and it defines two of the critical ankle joints—the talar and sub-talar (figs. 4.19 & 4.20). The large amount of cartilaginous surface—the area of interface with other bones—is indicative of its role as a negotiator of forces between adjacent bones. The lack of muscle attachment and therefore muscle control leaves the talus free to react to the forces passing through it, and its shape, in the context of its joints, shuffles those forces toward other bones and toward the appropriate soft tissues.

Looking back to the trabecular patterns, we see how the major lines all navigate their way toward the talus—up and forward from the calcaneus, up and back from the mid-foot (see fig. 4.1). I liken the talus to a traffic cop in the middle of a busy intersection having to negotiate traffic flows from

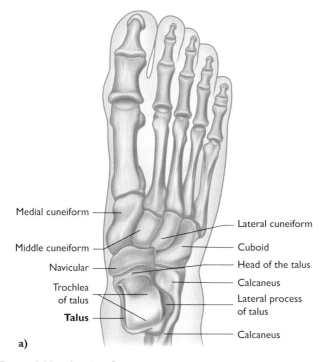

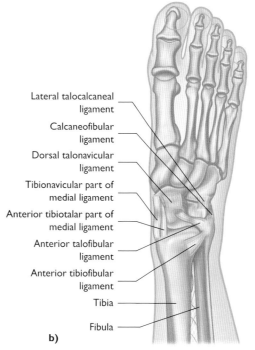

Medial cuneiform
Middle cuneiform
Navicular
Trochlea of talus
Talus

Lateral cuneiform
Cuboid
Head of the talus
Calcaneus
Lateral process of talus
Calcaneus

a)

Lateral talocalcaneal ligament
Calcaneofibular ligament
Dorsal talonavicular ligament
Tibionavicular part of medial ligament
Anterior tibiotalar part of medial ligament
Anterior talofibular ligament
Anterior tibiofibular ligament
Tibia
Fibula

b)

Figure 4.19. *(continued)*

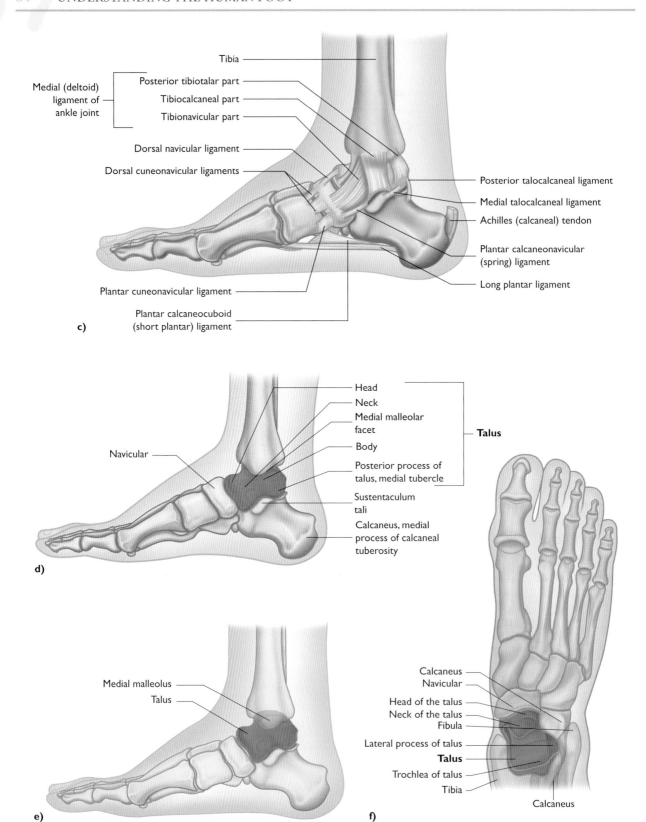

Medial (deltoid) ligament of ankle joint
- Posterior tibiotalar part
- Tibiocalcaneal part
- Tibionavicular part

Tibia

Dorsal navicular ligament

Dorsal cuneonavicular ligaments

Posterior talocalcaneal ligament

Medial talocalcaneal ligament

Achilles (calcaneal) tendon

Plantar calcaneonavicular (spring) ligament

Long plantar ligament

Plantar cuneonavicular ligament

Plantar calcaneocuboid (short plantar) ligament

c)

Navicular

Head
Neck
Medial malleolar facet
Body
Posterior process of talus, medial tubercle

Talus

Sustentaculum tali

Calcaneus, medial process of calcaneal tuberosity

d)

Medial malleolus

Talus

e)

Calcaneus
Navicular
Head of the talus
Neck of the talus
Fibula
Lateral process of talus
Talus
Trochlea of talus
Tibia
Calcaneus

f)

Figure 4.19. The talus sits directly below the tibia (a) and is encased by the two malleoli on either side (b). Although it has no muscles attaching to it, the talus is almost boxed in by bony structures on each aspect which are then wrapped together with strong ligaments that also help control the flow of forces during normal movement (b & c & fig. 4.22). The surface of the talus is 70% cartilage due to the large interfaces with the tibia above, calcaneus below, and the navicular in front (d–f). The head of the talus connects with the navicular and, as with the trunk of the upper body, the talar body and head are connected via the neck. The body of the talus provides plantar flexion and dorsiflexion and is wider at the front of the bone.

numerous directions. If we are lucky, the talus can keep this dance up with grace, elegance, and good timing. Movement chaos can happen when the ankle complex becomes jammed.

The size of both the calcaneus and talus is indicative of their weight-bearing roles: the talus is the first of the tarsal bones to receive weight coming down from the tibia and the rest of the body above, and the calcaneus takes much of the initial shock at heel strike. Think of the talus as the top of the pyramid (fig. 4.19d): it angles down and back to the calcaneus, and down and forward to the navicular via the neck matching the description we used for the trabecular pattern, indicating its role in force management. A simplified description is that the trochlea receives body weight from the tibia and divides it forward and back, but the reality is a little more complicated than that during gait. On heel strike, the calcaneus receives GRFs and sends them up to the talus and then, as the rest of the foot contacts the ground, the forefoot sends force back and up along the foot toward the talus. The talus is therefore positioned in the middle of a three-way flow of force—down from the tibia, forward and up from the calcaneus, and back and upward from the forefoot.

The talus' relationship to the surrounding bones guides its response to the ebb and flow of force, rather than being controlled by active muscle tension. The encasement by the malleoli either side, the tibia above, calcaneus below, and navicular to the front means the talus is well contained by bones and associated ligaments. As the talus is free from any muscular control, it can ride and guide the forces coming to it from each direction without having to wait for instruction or have its response directly overridden by aberrant muscle tones. Returning to the traffic cop analogy, we have all had the misery of waiting at junctions with temporary traffic lights that have not been programed to adapt

to traffic flow. At other times, we have been impressed by the traffic cop who reacts immediately to local conditions and minimizes traffic build-up.[3] Giving some degree of local autonomy to the talus seems to work for the busy ankle junction.

Below the talus is the important subtalar joint.[4] It is the interface between the talus and the calcaneus, and provides inversion and eversion of the foot. It is essential to differentiate between the movements of inversion/eversion and pronation/supination. Inversion and eversion are simple descriptors that involve predominately frontal plane movement. Pronation and supination describe an intricate sequence of events through the whole foot and ankle complex, of which inversion and eversion are only a part.

The talus and calcaneus interface in at least two areas.[5] The posterior subtalar joint is an almost direct line between the tibia, the talus, and the heel portion of the calcaneus. The anteromedial portion of the subtalar joint is between the talus and the sustentaculum tali (see fig. 4.20). The sustentaculum tali is a projection of the calcaneus, sometimes called "the waiter's tray" or, more officially, the talar shelf. Its name, however, means "suspender of the talus", which is exactly what it does.

The subtalar joint is quite complex as it has two sections which are curved in opposite directions (see fig. 4.20c) giving the joint motion in each of the three planes. As we saw in chapter 2, the alignment of the two joint surfaces has changed to become approximately 23° from the medial line of the body (i.e., it has laterally rotated from the ancestral condition, see fig. 4.20d). There can be individual

[3]And, of course, not everyone given the responsibility of managing traffic can do it with ease, but I hope you get the idea!
[4]We will explore the two ankle joints more in chapter 6 when we look at the arrangement of muscles.
[5]There are numerous variations of subtalar arrangements, both in the bone interfaces and in the various angles used to measure it. Those given here are considered the "normal" average.

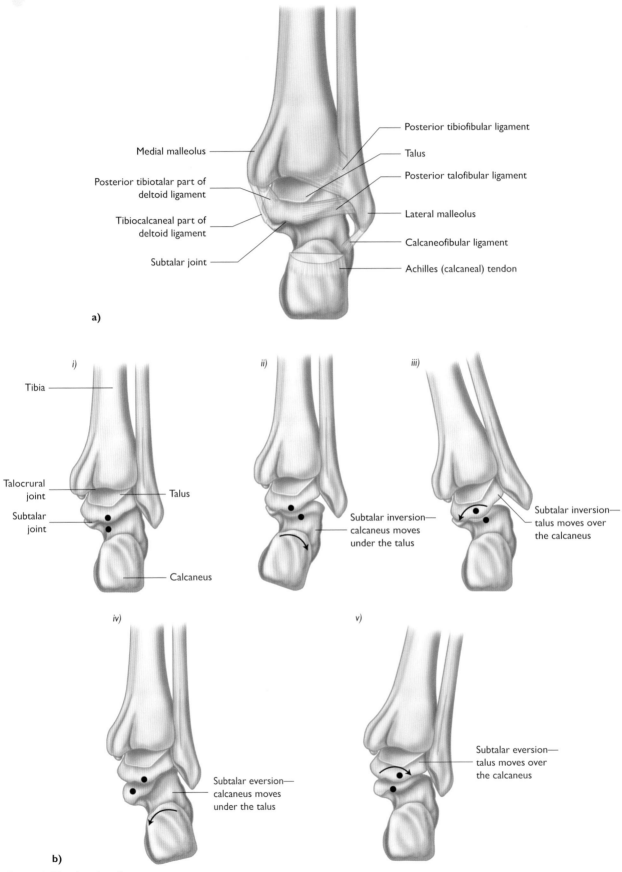

Medial malleolus

Posterior tibiotalar part of
deltoid ligament

Tibiocalcaneal part of
deltoid ligament

Subtalar joint

Posterior tibiofibular ligament

Talus

Posterior talofibular ligament

Lateral malleolus

Calcaneofibular ligament

Achilles (calcaneal) tendon

a)

i)

Tibia

Talocrural
joint

Subtalar
joint

Talus

Calcaneus

ii)

Subtalar inversion—
calcaneus moves
under the talus

iii)

Subtalar inversion—
talus moves over
the calcaneus

iv)

Subtalar eversion—
calcaneus moves
under the talus

v)

Subtalar eversion—
talus moves over
the calcaneus

b)

Figure 4.20.   *(continued)*

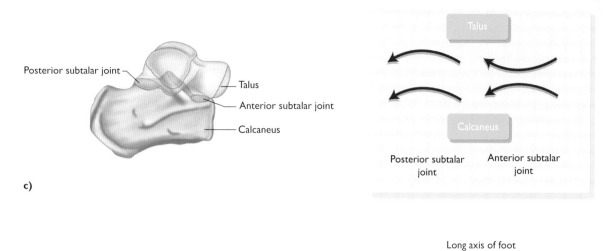

c)

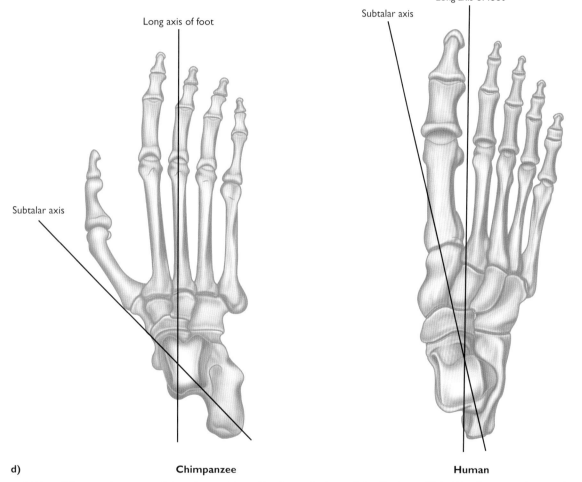

d)   **Chimpanzee**   **Human**

Figure 4.20.   *a) The superior aspect of the talus provides ankle plantar flexion and dorsiflexion and is held in place strongly to track on the parasagittal plane due to the position of the malleoli and the associated ankle ligaments, all of which provide medial-lateral stability. b) As the talus cannot move medially and laterally, inversion and eversion happen below the talus in the two joints between the talus and the calcaneus. Inversion and eversion can either be open-chain (foot moves from neutral (i) under the talus, ii & iii) or closed-chain (the talus moves over the foot, iv & v). c) The subtalar joint has two areas—anterior and posterior—which curve alternately to one another. d) A torsion of the human foot has occurred through evolution, which has led to the loss of an opposable big toe but brought the axis of the subtalar joint closer to the axis of the foot.*

variation from the 23° angle, which will affect various foot types and can be involved in a range of biomechanical issues. If the joint deviates medially, the foot-type will tend toward pronation, and a rigid supinated-type foot may occur if the joint angle is more than 23°.

It was probably the combination of tibial torsion and changes in the subtalar axis that gave us the human foot (see figs. 2.16, 4.17 & 4.20d), as discussed in chapter 2. The twist of the leg changed the axis of the subtalar joint, adducted the first ray, and brought the line of MTJs into the same plane to facilitate the sagittal progression over the four rockers.

CALCANEUS, TALUS, THE NAVICULAR, AND FORCE MANAGEMENT OF THE REARFOOT

Although we did not evolve from chimpanzees, the fossil evidence does show that it is reasonably safe to assume significant similarities between the modern human foot and our ape cousins. We can therefore use the comparison to appreciate the overall change in shape through the whole leg-ankle-foot complex. Fig. 4.20d shows how the body of the calcaneus has moved from being lateral to the talus in the chimpanzee foot to being closer under the talus bone in the human foot. The evolution of tibial torsion and the twist through the foot created the half-domed structure (remember again, the coupling between the lateral rotation of the leg and supination of the foot). The twist lifts the talus on top of the calcaneus. Or at least almost—look at fig. 4.21a and you will see how the talus is partly resting on the talar shelf,[6] the "waiter's tray" of the calcaneus. This offset is one of the mechanisms for the pronation response in gait.

The offset forces of GRF and body weight cause the calcaneus to tilt medially on heel strike. The talus follows (because it rests on the sustenaculum tali) and also rotates medially (fig. 4.21a & b). Just as lateral rotation of the talus creates supination, medial rotation is a trigger for the rest of the foot to pronate. The exaggerated view in fig. 4.21b shows how the medial rotation of the talus bone unlocks the sequence of tarsal joints. The unlocking of the half-dome arrangement assists shock absorption by the soft tissues, especially the ligaments and the intrinsic muscles of the foot.

The front of the talus, the head, is another rounded dome that projects slightly into the navicular bone. The *navicular* (Latin: little boat) is named for its resemblance to a boat. The bow of the boat is the navicular tuberosity, which can be easily palpated on most people and can be used to measure changes to the medial longitudinal arch during weight-bearing and movement (fig. 4.21d). The scooped out "deck" portion of the boat receives the head of the talus and facilitates rotation. Sadly, the nautical analogy is left behind for the naming of this "deck" in favor of the Latin *acetabulum pedis*—"cup of the foot". However, *acetabulum* is reminiscent of the hip joint and provides a useful image of the depth and rotational ability of this joint.

The medial talus, navicular, and calcaneal area forms the height of the foot's dome and receives a lot of stress because of its position between the foot and leg. The area requires a lot of soft tissue support to maintain integrity. A series of ligaments provide the first layer of support and, at first sight, they might seem intimidating due to the apparent complexity of their polysyllabic names (see figs. 4.22a & b). However, as with the trabecular pattern and the flow of stresses through the foot, there is a logic to their position and to their names (or at least to most of the names).

---

[6]The talar shelf is also commonly referred to as the sustentaculum tali.

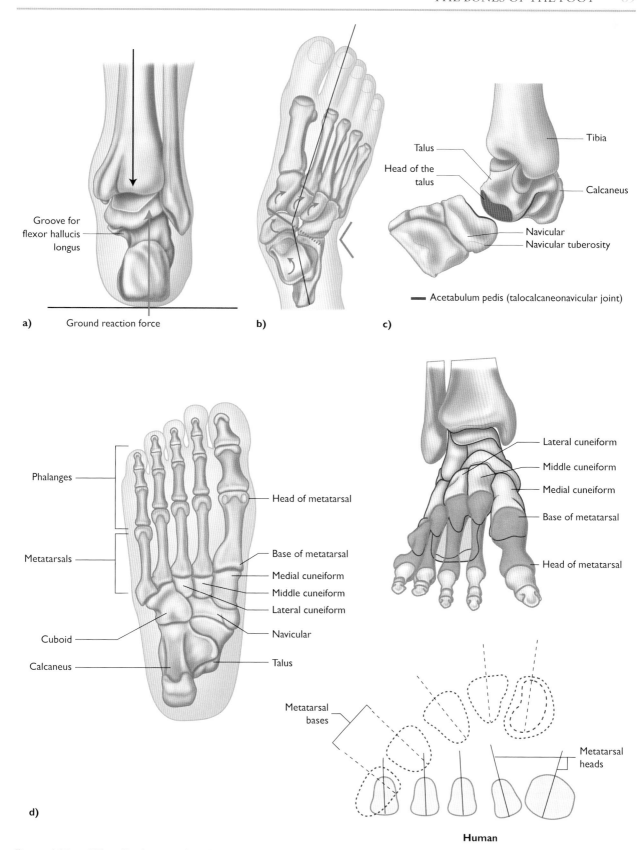

Human

Figure 4.21.   a) The offset between the calcaneus and talus causes an offset between the forces of gravity and momentum coming down the tibia relative to the GRFs coming up from the calcaneus during the early stages of stance phase. b) The offset causes the calcaneus and its talar shelf to tilt medially causing the talus to rotate, an action that unlocks the foot into pronation. c) The head of the talus rotates in the shallow socket of the navicular. The bony prominence (the "bow of the ship") can be palpated as it drops during pronation (see also fig. 4.26). d) The cuneiforms and metatarsal bases are wedge-like—wide at the top and narrow on the plantar aspect. The rotation through the foot opens the points of the bones to let the soft tissue absorb some of the force.

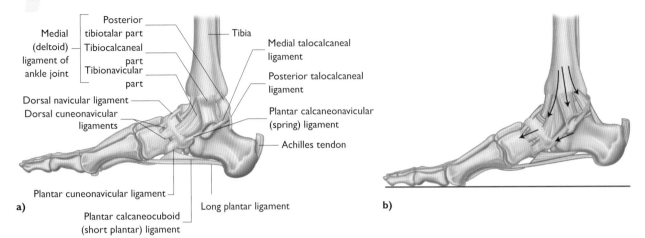

Figure 4.22.   a) Ligaments span the spaces between each bone to prevent separation and maintain joint integrity. The so-called "spring ligament" (or plantar calcaneonavicular ligament) also helps absorb some of the force during early stance phase as the foot pronates and the calcaneus and navicular bones start to move apart. b) This view shows the continuity of force passing through the dense soft tissues as the fibers align from one bone to the next along the medial aspect. The medial line of bones lengthens and separates during pronation as the inside of the dome drops. The deltoid ligament fans down from the tibial malleolus to support the bones of the dome from above as they drop and twist away from the tibia during pronation. (See also fig. 4.25.)

Perhaps the most famous ligament of the foot is the "spring ligament". Its name tells us a significant part of its role, and one could work out its position from the description of the pronation response above, as it makes sense to have a "safety net" under the area of high stress between the calcaneus and navicular. The official name for the spring ligament tells us exactly where it lies: it is the plantar calcaneonavicular ligament, a long spring that spans the gap between the ledge of the "waiter's tray" and the bow of the "boat". The spring ligament is assisted from above by a series of three ligaments, collectively the deltoid ligament, which join the tibia to the calcaneus, talus, and navicular. One can feel the strain through the area by palpating the navicular tuberosity as a client shifts their weight on and off the standing foot.

■ BONES AND JOINTS IN ACTION

It can be useful to consider this group of three bones—calcaneus, talus, and navicular—as a functional unit. Collectively they provide the major joints of the ankle and, through changes in joint axes, they allow the necessary coupling of rotation between the foot and leg. Working our way down:

- **The talar joint**—allows sagittal plane but limits frontal and transverse plane movement
- **The subtalar joint**—allows frontal plane movement but is limited in sagittal and transverse
- **The talonavicular joint**—provides transverse plane movement but is limited in both sagittal and frontal planes

When considering the joints, it is important to keep in mind that "limitations" are not necessarily negative. This is particularly true for the relationship at the ankle complex as its lack of rotation allows a reduction in muscle mass. Generally, if a joint has a movement available to it, there must be a muscle to create and control that action. The foot pronates and supinates through a series of predominately transverse plane motions. Limiting the rotation between the tibia, fibula, and talus allows us to resupinate the foot by rotating the bones rather than by contracting any muscles—as you felt in the turning exercise at the beginning of this chapter—your right foot supinated through bony coupling.

Palpate the heel to appreciate the bulk of the calcaneus' body and refer to the trabecular strain lines. The length of the calcaneal body serves several functions: it helps shock absorption, it lengthens the lever arm between the ankle joint and the heel for increased locomotor efficiency, and its tuberosity provides a rounded surface for the first of the foot rockers. On heel strike, the offset between GRF at the heel and momentum at the ankle joint creates a rolling action at the heel and forces the foot to plantar flex (fig. 4.23).

The landing of the forefoot then focuses the momentum onto the second rocker, the talar joint, and the tibia rolls over the trochlea of the talus in the sagittal plane. From a front or back view, however, the other offset of forces between the calcaneus and the talus causes the sustentaculum tali to tilt medially in the frontal plane, and the foot begins to pronate as it accepts weight during this second rocker phase.

The talus has quite a deep groove posteriorly that directly leads to another groove under the sustentaculum tali (see figs. 4.4, 4.24a & c, and 4.25a & b). This line is filled by the tendon of the flexor hallucis longus (FHL) that lifts and supports the medial portion of the foot's

dome. The FHL on the medial side of the foot is balanced on the lateral aspect of the foot by the tendons of the fibularii that follow a similarly grooved path behind the fibular malleolus and alongside the calcaneus to pass either side of the fibular trochlea—fibularis brevis above and longus below (see fig. 4.24b).

As we saw with the foot rockers above, the primary role of the foot is to assist forward movement and, although for other movements we often need to sway side to side in almost pure inversion and eversion, the foot needs medial-to-lateral stability to assist with forward propulsion. With the help of the various retinacula around the foot and ankle, the two bony prominences of the malleoli on either side of the talus help to stabilize it along the axis of the subtalar joint. The muscles, FHL medially and fibularii laterally, help control eversion and inversion respectively (see also chapter 6). The two muscle groups, the associated ligaments, and retinacula are almost like stabilizers on a kid's bike—they allow a little tilting left and right, guide and assist forward movement, and help prevent catastrophic tilting.

The tendons either side of the calcaneus help guide it through the changes during the gait phases. The most precarious of those are the few moments following heel strike. Ideally, the lateral aspect of the back of the calcaneus should hit the ground and then the natural forces help roll us forward. The danger occurs when the calcaneus strikes at an angle, as happened to me in my student days when trying to run across a road. Turning to look over my right shoulder to check for cars coming from behind me, I did not realize the effect this movement would have on my foot strike. As my body turned to the right, my left foot turned with me, just enough to land too far on the lateral aspect of the calcaneus, creating a mismatch between the joint alignment and my forward momentum. A lateral ankle sprain is a common injury and one that created quite a few compensations through my body as I

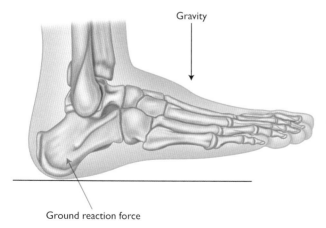

Gravity

Ground reaction force

Figure 4.23. *Striking the ground at an angle causes GRF to act posteriorly to the axis of the talar joint. The offset between the GRF and momentum causes the ankle to plantar flex.*

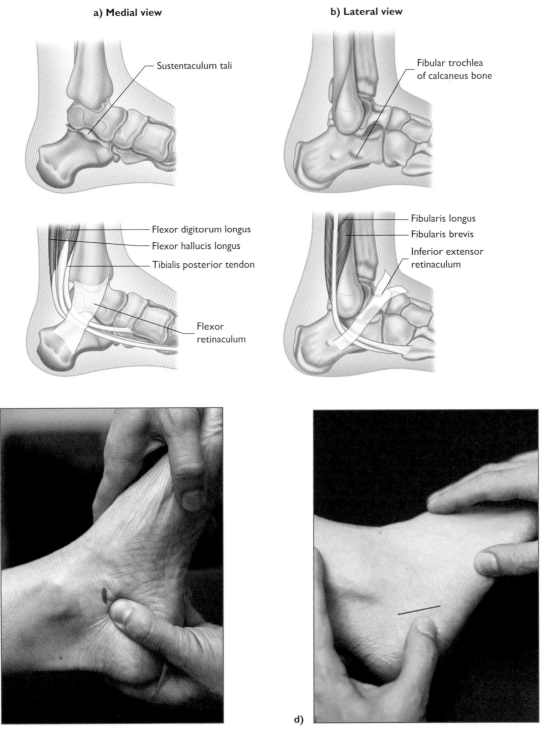

a) Medial view

Sustentaculum tali

b) Lateral view

Fibular trochlea
of calcaneus bone

Flexor digitorum longus
Flexor hallucis longus
Tibialis posterior tendon

Flexor
retinaculum

Fibularis longus
Fibularis brevis

Inferior extensor
retinaculum

c)

d)

Figure 4.24.   The tendons are guided around the ankle's pulley system by a series of bony landmarks. The flexor hallucis longus follows the channel below the sustentaculum tali (a) and the fibularii muscles are guided by the fibular trochlea (b). c) Use the malleoli as starting landmarks to explore the bony prominences around the calcaneus. About 1.5–2.5 cm inferior to the medial malleolus you should find the bump of the "waiter's tray". Check you are on it by inverting and everting the ankle; as part of the calcaneus, it should move the same amount as the rest of the heel. At the same time, you should feel the tensioning of the associated ligaments and, if you glide your finger or thumb anteriorly, you should also be able to feel the "bow" of the navicular. d) Below and slightly forward from the lateral malleolus, you should be able to feel another smaller bump, the fibular trochlea. Move your foot a little, and the tendons of the fibularii muscles should pop up as they pass around this "pulley".

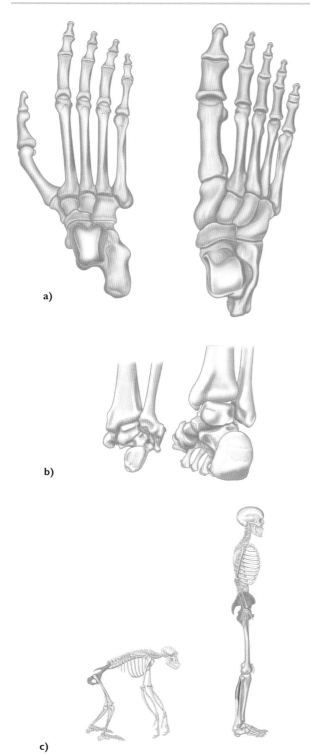

a)

b)

c)

Figure 4.25.   a) As a result of the torsion of the leg and foot, the human calcaneus and talus sit more directly below the tibia. b) The vertical arrangement of calcaneus, talus, and tibia has lifted the medial aspect of the foot to create the half-dome and facilitate efficient bipedality. The increased robustness of the calcaneus helps it absorb shock and form the heel rocker during early stance phase. c) The increased projection posteriorly allows the soleus muscle to support the slight forward lean of the tibia during quiet upright stance.

limped around university, struggling to get my final thesis printed and delivered on time.

TO HEEL STRIKE OR NOT?

When pointed out, it is an obvious aspect of musculoskeletal anatomy that our joints, their associated muscles, and our natural movement patterns all tend to align with one another. There is a natural tracking of the flow of energy from muscles acting across joints to create movement, and there is a return flow of momentum moving through the joints, which can then be controlled—maintained, decelerated, or accelerated, according to need—by the muscles. By seeing the interaction of movement and anatomy, we can interpret "normal" function.

In these days of education by social media, a few "experts" have popped up to preach the benefits and naturalness of forefoot walking. Even back in 1952, long before the internet provided a platform for different ideas, Morton lamented the fact that every so often the idea of forefoot-to-heel walking raises its head. Its proponents usually try to reference the front-to-back strategy as somehow being more natural. The rationale varies from the forefoot being better designed to deal with shock absorption, to the fact that adopting the strategy will give one larger, better-developed calf muscles. Morton dismissed forefoot walking with a simple statement—"it is not observed in primitive cultures."

Forefoot striking during walking is an option and is necessary for side-stepping, stepping down, or to check the security of the next rock when bouldering. There are many times when we can use the strategy appropriately, but, for a repeated rhythmical forward gait, heel striking is more efficient and perfectly natural (Webber & Raichlen 2016). To the uninformed, the common experiment to prove that forefoot striking is better than heel striking is to heel strike barefoot with your fingers in your ears so you hear a thud—supposedly a bad thing. Yes, you will hear a thud. The noise proves that you have heel struck and that you did it with a relatively straight, stacked series of bones— and in doing so you provided yourself with a significant amount of energy efficiency during locomotion. Habitual forefoot striking will give you larger, stronger muscles, but is that a good thing? It might be, but it is not indicative of an efficient or common strategy.

The human calcaneus is the largest of the tarsals and has numerous features to assist our unique style of gait. It is larger, more robust, and projects posteriorly more than the heel bone of any other primate. Its large size, along with its strong, dense fat, probably assists shock absorption at heel strike, and its further posteriorly extension helps us balance while upright (fig. 4.25c). One of the main reasons other animals struggle to walk on two legs is that it requires anteroposterior balance. Pitching forward on all four limbs removes this pressure, so too would counterbalancing with a tail, or having a series of bends in the joints of the legs and trunk. The latter strategy, adopted by many species, such as cats and dogs, requires an elevation of the calcaneus. However, our plantigrade, straight-limbed posture requires some bony extension to the back.

Of course, the foot is longer in front of the talar joint than behind, causing our center of balance to be slightly in front of the joint line. This anterior shift of body weight puts some work into the posterior compartment, particularly the soleus muscle which, thankfully, contains a high proportion of endurance-friendly, slow-twitch fibers. The combination of relatively straight bone alignment with only a slight angle at the ankle joint, and a fatigue-resistant slow-twitch muscle, allows us to stand reasonably comfortably for prolonged periods.

The sustentaculum tali of the human calcaneus is horizontal at rest, unlike the medially tilted sustentaculum tali of the chimpanzee. The lift and support given to the talus by the horizontal "waiter's tray" allows the talus and tibia to sit almost vertically above the calcaneus for efficient bony alignment, while the offset between the talus and calcaneus lets the calcaneus tilt to dissipate some of the shock at heel strike. As mentioned above, the offset means that gravity and GRFs acting through the tibia and calcaneus cause the calcaneus to tilt, the sustentaculum tali to incline medially, and the talus to slide along the surface to unlock the mid-foot. Unlocking the foot sends force into the soft tissue and helps divide the shock absorption role between different types of tissue.

A pure forefoot strike would place most of the force on the soft tissues and reduce the load on the bones. The change in striking style from heel to forefoot alters the load distribution, which is why forefoot striking leads to larger calf muscles. The extra load is also felt by anyone transitioning to mid-foot or forefoot running, where soft tissue injuries can occur if care is not taken to transition gradually.

As we saw above, the horizontal sustentaculum tali that supports the medially placed talus creates a movement bias to the medial aspect of the foot. Under the normal loading of heel strike, the foot's design creates a medial tilt of the calcaneus, which must be corrected to resupinate and lock the foot again before toe-off. Several features help correct the medial tilt and resupinate the foot. The first is the soft tissue. We will explore the soft tissues in chapter 5, but it is worthy of first mention here.

When exploring the two bony prominences either side of the calcaneus, you may have noticed that the sustentaculum tali is much larger than the groove provided for the two fibularii muscles on the lateral aspect of the foot. The FHL follows the strong furrow along the back of the talus and under the sustentaculum to provide lift to the tray when the muscle is tensioned. The FHL has much more purchase and control of the calcaneus than the lateral fibularii, with their much smaller groove. Likewise, the soleus, which joins the gastrocnemius to form the Achilles tendon and attaches to the top of the calcaneus, has more tendinous fibers on the medial aspect of the bone, which help to invert it as the muscle tensions. These prime supinators—FHL and soleus—are assisted by the rest of the deep posterior compartment—tibialis posterior and flexor digitorum longus—to help give "force closure" to the foot.

"Form closure" of the foot is assisted by the return to horizontal of the sustentaculum tali. The return of the talus to horizontal is driven by its position between the malleoli. As we discovered in the rotating exercise above, the talus rotates in concert with the tibia and fibula. When one lower limb is swinging forward, the bones of the standing leg laterally rotate in response. This lateral rotation of the standing leg rotates the talus laterally to aid the soft tissues' lift of the foot into supination—both systems, bone and muscle, working in harmony.

■ THE NAVICULAR'S ROLE IN PRONATION AND SUPINATION

All three bones of the rearfoot, the calcaneus, talus, and navicular, are coupled together not only by their bony architecture but also by their ligaments.

The spring ligament spans from the sustentaculum tali to the navicular tuberosity, coupling movement between the calcaneus and the navicular. This is crucial for both pronation and supination, as it allows the appropriate movement of the talus. When the calcaneus tilts in response to heel strike, the spring ligament will pull the navicular with it, allowing the talus to turn in the navicular's socket and create pronation. If medial rotation is driven from the tibia and fibula to the talus, the talus rotates

within the acetabulum of the navicular bone and the movement will stiffen the adjoining ligaments to couple the movement and also causes pronation.

In this way, talar rotation is tied to navicular movement in either direction—from ground reaction forces below or from rotation of the leg from above.

The navicular's position and connections to the other bones make it a useful proxy for measuring the degree of pronation through the foot. Although the literature is ambivalent on the use and interpretation of navicular drop, navicular drop can be useful for building a picture of the foot's overall ability to move and adapt (see fig. 4.26).

While it is important not to pathologize bad mechanics, it is essential to build a picture of a client's functional abilities and restrictions to fully understand a presenting pathology and give case-specific interventions. These will be explored more in chapter 8, but for now it is enough to understand why one performs the related tests. If the navicular tuberosity is too low or drops significantly, the joints may be held permanently in an opened position and strain is received directly into the soft tissues. If the navicular cannot rise following pronation or if it is slow to do so, the failure of the sustentaculum tali to lift may leave the foot in a relatively pronated position, causing the foot to toe-off without true "form closure". Failure to reach the rigid lever condition, without both form and force closure may also put more strain onto soft tissues because of the lack of bony support. Conversely, if the navicular cannot drop, for whatever reason, the soft tissues will not lengthen, and the bones and joints may receive more than their fair share of force.

As mentioned in the discussion regarding forefoot striking, bulky calves are a result of a higher percentage of load being redirected from the skeleton to the soft tissues. A properly functioning foot should be able to divide the

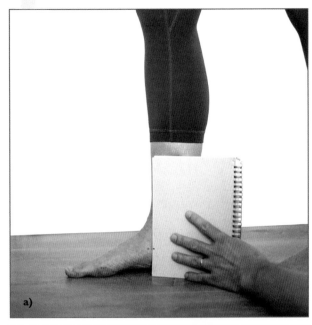

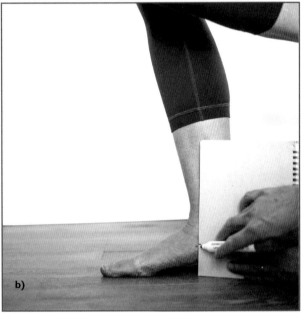

Figure 4.26. *Navicular drop is determined by comparing the height of the navicular tuberosity in non-weightbearing (a) to weightbearing (b).*

load fairly between the two systems—bone and soft tissue—to prevent overuse of either. Heel striking during walking should achieve this easily.

■ CUNEIFORMS AND THE TRANSVERSE ARCH

The navicular links to the row of three cuneiforms—medial, middle, and lateral

(fig. 4.27a). From the Greek, *cuneus*: wedge-shaped, the word describes the form of these bones perfectly. Their wedge-like arrangement, wide on top and pointed inferiorly, helps form and maintain the transverse arch. Generally considered to act like bony keystones for the transverse arch, the cuneiform array also provides stability for the overall shape of the foot. A recent study demonstrated how the transverse curvature of the cuneiform to cuboid line increased foot stiffness for toe-off. In their paper, Venkadesan et al. 2020, point out that ground contact with the forefoot and the forces acting around the ankle complex place significant bending stress through the length of the foot. The transverse arch therefore creates another "form support" mechanism for the length of the foot adding to its overall stability.

Fig. 4.27b shows the difference in arch curvature between other primates (macaque, grivet monkey, chimpanzee, and gorilla) and various species of upright bipeds (which may or may not be ancestral to *Homo sapiens*). From the chart, it appears that upright gait benefits from the transverse arch, both as a potential shock absorber for heel strike and in its ability to provide stiffness. Venkadesan's paper argues that while much attention has focused on the importance of the medial longitudinal arch, the longitudinal line of bones is actively assisted and supported by the foot's transverse dome. The transverse arch has dual—and seemingly conflicting—roles in that it allows opening and adaptation of the foot at one phase and provides stability during another. However, this serves to emphasize the usefulness of our half-dome model as it is the 3D curvature, not the individual arches, that provides the natural stiffness.

As usual, there is an interplay between bony (form) and muscle (force) support to prevent the foot from buckling during the rise of the heel in preparation for toe-off. The switch between the two functions of the cuneiform arch (shock absorption and stiffness) is provided by the rotation of bones, especially rotation of the

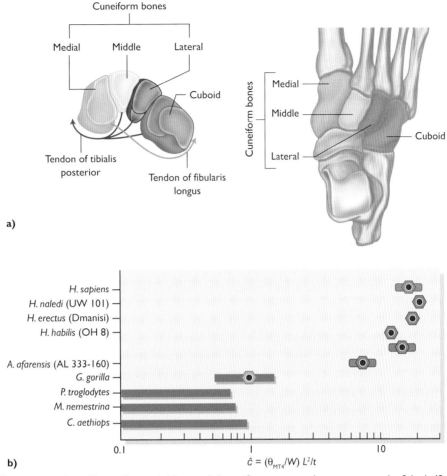

Figure 4.27   a) The transverse line of bones from cuboid to medial cuneiform supports the transverse arch of the half-domed foot. The arrangement is supported by the wedge-like interfaces and by the compressive force of several tendons, notably tibialis posterior and fibularis longus, which act as a sling across the plantar aspect. b) Median curvature of the transverse arch on a logarithmic scale of a few species allows easy comparison between other primates (gorilla and chimpanzee), early bipeds (Australopithecus afarensis, Homo habilis, Homo erectus, and Homo naledi) and modern human (Homo sapiens). (Adapted from Venkadesan et al. 2020.)

rearfoot complex, and by the arrangement of soft tissues creating a sling around and under the cuneiforms (fig. 4.27a), most notably the tendons of posterior tibialis and fibularis longus. The inferior view (see fig. 4.28) highlights many ligamentous connections between the calcaneus, navicular, and medial cuneiform. As we know from looking at the spring ligament, ligaments provide stability, mobility, and elastic potential, but they also couple movements between bones—if a bone moves in one direction, its neighbors get dragged along for the ride.

As the talus medially rotates on the sustentaculum tali, the spring ligament tensions and the gap between the talus and navicular opens. But the ligament also pulls the navicular in the same direction. The talus, navicular, and the medial cuneiform medially rotate, but their associated joints are laterally rotating (see side bar, page 100). Lateral rotation through the tarsal joints (caused by the proximal bones medially rotating), opens the joints and causes the ligaments to strain—like a team of firefighters holding a trampoline for the jumpers at the base of a burning building—to tension the material between them, they must move apart.

The cuneiforms abut onto the cuboid and this row of five bones—the navicular, the three cuneiforms, and the cuboid—form the mid-foot (please note that I added the navicular into the discussion of the rearfoot for functional rather than anatomical reasons). The cuboid, so-called because of its squared shape, spans

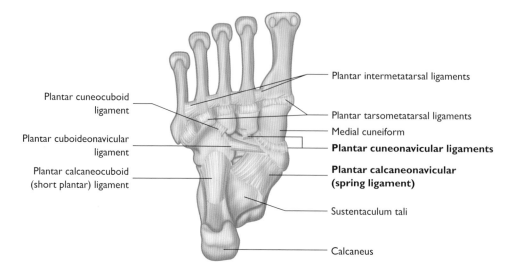

Plantar cuneocuboid ligament

Plantar cuboideonavicular ligament

Plantar calcaneocuboid (short plantar) ligament

Plantar intermetatarsal ligaments

Plantar tarsometatarsal ligaments

Medial cuneiform

Plantar cuneonavicular ligaments

Plantar calcaneonavicular (spring ligament)

Sustentaculum tali

Calcaneus

Figure 4.28.   As we saw in fig. 4.19, pronation is partly decelerated by the ligaments as the bones move apart. Supporting the bones above them, the plantar ligaments are crucial in preventing the foot's collapse. As they lengthen (strain), they absorb energy which can then be re-used to assist the return movement.

between the two transverse compound joints of the foot.

As shown by their use for amputation and propensity for severe dislocation, the midtarsal joint and the tarsometatarsal joint that sit on either side of the cuboid, are potential weak points in the ability of the foot to achieve a stable rigid lever. However, a projection of bone has evolved that interlocks with the calcaneus to "interrupt" the line across the midtarsal joint and provide a one-way locking mechanism for the midtarsal joint (fig. 4.30)— locked on supination, unlocked in pronation. It has generally been thought that this uniquely human, calcaneocuboid joint helps prevent the midtarsal break that occurs in primate feet (fig. 4.30b), but it is not enough on its own and other support from soft tissue is still required (Holowka and Lieberman 2018).

The midtarsal break—the lack of form closure in non-human primate feet— can still be present in some human feet, despite the calcaneocuboid joint (fig. 4.30c). Although it may not necessarily lead to a pathology, a midtarsal break prevents the rigid lever from forming and will put extra load onto the tissues at toe-off.

The tarsometatarsal joint is the line between the cuboid and cuneiforms proximally and the metatarsals distally. As mentioned above, this line is not as straight as the midtarsal joint and, while more prone to injury, is a less common choice for surgical amputation. The medial portion of the joint line is interrupted by the

Palpation of the Cuboid

Find the styloid process at the base of the fifth metatarsal and explore the tissues proximal and superior to it. Proximal to the process is a gap above which one should be able to feel the cuboid bone.

Feel how the cuboid is lifted to form the lateral longitudinal arch and provide a passage for the tendon of the fibularis longus.

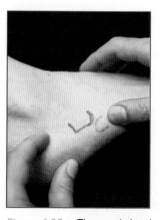

Figure 4.29.   The rounded end of the fifth metatarsal (marked in green) can be easily palpated and should align with the fibular trochlea and the posterior aspect of the lateral malleolus. The cuboid (red) is suspended above the thick fat pad which should be easy to find.

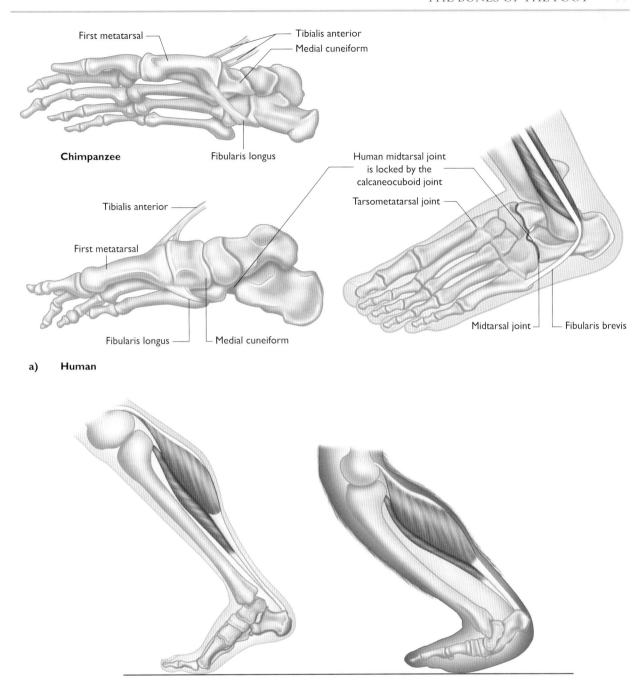

First metatarsal
Tibialis anterior
Medial cuneiform

Chimpanzee

Fibularis longus

Tibialis anterior

Human midtarsal joint
is locked by the
calcaneocuboid joint

Tarsometatarsal joint

First metatarsal

Fibularis longus
Medial cuneiform

Midtarsal joint
Fibularis brevis

a)   **Human**

b)   **Human**   **Primate**

Figure 4.30.   a) Along with the torsion of the human foot and leg, the cuboid has lengthened and is held in place by the styloid process of the fifth metatarsal. The transverse arch and associated midtarsal joint are further supported by the overlapping calcaneocuboid joint for form closure. Force closure and support is provided by tension of the fibularis brevis. The lack of a calcaneocuboid joint allows the primate foot to collapse and prevents it from acting as a rigid lever (b).

difference in length between the medial and middle cuneiforms; laterally, the joint line is overlapped by the styloid process, a projection of the fifth metatarsal (see figs 4.32 & 4.33). Each of these waves in the joint line provide more stability to this distal interface between the tarsals and metatarsals.

As we saw above, the foot's transverse arch is partially suspended by the series of wedge-shaped cuneiforms but also supported by the two fibularii muscles. Along with the tibialis posterior (see fig. 4.27a), the two fibularii muscles support the arch from either side of

Real and Relative Motion

Description of movement requires accuracy and consistency, neither of which is always easy. One convention I try to adhere to through this text, is that of naming bone (real) or naming joint motion (relative).

The movement of bones is referenced according to the normal anatomical position so bones can move medially, or laterally, invert or evert, etc. Relative motion is used to describe the relationship between bones, i.e., joint motions, and they are referenced according to the position of the distal bone relative to the proximal bone in the limbs and according to the superior bone when describing motion of the spine.

Developing fluency with real and relative motions requires some time and practice, but a good start is to be accurate with whether you are describing the movement of a bone, or the motion at a joint.

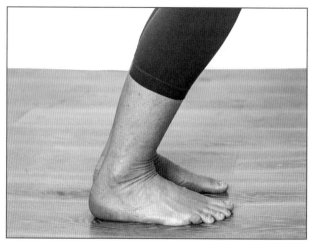

Figure 4.31. *A simple knee bend can expose the fibularii tendons as they pass along the lateral aspect of the foot.*

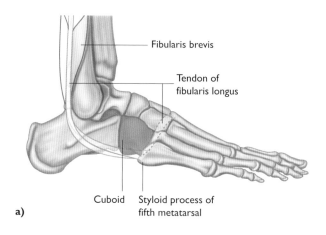

Fibularis brevis

Tendon of fibularis longus

Cuboid   Styloid process of fifth metatarsal

a)

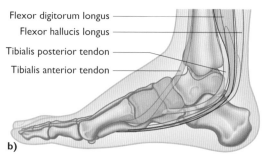

Flexor digitorum longus
Flexor hallucis longus
Tibialis posterior tendon
Tibialis anterior tendon

b)

Figure 4.32. *a) The cuboid is supported by the styloid process of the fifth metatarsal, which is held in place by the fibularis brevis. The tunnel created under the cuboid provides a pathway for fibularis longus to pass across to the medial aspect of the foot. b) The medial portion of the foot, the navicular, and medial cuneiform, in particular has less natural, architectural support from the bones and requires more lift from the soft tissues. The extrinsic muscles that give some control are the tibialis anterior, tibialis posterior, flexor hallucis longus, and flexor digitorum longus.*

the foot. Fibularis longus crosses the bottom of the foot to attach onto the medial cuneiform and pull it across to hold the wedge-shaped bones together. Fibularis brevis attaches to the styloid process of the fifth metatarsal and draws the fifth metatarsal back toward and slightly under the cuboid (figs. 4.31 & 4.32a). Keeping the fifth metatarsal and cuboid in place creates a channel that allows fibularis longus to pass below the cuboid on its way across to the medial aspect of the foot to attach into the medial cuneiform.

The medial cuneiform and navicular (fig. 4.32b) are well supported by various tendons that we will explore in a later chapter. In their place at the apex of the half-dome and in an area of strong force interface, the medial cuneiform and navicular require the combination of muscular as well as the ligamentous support mentioned above to keep their integrity.

The three cuneiform bones vary in length from front to back (fig. 4.33a). The length of the shorter middle cuneiform is compensated for by the longer second metatarsal, which is inset along the tarsometatarsal joint line. The medial cuneiform is the longest of the three and projects beyond the base of the second metatarsal giving the medial cuneiform a joint with both first and second metatarsals. The lateral cuneiform quite neatly joins with the third metatarsal, while the chunkier cuboid interfaces with the bases of both fourth and fifth metatarsals.

The distal face of the medial cuneiform, the portion that meets the first metatarsal, is aligned slightly medially. This alignment is a partial hangover from the abducted great toe of our ancestors, a feature still present in the chimpanzee foot (fig. 4.33b). This would not be a problem if we still had abducted, grasping big toes, but we have evolved to arrange the major hinge joints along our predominant sagittal progression. To allow a sagittal alignment and bring its head to rest flat on the ground, the first metatarsal evolved with a twist and some lateral torsion (Tamer and Simpson 2017, see fig. 4.34); we saw a similar process with the tibia. This lateral torsion of the first metatarsal and the medial alignment of its tarsometatarsal joint makes us susceptible to bunions. The dreaded hallux valgus has numerous possible causes—genetic, footwear, misuse, lack of strength, etc.—but it really comes back to a time when we preferred to hold onto things with our feet rather than squeezing them into tight-fitting shoes.

It is not only the first metatarsal that must twist itself to maintain purchase on the ground, the rest of the metatarsals also torsion—but they twist in the opposite direction (see fig. 4.34b).

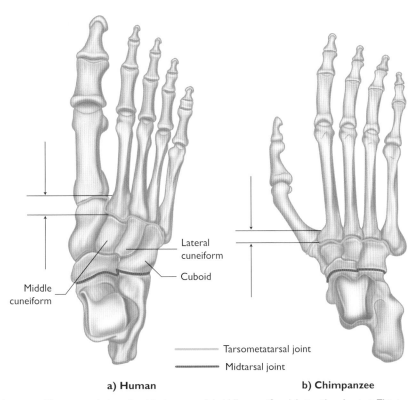

Lateral cuneiform

Cuboid

Middle cuneiform

Tarsometatarsal joint

Midtarsal joint

a) Human   b) Chimpanzee

Figure 4.33.   a) The three cuneiforms vary in length, with the second (middle cuneiform) being the shortest. This is compensated for by a longer second metatarsal to ensure a relatively even placement of the first and second MTJs. The lengthened medial cuneiform provides another locking mechanism due to breaking the joint line across the tarsometatarsal interface. b) In comparison, the chimpanzee foot has a shorter medial cuneiform that directs the first metatarsal medially and, also provides less overlap of the bones. The lack of interlocking bones provides more movement possibilities but inhibits inherent stability of the foot.

The change of use from grasping to supporting us against gravity required the metatarsals to make a few adjustments on their journey from base to head. Rather than facing toward the big toe, they have to torsion medially to plant on the ground. The lateral torsion of the first metatarsal and the medial torsion of the others allows all the metatarsal heads to rest on the ground in a relatively straight line (fig. 4.34b).

ACHIEVING TOE-OFF

Although the metatarsal heads rest on the ground, their joint line creates a shallow curve when viewed from above (figs. 4.35 & 4.36a). One aim for locomotion is to have final toe contact along the "transverse axis", i.e., along the heads of the first and second metatarsals—referred to as the "high gear" toe-off. The alternative "low-gear" is the oblique axis, the line along the lateral three metatarsals. The "gearing" refers to the lever length back to the ankle—since the first and second metatarsals are longer, they are further from the ankle joint than the other metatarsals. The greater distance from MTJs to ankle, on a rigid, supinated foot, creates a more powerful toe-off.

Increased power is only one factor for toe-off, alignment of the final contact points also affects the tracking of force into other joints further up the mechanical chain. The transverse axis is aligned to the talar joint, the knee joint, and the strong tissues of the front of the hip (see *Born to Walk* for further exploration).

Other primate feet show a strong change of direction around the metatarsal heads compared with the human foot (fig. 4.36a–d). An increased parabola is indicative of the primary grasping function of apes' feet—the grasping primate foot uses opposition between the big toe and the rest of the digits. The primary role of the modern human foot is bipedalism, making forward propulsion the prime design directive. As the human big toe has adducted, we can now toe-off on the relatively stable base of the first and second MTJs (see fig. 4.37).

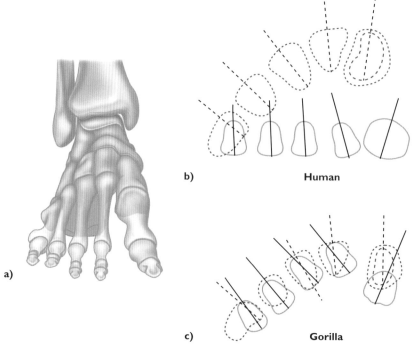

b)   **Human**

a)

c)   **Gorilla**

Figure 4.34.   *The lifted dome arrangement of the human mid-foot (represented with hatched outlines, (a) requires torsion through the metatarsal shafts to place all the metatarsal heads on the ground. Contrasting the long axis of the metatarsal bases (hatched lines in b & c) with the long axes of the heads (solid lines in b & c) indicates the direction and amount of torsion for each bone.*

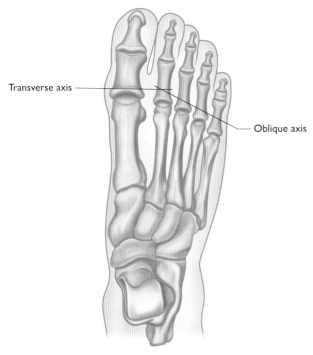

Transverse axis

Oblique axis

Figure 4.35.   Allied to the parabola below (fig. 4.36), the two axes of the metatarsal heads relate to the foot and ankle's position at toe-off. A so-called "high-gear" toe-off is achieved along the transverse axis in contrast to the "low-gear" of the oblique.

The relative positions of the first and second metatarsals were one of the most critical metatarsal features according to Morton, as they provide the last points of contact before toe-off. As we come up into toe extension

in preparation for toe-off, there should be a stable contact with the ground with at least two points of contact—the first and second MTJ. The MTJs are predominately hinge joints, so as they fold back into extension, they align with the talar, knee, and anterior hip joints. Some could even take that line of force further into the spine and the control of the resultant spinal extension by rectus abdominis (see fig. 4.37).

Morton was so obsessed with this feature that he dedicated a significant part of his 1935 text to it. He identified a tendency for the second metatarsal to be relatively longer than the first and this condition has since been named after him—Morton's foot (see figs. 4.36e and 8.11). This eponymous issue has numerous causes and just as many related pathologies. Morton blamed many of the cases he saw on less than adequate footwear and had strong views regarding the choices made by many women of his day: *"High-heeled shoes are to be regarded as a powerful and vicious factor in the development of foot disorder…the restriction of their use to evening hours would very nearly eliminate their baneful influence in producing disorder."* (1935, page 174).

Long second metatarsal

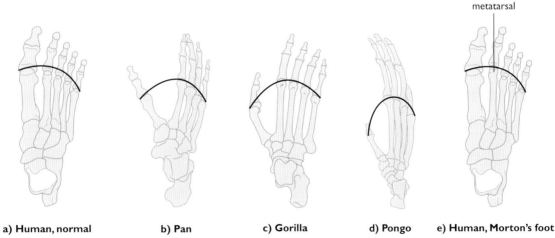

a) **Human, normal**   b) **Pan**   c) **Gorilla**   d) **Pongo**   e) **Human, Morton's foot**

Figure 4.36.   The shallow parabola along the human metatarsal heads (a) has been created by a suite of anatomical changes as explored above. Bringing the first and second metatarsals in line facilitates a predominately sagittal plane toe-off. The shallow human parabola contrasts with the greater curvature of the other apes (b–d). However, a relatively longer second metatarsal, a so-called Morton's foot, can affect foot functioning and alignment at toe-off (e).

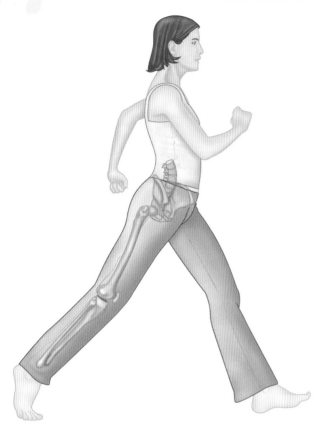

Figure 4.37.   *The first and second metatarsal joint placement allows forward momentum to act through many of the joints of the body to bring them into extension.*

Leaving any implied sexism aside, Morton saw the cramped toe boxes and elevated heel as culprits in creating malalignment by forcing the big toe into adduction (fig. 4.38) creating the renowned bunion bend at the first MTJ. The bend is caused by adduction of the phalange, which in turn encourages abduction

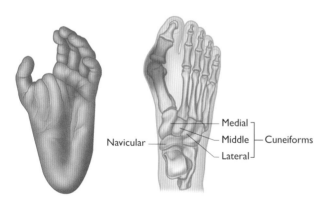

Figure 4.38.   *The medially facing facet of the medial cuneiform contributes to the abducted and grasping great toe of other primates. The human cuneiform retains a medial tendency making us prone to hallux valgus.*

of the first metatarsal. Developing a bunion can therefore cause a *functional* Morton's foot, one which is a developed, as opposed to a *structural* offset (when the two bones have grown to offset joint positions).

The position and alignment of the MTJs are not just factors of metatarsal length, they are created by the cumulative effect of the line of bones associated with each toe. Directly proximal to the great toe is the first ray, a line of bones consisting of the first metatarsal, medial cuneiform, and navicular. The neighboring second ray consists of the second metatarsal, middle cuneiform, and navicular.[7] The position of the MTJs associated with each line is a function of the relative lengths between each bone in that line. When we compare the first ray with the second, we see that the second metatarsal is structurally longer than the first, but it is inset back against the middle cuneiform, which is much shorter than the medial.

Comparing the chimpanzee foot with the human, we can see that the human foot has a longer medial cuneiform (see fig. 4.36). This adaptation was necessary to lift the human inner arch but still allow the MTJ contact with the ground. The medial cuneiform's elongation has also added extra security along the tarsometatarsal joint line because of the increased inset (see figs. 4.33 & 4.36). Comparing joint position for the presence of Morton's foot is therefore not a comparison of metatarsal length but rather an evaluation of the cumulative length of each ray (fig. 4.39).

If the second MTJ is further forward than the other MTJs, the foot may seek extra stability by dropping or twisting to plant either the first or third MTJ alongside the second as the foot lifts into the toe rocker phase. Rolling medially or

[7]It should be noted that there seems to be no real consistency over how many bones should be included in the "ray". Some use only the metatarsal and cuneiforms, others add the navicular, and others add the calcaneus.

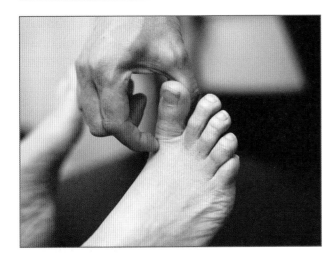

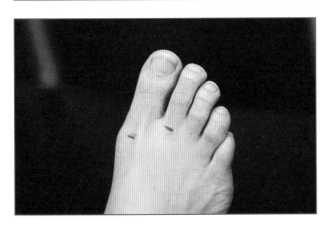

Figure 4.39.   Find the joint line for the first and second MTJs by extending the first and then second MTJs (a & b). Without moving the skin, make a mark along the joint lines and then compare the positions with the joints in neutral (c).

laterally on the "ball" of the second MTJ can be easily observed from behind the walker as the affected heel swings to one side or the other as the foot comes into toe extension. This focuses forces onto one point of contact rather than

two, placing extra pressure under the head of the second metatarsal, which may affect bone stress. It also places additional load on the skin, which usually develops extra callusing.

Callus patterning can be indicative of the movement adaptation used by the client. A straight line of calluses suggests a sagittal progression placing extra stress on the second MTJ area; a circle is indicative of a rotational strategy, which is usually an attempt to land one of the neighboring MTJs for extra stability.

The first metatarsal is the shortest and thickest of the row of miniature[8] long bones, but a few unique features afford it extra functional length. The most obvious is the presence of two sesamoid bones (so-called because they resemble sesame seeds!) under the metatarsal head. The two sesamoids are placed within, and partly controlled by, the flexor hallucis brevis tendons. This arrangement allows the sesamoids to track along with the movement of the overlying metatarsal head and gives the metatarsal head a platform to roll on as the joint goes into extension (see fig. 4.40).

Extension of the first MTJ is a complex action: it requires the rolling action of the metatarsal head over the sesamoids but because of its increased robusticity, the head of the first metatarsal has a larger joint surface, which increases the radius of movement into extension. Crucially, to allow enough movement to take place at the joint, the first metatarsal must take advantage of a third feature, its ability to plantar flex.

As the heel lifts, the MTJs are forced into extension because of their contact with the ground. The MTJs act like a hinge during this motion, but, as the heel lifts, the fibularis longus draws the first metatarsal back and down to open the first MTJ and provides

---

[8]The metatarsals are classed as long bones even though they are relatively short when compared with the likes of the femur and humerus.

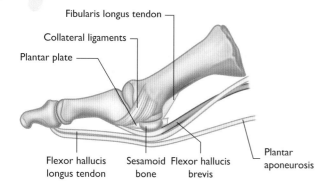

Fibularis longus tendon

Collateral ligaments

Plantar plate

Flexor hallucis longus tendon

Sesamoid bone

Flexor hallucis brevis

Plantar aponeurosis

a)

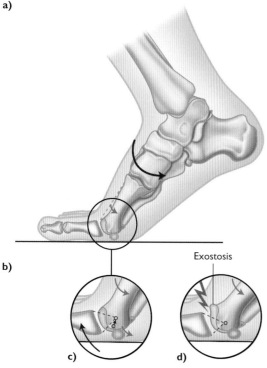

b)

Exostosis

c)

d)

Figure 4.40.   Extension of the first MTJ, (a), requires a series of coordinated events. As the heel lifts, the joint extends from 0–20° (b), from 10–50° the first metatarsal has to be "drawn" back through a plantar flexion partly created by the fibularis longus (c). The first metatarsal plantar flexes by slightly rolling back over the sesamoids, an action that helps create more joint space for the bones to glide further into extension (c). Failure of this system creates "jamming" of the bone surfaces potentially leading to exostosis (bone growth) which further restricts joint mobility (d).

extra range of motion. The posterior glide of the metatarsal head is possible because of the two sesamoids. The smooth upper surfaces of the sesamoids allow the metatarsal head to glide back, and their correct placement beneath the first metatarsal head is of crucial importance—a factor often affecting and affected by muscle imbalances or incorrect mechanics.

Lack of big toe extension can also lead to many adaptations, such as reduced stride length or turning the feet in or out to avoid the joint (we will explore some of the reasons for loss of extension in chapter 8). The latter example can also lead to callus formation that can indicate the preferred compensation strategy. Reading calluses is not as difficult as it may first seem, as they simply show which areas are under extra stress. They are rarely diagnostic by themselves, but can be useful indicators of areas experiencing high levels of stress.

As we saw above, callusing along the line of the second metatarsal head can be a sign of Morton's foot, but a hypermobile or unstable first ray could also cause the callusing pattern. Both conditions put extra stress on the second metatarsal and can lead to its hypertrophy. It is common for a longer second and a hypermobile first ray to be present in the same foot. The hypermobility of the first ray exacerbates the problem of trying to find a stable base for toe-off and can have significant effects through the rest of the mechanical chain.

Numerous factors determine the position at toe-off—ankle mobility, tibial torsion, toe stability, and range of motion, among many others. It is important to track issues upward and downward through the body to find the actual culprit, as the callus pattern created by any one of those factors can look very similar. The purpose of this text is not to delve into the ever more complex world of differential diagnostics but to establish the base of understanding from which the significance of each test will be much easier to grasp.

DISTAL TRANSVERSE ARCH

There is some debate over the terminology of the transverse "arch". Some references will list the proximal and distal transverse arches; some only list the proximal. As discussed, there is no doubt over the architecture and the importance of the proximal arch created across the foot from cuneiforms to cuboid. The distal arch does not have the same bony support, and therefore is not listed as an arch by some. Instead it relies on a series of soft tissues that play important roles during pronation and supination.

Pronation has two primary benefits—shock absorption and helping the foot adapt to the terrain. The slight opening of the joints during pronation gives the foot more flexibility to curl around the contours of the walking surface, and in chapter 7, we will also see that the spread of the foot helps the intrinsic muscles produce more force. Adaptation of the forefoot is made easier by the relative separation between the metatarsal heads that are spanned by a series of short tissues that allow a natural freedom to the distal bones.

The metatarsals are stable proximally (because of the close-pack position) and mobile distally. To maintain their connection but facilitate movement, the fibrous joint capsules of metatarsal heads are tethered together by the deep transverse ligament (see fig. 7.14). This soft tissue connection allows mobility of the metatarsal heads, which adds some overall range to the movement of the toes. The progressive increase in mobility through the foot from proximal to distal reflects the carpal and metacarpal arrangement in the hand.

PHALANGES—THE TOES

The transition joints from metatarsals to phalanges (MTJs) are not simple hinge joints providing pure flexion and extension, they are slightly rounded and classed as condyloid joints. One can easily see the implication of that by flexing and extending the toes. As with the fingers of the hand, the toes adduct as they flex, curling in as if grasping; and, as the toes extend, they abduct as if letting go—a valuable benefit for those who have to use their feet in place of their hands, as it enables the control and release tools.

There are 14 phalanges in each foot, two for the big toe and three each for the rest. The big toe therefore only has one interphalangeal joint while the others have two each—a proximal and a distal. Acting as relatively simple hinge joints, the interphalangeal joints require a complex arrangement of soft tissues to control their movement, and we explore them in chapter 7.

SUMMARY

The bony architecture and the foot's function are closely intertwined, and a full appreciation of the foot requires an understanding of both. The foot is a functioning whole that must deal with the high forces created during locomotion. From dissipating the shock of the first contact, through molding to contoured surfaces, and back to a rigid lever again to manage and direct forces for toe-off, all require numerous working parts coming together as a functional whole. Understanding the whole involves an appreciation of the parts, but their shape only makes sense in the context of their function. Round in a circle we go!

Gravity, momentum, and GRF all act through the foot's unique architecture to help switch it back and forth between pronation and supination. The various vectors of force acting through the shaped bones create a reasonably predictable response.[9]

We have now put most of the elements in place for you to understand why your left foot pronated and your right foot supinated in the exercise at the beginning of this chapter. As you turn your body to the right, the trunk and pelvis will follow your head to the right. Turning the pelvis will cause your femurs to also rotate to the right but your left is turning

[9]Please note that the "chain reaction" can be overridden by the soft tissue and nervous system interventions: we are not fully at the mercy of bones, forces, and muscular reactions. The purpose of this book is to outline and familiarize ourselves with the general patterns.

medially and the right is turning laterally. The two tibias will follow the femurs above them causing the fibulas, and therefore the malleoli, to rotate as well. As we saw above, the rotation of the malleoli is linked to the rotation of the talus of each foot through the mortise and tenon relationship.

The medial rotation of the left talus encourages the calcaneus to medially tilt and starts the series of events that unlock the foot's bony architecture. Meanwhile the bones of the right foot are brought together, close packing into a more compact and rigid structure—a reaction caused by the coupling between the laterally rotating malleoli and the rear foot. The close-packed, supinated position provides stability to the foot and allows it to manage the forces associated with toe-off. Achieving a high gear toe-off with a supinated foot also brings the MTJ and talar joints into alignment to allow the movement to track upward into the rest of the body.

The supinated, rigid lever is required at toe-off and is supported by a range of features:

- the alignment of the first and second MTJs
- the irregular compound joints across the foot
- the wedges of the transverse arch
- the support of the talus from the sustentaculum tali
- the coupling of rotation between the malleoli and the talus

Familiarity with these form relationships will set us up for the following chapters that describe the force reactions provided by the myofascia. The form of the bones provides the pathways for the muscles and their tendons, the tensioning of these soft tissues help maintain the integrity of the compound "rigid lever". Although we have mostly dealt with the bones and the soft tissues in separate sections, they must be visualized together to make sense of the complete system. Our next chapters will help put them into context first by seeing the advantages given to us by the soft tissue in general (chapter 5) and then exploring some of the true functions of the individual muscles (chapters 6 and 7).

5

SOFT TISSUES AND THEIR FUNCTIONS

Never forget that you may not have learned the function of a muscle if all you know is its action.

—Jack Stern 2003

▪ INTRODUCTION

Traditionally, anatomy texts give the impression that muscles are the prime movers of the body, but the true story is much more interesting. When exploring bones in the previous chapters, we concentrated on gravity and GRF and now, as we integrate the soft tissues into the picture, we must add a third force, *momentum*.[1] We will see below that muscles are far more variable in their actions than we have been led to believe: they can function in different directions at different times; they can "contract" without changing length; and muscle fibers can even shorten while the tissue around them lengthens. Once momentum is involved with movement,

muscles work in concert with surrounding collagenous tissues to optimize efficiency by recruiting elastic energy and varying stiffness levels.

So many of us have suffered from a disconnect between the anatomy we are taught and what we find in clinic and in the "real-world". Muscle "actions" must be listed to pass exams, but often they do not match what happens when we see people move. The mismatch between what we learn and what we see has led to the creation of a lot of "anatomy stories"—the imposition of textbook anatomy onto movement. At best, these stories are limited, and often just outright wrong. If only we started our study from movement and then looked at the anatomy, life would be much simpler.

As we have seen through this text so far, one of the major problems has been access to a language to describe what we see. Thankfully, there are many good tools and useful vocabularies that can be recruited to help us fully grasp and understand the anatomy of movement. However, many of these tools have been poorly taught or underexplored during our education which then lacks the three-dimensional context to

---

[1]While *momentum* can be officially defined as mass x velocity, I use it here in the everyday sense to describe one's movement, to avoid overloading with unnecessary equations. There are plenty of references available for those who wish to investigate further.

bring anatomy alive. Each of the concepts below is worthy of its own textbook and there are many helpful resources out there if you want to go further. My intent here is to ensure a solid grounding from which you can use each vocabulary to empower a deeper appreciation of how movement and anatomy interact through the body.

Our feet are the first and last points of contact with the ground during our most common movement pattern, gait, and their soft tissues manage significant levels of stress. Feet must dissipate some of that force, but they can also recycle and repurpose some of the force to reduce muscle workload. However, before we can really grasp the true functions of our feet there are a few basic aspects of functional anatomy we need to understand. In this chapter, we will explore open- and closed-chain movement, the role of momentum, force-length and velocity relationships, muscle architecture, and how function can be interpreted from muscle form. Through this chapter we will begin to appreciate the many dynamics afforded by the fascial tissues, not just the fascia associated with each muscle, but also their compartments.

Now, that is a lot. You might have heard of—even suffered through—some of these elements before, but this chapter brings them all together to demonstrate the interactions and implications of each concept. Although the terminology may seem tedious at times, building some degree of fluency with each concept is important and each word will support your understanding of the larger idea it represents. If this material is new to you, I recommend reading this section quickly once, carry on to the rest of the book and then return to this section with a new vision and understanding.

Of all this book, this is my favorite chapter. I hope it will be yours too.

■ "ACTION" IS NOT ALWAYS "FUNCTION"

As Stern alludes to above, the actions we learn and the functions a muscle performs are not always the same—they can be, and when that happens it makes things pretty easy. But to grasp the wider picture of what is happening through the body in everyday movements we must lose a few prejudices—often prejudices we did not even know we had—and be able to see the muscle in context of its environment. Morton talked a lot about "interaction" and how the body is best considered as a complex ecosystem in which any change in one tissue, or one area, will have an effect everywhere else. If we accept the idea of the body as an ecosystem, especially when it is moving, then we can begin to see the inherent complexity.

We can take the "ecosystem" idea a step further. Ecology is defined as the study of organisms and their interactions with their environment. As we saw in chapter 2, our drive to bipedalism is often assumed to be a reaction to climate change and the reduction of tree coverage. As the environment became hotter and trees more dispersed during the late Miocene, having an efficient mode of locomotion that also helped reduce exposure to sunlight and gave a better view over the top of tall grass may have helped drive our upright stance. Not only is the human body an ecosystem, but also its shape and function are altered by the wider ecosystem it is part of.

A problem with complex systems is how to monitor, measure, and describe the outward ripples caused by a change of any one variable. Think of the over-used story of the Japanese butterfly flapping its wings causing a tsunami in San Francisco; would anyone be able to list the interdependent factors involved? This question mirrors one of the issues, I think, within the field of biomechanics, as too often terms are presented that appear linear—if X, then Y. This approach does not hold in reality as there are many other intervening variables between X and Y. Due to the complexity of the human system, we must become comfortable with not knowing every answer but strive to develop fluidity in how we interpret forces and reactions through our system.

Breaking away from the "action is function" prejudice of anatomy texts is the first important step to take. An easy example of how we have imposed the X then Y anatomy stories onto our understanding of soft tissue is the "action" of the gluteal muscles. Collectively known as the ABductors, in function, they are just as likely to be preventing ADduction as creating ABduction. If we stand on one leg, there is an offset between the support received from the standing limb and the downward force of the body's center of gravity. That displacement, similar in essence to the offset between talus and calcaneus in the previous chapters, requires control, and the control is provided by the gluteal group (fig. 5.1).

During the stance phase of gait, the gluteals are not abducting, they are preventing adduction—they are stopping the pelvis from dropping down too much on the swing leg side. Control of adduction is a role they fulfill with every alternating step and is necessary because of the offset relationship between our center of gravity and GRF. These offset relationships might seem like weak points in the system at first, but each of them has a purpose and, as we will see, provides functional benefits once momentum is added.

Momentum helps us get places but must also be controlled. Our synovial joints are almost friction-free, so once we start moving, a regulating mechanism is required to prevent us having constant acceleration and missing our target. It can be difficult to see initially, but muscles can both provide and control the body's momentum. Muscle contraction is required to break inertia and get us going,

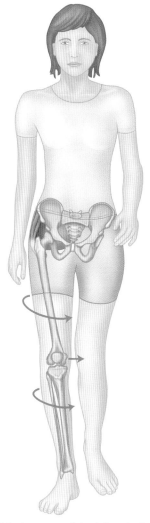

Figure 5.1.   *While they can and do abduct the hip, the gluteal muscles are just as often recruited to decelerate and control adduction and rotation of the hip during gait. Their role in maintaining lateral stability of the pelvis as the other leg swings forward assists our bipedal gait.*

but we also require muscle tension to control the movement—a similar function to the abductors controlling adduction. Morton's image of the work of muscles adjusting like a person controlling a wheelchair is particularly apt: at some stages, the muscles actively work to create movement; sometimes they work to resist movement; and sometimes they can quietly adjust back and forth to maintain the right momentum.

To give context to this idea of the control of momentum, we can take the example of the first of the four foot rockers, the heel rocker.

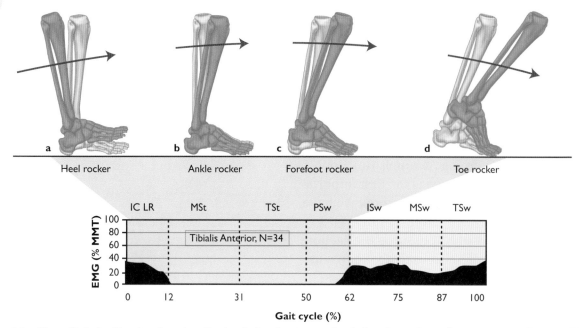

Heel rocker   Ankle rocker   Forefoot rocker   Toe rocker

Figure 5.2. *The ankle is dorsiflexed at the point of heel strike but then is immediately forced into plantar flexion on contact. From the EMG readings, we can see that tibialis anterior is active during the swing phase (62–100%) and acts to draw the foot into its dorsiflexed position in preparation for heel strike. Immediately following heel strike (0–2%) the ankle plantar flexes but tibialis anterior is still active to give a controlled descent of the foot. (Adapted from Perry and Burnfield 2010.)*

The ankle joint plantar flexes rapidly following heel strike; failure to control that movement results in foot slap, a common outcome post-stroke when neural control of the tibialis anterior can be lost or inhibited. In this example, the lost function of tibialis anterior was not to create dorsiflexion but to decelerate and control plantar flexion, a controlled lengthening of the muscle (fig. 5.2).

> **My preference is to call both ends insertions or attachments, muscular or tendinous, as the case may be, and drop the term *origin* altogether.**
>
> —T.S. Ellis 1889, *The Human Foot*

When you first learned anatomy you might have thought yourself to be uniquely frustrated but, as you can see from the above quotation, there were complaints about the notion of muscle origins and insertions as long ago as 1889. In spite of Ellis' complaints, many texts still use the concept of a concentric action bringing the "insertion" toward the "origin",

and the reverse for an eccentric contraction, while the isometric contraction makes no change in the distance between the two points of attachment. It is important for us to remember that anatomy texts (and anatomy tests!!), stubbornly insist on prioritizing concentric contractions over any other form of contraction.

Many standard references list origin, insertion, and actions because they are portraying an imaginary body floating in space with apparently free-floating limbs. The benefit of doing so is that complicating factors (gravity, GRF, momentum, etc.) are removed from the equation and the actions are relatively straightforward. A result of using the "floating body" is that when one muscle is "contracted" the lightest body part moves in response. This false theoretical arrangement used in standard anatomy listings of "actions" is not stated at the beginning of any text I have read. Each anatomy text should come with an introductory warning that all muscle actions refer to an open-chain response from a contraction of a single muscle from anatomical position.

"Open-" and "closed-chain" is a vocabulary used to differentiate between the positioning of the limbs. In open-chain movements, the limbs are unanchored and therefore move more than the trunk—these movements are similar to those described in anatomy books as the "actions" of the muscles. This contrasts with closed-chain movements, in which the limb is anchored somehow (such as the foot being on the ground), and the trunk moves relative to the limb.

We saw an example of closed-chain movement earlier when investigating the foot rockers. With the foot temporarily "anchored" on the ground, the body moves over the top (fig. 5.3). However, once the foot is released at toe-off, the limb movement becomes an open-chain reaction as the limb moves ahead of the trunk ready for the next heel strike. The gait pattern is therefore an alternating sequence of open- and closed-chain reactions.

As the body progresses over the foot, the muscles of the leg must control the movement and prevent the body over-accelerating. One way to visualize muscle activity during movement is to use electromyography (EMG) readings (see fig 5.4) as they can tell us exactly when a muscle is switching on and with approximately how much force. However, what they can't tell us is the direction of length change, or if there is any at all, within the muscle fibers. The EMG signals only tell us that the muscle is working, not whether they are working concentrically, eccentrically, or isometrically. To have an indication of length change we need to cross-relate the EMG signals to the movement at the muscle's related joints during the gait cycle.

The readings in figure 5.4 show the plantar flexors switch on as the talar joint dorsiflexes and they continue to be active—controlling dorsiflexion—until prior to toe-off (mostly between 12% and 50% of the cycle). The EMG readings do not make sense if we restrict ourselves to textbook "actions", however they do make sense when we consider them in context of their real-life function (more of which we will explore in chapter 6).

To understand the role of the plantar flexors during gait, we must break the stance phase

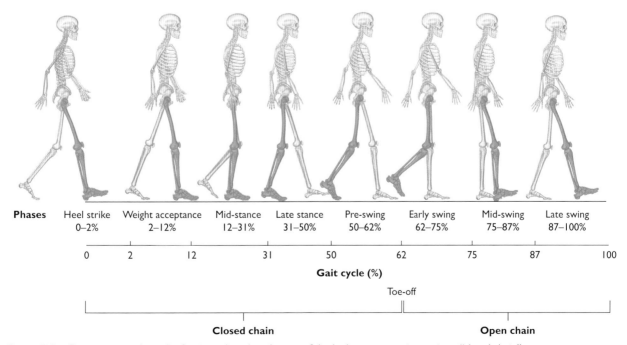

| Phases | Heel strike 0–2% | Weight acceptance 2–12% | Mid-stance 12–31% | Late stance 31–50% | Pre-swing 50–62% | Early swing 62–75% | Mid-swing 75–87% | Late swing 87–100% |

0   2   12   31   50   62   75   87   100

Gait cycle (%)

Toe-off

Closed chain   **Open chain**

Figure 5.3.   During stance phase the foot is anchored as the rest of the body moves over it creating a "closed-chain" movement. When either leg is free to swing forward, the movement returns to being "open-chain".

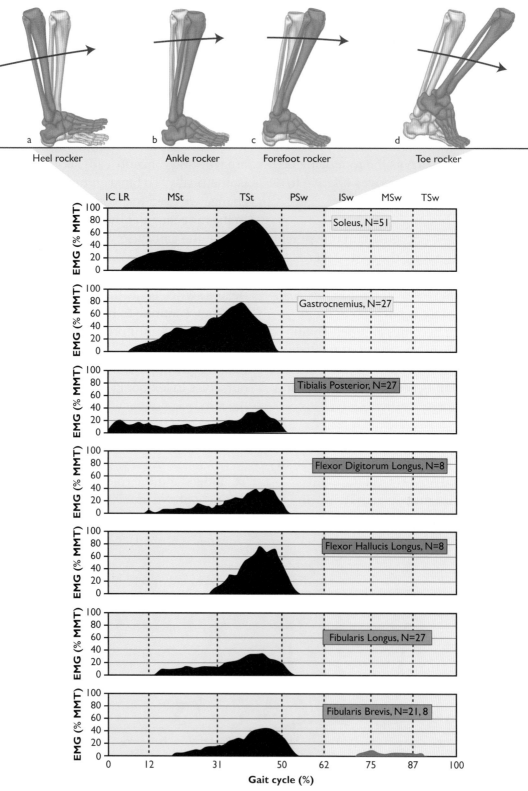

Figure 5.4.   *We will further investigate the functions of the plantar flexor group as we progress in the text, but for now it is important to see the main plantar flexors (soleus, gastrocnemius, and tibialis posterior) are active and lengthening during stance phase and the ankle's progression into dorsiflexion (0–12%). The long toe flexors are active as the toes extend (31–62%) and the whole group is active once the heel lifts (31%) to prevent the foot and ankle from collapsing. We will see that the tension between heel lift at 31% and toe-off at 62% provides part of the force closure support for supination. Electomyographic readings such as these come alive as one gets used to correlating the muscle activity to the joint movement but that does require time and practice whilst also losing the textbook bias toward concentric actions. (Adapted from Perry and Burnfield 2010, N= number of subjects sampled.)*

down into its sections as the muscles' function changes part way through, a fact that is often confused. Following heel strike, the planted foot closes the mechanical chain on that side, while the other leg swings through in an open-chain movement and creates momentum for the body. Momentum from the swinging limb drives the planted foot into dorsiflexion and eventually the heel lifts and the ankle plantar flexes.

The plantar flexors are all active during each of those movements. At first, they decelerate or control the active dorsiflexion through to the forefoot rocker when the heel begins to lift. Once the heel is lifted, the plantar flexors remain active to prevent dorsiflexion and the collapse of the foot as the body weight progresses forward in preparation for toe-off.

Once the heel lifts, the ankle begins to plantar flex and this is regularly interpreted as a direct result of the activity of the plantar flexors. I disagree—a little. I think it can happen that way, but I believe it also happens because of momentum and the reaction of the hip joint. The planted heel lifts in response to the momentum provided by the swing of the other leg and by arriving at the end of the available hip extension on the stance side. This takes a little experimentation to feel, so try the exercise below and then re-read the description of what is happening.

Exercise 5.1.

1. **Stand in neutral on a surface that provides some resistance or in soft soled shoes. Step forward with one foot—step as far as is comfortable and notice what happens with your back foot—did your heel lift?**
2. **Find a step-length in which your heel almost begins to lift but where you can manage to step forward and the back heel can comfortably remain in place; just far enough to create a point of bind in the tissue at the front of the hip. Do not force the heel to stay there, just let your body**

respond with its own natural reactions as you progress into the next action.
3. **From that position, with your trunk and head up as if taking a step, bend your forward knee to let your body weight move forward.**
   • **What happens to your foot as your bodyweight moves ahead?**
   • **What is happening at your hip joint on that same side?**

Do you feel how the bend of the forward knee "requests" more hip extension of the back hip? Once any available movement in the hip is used, the back heel begins to rise. I accept I am leading you to my own conclusions and bias, which is that the back heel is not being pushed up by the plantar flexors, it is being pulled forward by the naturally limited hip extension.

Plantar flexion during stance phase is not necessarily a direct result of plantar flexor contraction. The plantar flexor group stays active to prevent the ankle and foot from collapsing as it rises and creates the rigid lever. Admittedly, the rise of the heel can be driven by the active contraction of the plantar flexors, which, in my clinical experience, results in a characteristic bounce in the walk, in contrast to the smooth progression of those who use a less active and more reactive strategy.

Understanding the soft tissue of the foot and leg (and, really the rest of the body too) requires a flexibility in how we recognize the effects of muscle tension. We must be content to accept that the fluid relationship between cause and effect as a reaction (in this case, plantar flexion) could come from several different sources. So far, we have seen the differences made by open- and closed-chain movement. With the introduction of momentum, we also see how the influence of a muscle can travel beyond its associated joints.

During locomotion, there is a reciprocation between the ankle, knee, and hip as they act as a unit (see fig. 5.5). Through the early part

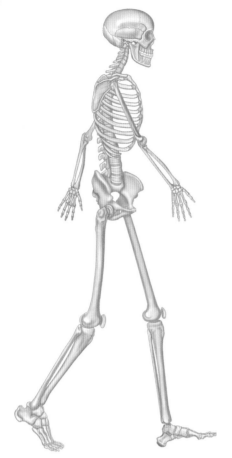

Figure 5.5. *Anchoring one foot on the ground as the other leg swings forward creates two opposing forces acting through the pelvis. The pelvis is drawn forward on the swing side and held back on the stance side. The natural reaction of the stance limb is to extend both the knee and hip in response to momentum with the result of adding extra stride length. The final position of the stance limb before toe-off is a combination of toe extension, ankle plantar flexion, knee, and hip extension, which has all resulted from anchoring the stance foot as the other swings forward.*

of stance phase, the plantar flexors decelerate the tibia and fibula as the ankle dorsiflexes. The other leg swings forward and provides momentum that draws the pelvis forward with it. As one foot is anchored on the ground in closed-chain, the other foot propels forward and generates opposing forces that act through the hips, causing the pelvis to rotate and tilt, and the hip on the stance side to extend. It can be argued that the hip extension has been caused by the contraction of the same side plantar flexors.

If the plantar flexors did not decelerate the tibia and if there was no friction between the ground and the stance foot, the stance leg could, theoretically at least, move forward in time with the swing leg. The resistance offered by the plantar flexors slows the stance limb relative to the swinging leg and the difference in speeds between the two limbs results in the extension of the hip. In this case, hip extension is driven by the muscles of the calf. Our naturally limited hip extension (12–16°) then causes the heel to lift and creates further plantar flexion and toe extension.

We could be seen to be playing with words and concepts, but it is interesting to consider that the plantar flexors, in a closed-chain forward movement such as walking, assist hip extension. The hip returns the favor by driving forward to raise the heel. In this context, the plantar flexors are hip extensors and the hip flexors (and all the other tissues crossing the front of the hip) are ankle plantar flexors and toe extenders (review fig. 5.5).

MUSCLE CONTRACTION AND ELASTICITY

The plantar flexors are a hard-working group of muscles but, thankfully, they are designed for the job. Not only must they hold the body temporarily aloft with each step, but they must also decelerate each landing during a run, jump, skip, or hop. Each of these activities multiplies the mass that must be controlled (fig. 5.6), but the plantar flexors possess many features to help manage the heavy workloads during walking, running, and landing. The most obvious of these is the amount and type of collagenous tissue they possess. From the long, thick Achilles tendon, and the thick aponeurosis of the soleus, to the much longer and slender tendons of the toe flexors, each structure plays an important role in active force management. But there are other important aspects within the muscle design themselves, such as fiber direction and length.

This section will review a few anatomical features of the myofascia and discuss the

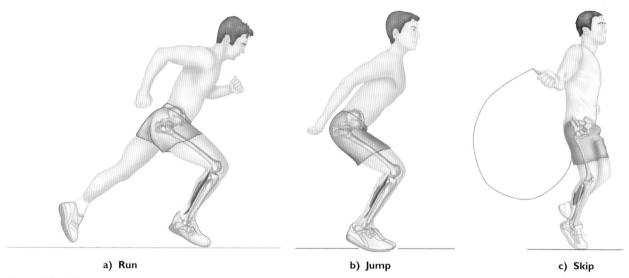

a) **Run**   b) **Jump**   c) **Skip**

Figure 5.6.   Many activities require rapid dorsiflexion to decelerate which puts stress into the plantar flexors. Due to their resultant strain, the plantar flexors can then respond by pushing the body up or forward with increased force and efficiency.

benefits and limitations that come with each characteristic. Appreciating and understanding the roles each tissue plays should help visualize the interplay between the pieces of the movement puzzle. No muscle has only one role, and each must accommodate constant changes in degree and direction of force. As we saw with the tibialis anterior and the plantar flexors (see figs. 5.2 & 5.4), to understand what is happening in the tissue we must place each force in context simultaneously. Only when we have movement and the force environment in context, are we able to interpret muscle activity. Limiting ourselves to textbook actions restricts our understanding; we must build a fuller, richer, and more accurate representation of muscle activity.

Muscles can contract concentrically to break inertia and create momentum, but once we start moving, we must also have a way to control that momentum. The "eccentric" role of a muscle can prevent us from succumbing to gravity and falling, or from accelerating without control. Muscle work, either the positive work of concentric contraction or the so-called negative work[2] of deceleration, is

metabolically expensive. Active lengthening and shortening of the muscles require repeated processing of adenosine triphosphate (ATP) and the various other chemical compounds that make up muscular metabolism (see fig. 5.7). Each locking and unlocking of myosin and actin cross-bridges creates a turnover of ATP, which must be replenished at a metabolic cost. Minimizing the number of cross-bridge turnovers, i.e., concentric and eccentric contractions, reduces the metabolic turnover of calories, a potentially life-saving strategy for any organism.

We saw the body's drive to optimal weight/ strength balance in chapter 3 when considering bone, a dense and costly tissue to produce and to move. Muscles and their associated mechanoreceptors also appear to follow calorie management strategies by combining the effects of muscle fiber length and direction, as well as elastic tissue properties. As with many physiological processes, none of these is a discrete feature, all of them overlap and each tissue has numerous roles to fulfill during movement. When working effectively, the proprioceptive system should be able to monitor the forces acting through the system

---

[2]Negative work, the act of deceleration, is not necessarily concentric or eccentric. It can be either depending on the forces involved.

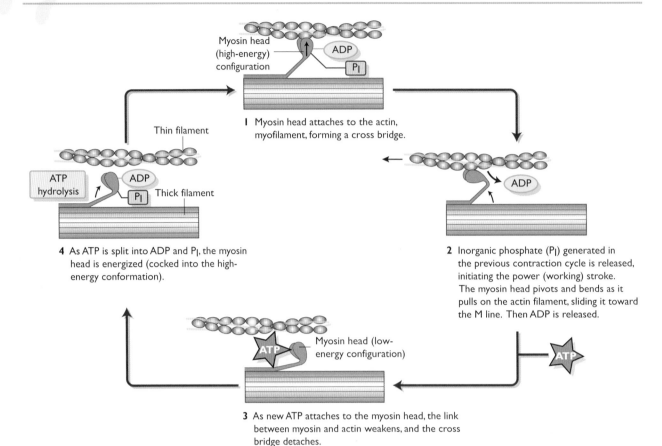

Figure 5.7.   *The sliding filament theory of muscle action demonstrates how the interlocking of myosin and actin filaments facilitates lengthening and shortening of the muscle fibers. Alternating locking and unlocking of the filaments requires energy exchange as part of the metabolic cost of muscle action. (Adapted from Pearson Educational 2006.)*

and adjust muscle tone and length to optimize the use of each characteristic.

For example, when watching someone move, we may think that a muscle is lengthening as the joint it crosses opens. However, numerous researchers have found that when the movement has a momentum that is repetitive and rhythmical, such as flat walking and running, the muscle remains close to isometric. This quasi-isometric condition of the muscle allows the energy of momentum to lengthen the collagenous tissues across the joints. Collagen-based tissues can capture a portion of the kinetic energy from momentum and store it as elastic energy ready to be used for the return movement, in the same way as one pulls back the elastic of a catapult to propel a ball toward its target. Using momentum to provide elastic energy in this way decreases the number of

cross-bridge linkages made by the muscles, thereby reducing overall calorie use.

We are given a more understandable insight in the specialized qualities of muscle tissue, and how those qualities have been devised for the saving of organic energy without sacrifice in functional proficiency.

—Morton 1952, page 244

The recycling of kinetic energy by collagenous tissues has attained a lot of attention over the last few years, partly due to the work of McNeill Alexander, Kawakami, and Fukunaga, among others. In the past, when we saw a musculotendinous element lengthen, it was commonly assumed to be an eccentric lengthening of muscle fibers. We now know that the muscle fibers may remain isometric as the tendons lengthen (by up to 10% of their original length). However, even that is only one characteristic of the system's interactions.

Using real-time ultrasound, various researchers, notably Lidstone et al. 2018, have shown that the muscle fibers can act eccentrically, isometrically, or concentrically as the whole musculotendinous unit (MTU) lengthens. At first sight this seems counterintuitive, but the muscles appear to lengthen or shorten to accommodate the amount of momentum to be controlled, as well as the overall tissue stiffness required (stiffness is explored further below). With this piece of knowledge in place, we can visualize the muscle fiber acting to guide and regulate tissue length from inside an elastic bag. The inherent elasticity of the fascial bag allows the muscle fiber contents some degree of autonomy over its direction of movement. The muscle can either rein in, let out, or remain the same length dependent on movement demands; just like guiding Morton's wheelchair.

One difference Morton liked to point out between skeletal muscle and the smooth muscle that surrounds many internal organs, is the collagen content. Skeletal muscle has more collagen fiber content because it is subject to stretch by external forces. Cardiac and smooth muscle fibers are rarely stretched in the same way and do not have to deal with the high loads experienced during movement—the visceral organs are protected by the various layers of well-lubricated serous fascia that allow mechanical forces to pass around them via the abdominal and thoracic walls (fig. 5.8).

The musculoskeletal system is designed to carry mechanical stress and strain. The terminology can be confusing, but as we saw in chapter 3, a simple definition of stress is as a measurement of force applied to a material; the material's response to the stress is referred to

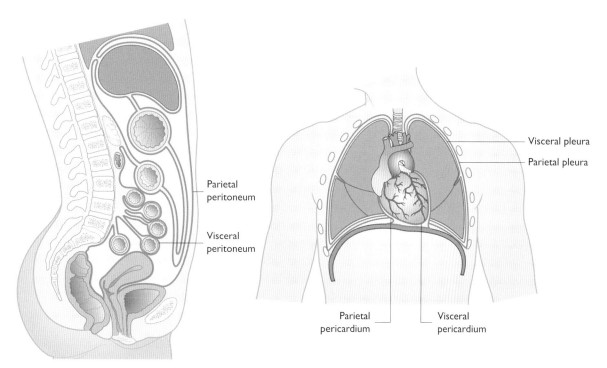

Parietal peritoneum

Visceral peritoneum

Visceral pleura

Parietal pleura

Parietal pericardium

Visceral pericardium

Figure 5.8.   *The internal organs are contained within layers of serous membranes that allow relatively independent movement between the thoraco-abdominal contents and the outer musculoskeletal locomotor system. The layered arrangement reduces external mechanical stress reaching the visceral tissues.*

as strain—the material is strained by the stress applied to it. Importantly, in biomechanics, the reaction is referred to as strain.

To give further context for the vocabulary, explore the graph in fig 5.9. Stress is traditionally plotted along the y axis and strain along the x axis. The graph shows a linear relationship between the two measurements: when one increases, so does the other at the same rate. Lines A and B represent two imaginary materials that respond to stress with a different ratio; an increase of two units of stress lengthen "A" twice as much as "B". It does not matter where along the line we are, if we increase the stress by two units, the strain increases by two units along line "B" and by four units on line "A". Material "B" is therefore more resistant to lengthening than "A". Another way to express the difference is that "B" is stiffer than "A", as "A" lengthens more under the same force.

As we saw in chapter 3, stiffness has an official definition—it is the ratio between stress and strain. Each material has a different degree of stiffness depending on its material make up (see also fig. 3.4). For example, elastic bands are much less stiff than string. Pull on a piece of string as hard as you can and it will not lengthen much; apply the same stress to an elastic band and it will probably stretch beyond its capacity and snap.

Apply enough stress to any material and it will eventually break, but the amount of lengthening each material is capable of also varies. Often, very stiff materials, like concrete for example (Fig. 5.10a), can withstand high stresses but do not lengthen (strain) much before they break. Contrast that to an elastic band that can stretch a couple times its own length before snapping. Neither property is good or bad, it depends on the needs of the area. Some areas require more stability and therefore take advantage of stiffer materials and some require more mobility with less stiffness. One strength of biological tissue over man-made material is its ability to alter stiffness according to its length.

When exploring characteristics of bone, we saw how biological materials do not follow the simple straight-line relationship between stress and strain. Most biological structures get stiffer the further they strain. The J-shaped curve in fig. 5.11b illustrates how tendon, for example, is easily lengthened (remember, strain is a measurement of change of length) in the early stages, just like the elastic band. The gradient of the curve changes and, at the latter stages, more closely resembles the stress/strain line of concrete. The J-shape curve illustrates how tendon lengthens easily initially but becomes more resistant to change the longer it gets.

When the tendon is shorter it is less stiff; as it lengthens it becomes stiffer. The degree of tissue stiffness plays an important role in movement as it relates to mobility, stability, and elasticity. In anatomy and

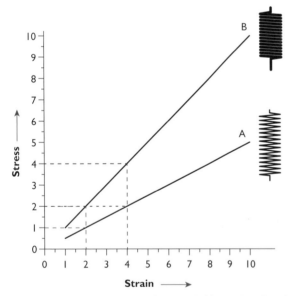

Figure 5.9.   Traditionally stress (force divided by area) is plotted along the y axis and strain (change in length) along the x axis. The two lines ("A" and "B") represent materials of different stiffness as they respond differently to increases in stress. To increase the length of both lines by two units requires twice as much stress to be applied to material "B". At a glance, the steeper gradient of line "B" demonstrates its greater resistance to lengthening. B's greater stiffness is demonstrated by the series of dotted lines—to change length from 2 to 4 units (x axis) requires only 1 unit of strain applied to material "A" but 2 units of strain applied to material "B" (y axis).

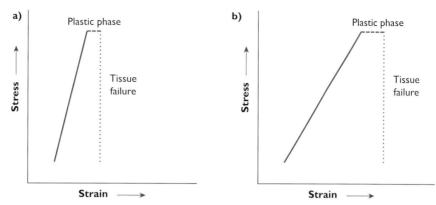

Figure 5.10.   a) Stiffer materials, such as our imaginary concrete, will lengthen less (measured along the x axis) but require more stress (measured on the y axis) to be applied before breaking. Stiffer materials tend to have shorter plastic phases—where the material can lengthen further but can no longer return to its original state. Materials with short plastic phases are usually referred to as brittle. b) Less stiff materials can experience more deformation before entering the plastic phase (when they are no longer able to return to their original form) and into tissue failure. They can lengthen further and still return to their original length—hence they are described as elastic (the ability to deform and return to normal). To give a real-word example, bones of older people tend to be more brittle and will deform less before breaking compared with those of their young grandchildren. The elasticity of bone and soft tissues will change through life and as a result of quality of diet and amounts of exercise.

engineering, the term *stiffness* is neutral, it is just a characteristic of the material under investigation. There are times when a high degree of stiffness is favorable and other times when we need the tissue to easily lengthen.

It makes sense that our tissues become naturally stiffer when exposed to higher stresses. If we take the example of skipping when the foot lands, the plantar flexors lengthen and their collagenous tissues *strain*, but they also increase their *stiffness* to resist lengthening further. This makes our tissues adaptable, as our bodies are not exposed to uniform conditions all the time. We can skip at different speeds and heights, in different climates and temperatures, and the beauty of biological materials is that they can adapt to these different conditions.

Lengthening tissue requires energy and some of that energy is captured by the tissues—this is energy then helps the tissue return to its original length, a dynamic we recognize as *elasticity*. Elasticity plays a vital role in many of our movement efficiency mechanisms as it allows the recycling of kinetic energy from momentum.

Efficiency is further enhanced when we can balance the momentum of the movement with the tissue stiffness for optimum energy capture. As we see in fig. 5.11b, the early and late stages of lengthening do not capture much energy. Enough stress must be applied to the tissue to strain it into the middle portion of the stress/strain graph where the greatest gains can be made but without lengthening the tissue too far toward its plastic phase and point of failure.

There are numerous intrinsic factors that affect tissue stiffness, no doubt you will have directly experienced some of these yourself. The list is almost endless, but the major variables include temperature, hydration, age, tissue type, hyaluronan content (a hydrophilic lubricating element of fascial tissue), hormone variations, and collagen types (there are numerous forms of collagen in the body and each has a different degree of stiffness, Zügel et al. 2018).

Every movement requires varying degrees of stiffness through the whole-body system and between individual body parts. Too much stiffness decreases range of motion; too little causes instability and relative hypermobility. The body must alter and adjust the stiffness

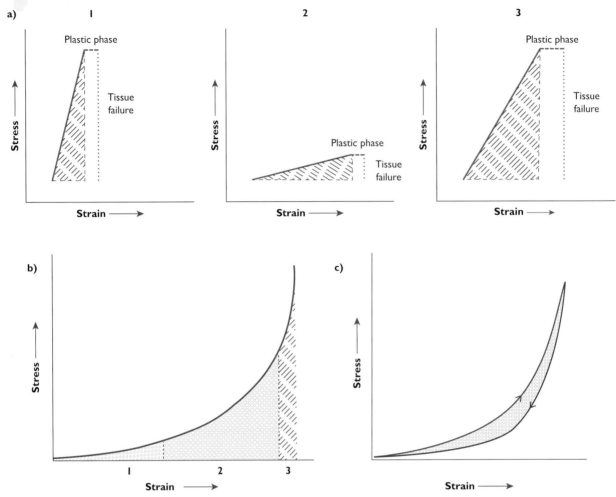

Figure 5.11.   *The area below the curve indicates the amount of potential energy created when a material is deformed. a) If the tissue has high stiffness and does not lengthen, little energy will be captured (1). Similarly, if the tissue lengthens easily under low stress then little energy must be applied to the material. (2) An average degree of stiffness will allow the capture of more energy but it is a compromise between the stability given by stiff tissues (3) and the mobility offered by the easily lengthened tissue (1). b) Natural materials, such as tendon, can use the benefits of low, high, and medium stiffness levels by having a variable degree of stiffness as they lengthen. In the early phase of lengthening (1), little strain is required and not much energy (shown as triangles) is loaded into the tissue. The situation is similar toward the end of lengthening (3) when the tissue becomes stiffer and therefore offers more protection to the joints. More energy is required to lengthen the material toward its end of range and, because of the small degree of extra length, less energy is added for the return movement (hatched area). It is in the middle phase (2) where the most energy is loaded into the tissue for its return (circles). c) Not all of the stored energy is returned in the recoil as energy is lost due to friction and production of heat. The lost energy, known as hysteresis, is variable and depends on numerous factors including timing of loading and unloading, tissue health, and tissue viscosity.*

according to demand on local areas. Take the foot during stance phase, for example. At toe-off the foot is required to act as a "rigid lever", a platform to manage the forces of momentum, GRF, and body mass. We saw that the bones act together to alter the "stiffness" of the foot as they unlock and lock again, but the soft tissue also adapts to the change in demand as the positions and the role of the foot switches from mobile adaptor to rigid lever through the stance phase.

The soft tissues must respond to the extrinsic demands of movement, and, although gravity is constant, GRFs, momentum, and body position change continually. Successful movement requires constant surveillance of tissue demand—how are the forces acting through the body? How is the body responding? Is the body getting closer to its goal? Is it moving efficiently?

In a feedback loop like the one used by the osteocytes to guide bone modeling, the monitoring of each of those questions is the role of the mechanoreceptors, part of the body's proprioceptive system. Mechanoreceptors have direct and indirect communication to the muscles, which then adjust their tone to affect overall stiffness in the area according to a complex algorithm with many variables.

One can think of the muscles constantly drawing in or letting out in reaction to need. If they need to create movement, they pull in a lot through concentric contraction. Conversely, if an antagonist pulls in, they must eccentrically "let out" at a rate matched to that concentric contraction to give a controlled movement. As momentum acts through the tissue, the muscle fibers appear to react in response to the forces to ensure progression toward the movement goal. Muscle tissue is an active "stiffness adjusting system", able to shorten, lengthen, or remain constant according to need (Sawicki et al. 2009).

Constant proprioceptive monitoring might seem like hard work but, according to the work of Prof. Huijing et al. (2003), the information appears to be processed locally without a continuous need to signal to the spinal cord or brain.

Fine adjustments to muscle fiber length and tone directly affect the elastic and stiffness properties of their associated collagenous tissues. In an optimized system, the muscle will undergo minimal change of length, momentum will stiffen and load energy into the tendons and surrounding collagen, providing several benefits to the overall system, including efficiency. The best return of elastic energy happens in the mid-range of the tissue's length—think of one end of the range as like the elastic band and the other end like concrete (as seen in fig. 5.11b). Working in the mid-range requires a reasonable amount of force to lengthen the tendinous elastic

tissue, which means that kinetic energy is then available to assist the return movement.

TISSUE STIFFNESS AND FORCE OUTPUT

Elastic energy is not the only advantage within this process, as muscle fibers can also operate within their optimal length range. Muscle fiber creates less force at either end of its length range (see fig. 5.12), lengthening the tendinous collagen fibers through momentum lets the muscles remain within their optimum force/length relationship and therefore able to provide optimum force—especially toward the end of joint range when control of movement is particularly needed. Using momentum to lengthen the collagenous tissues also allows the muscle fibers to stay close to an isometric state and burn fewer calories.

Sports activities use the momentum of countermovement as a common strategy to add power and increase efficiency. Many benefits are gained through the myofascial natural dynamics by first moving in the opposite direction for a throw, a jump, or any other movement that requires additional force. Muscle force production is reduced by increased speed of contraction (see fig. 5.13) but, by loading the elastic tissue, some of the required velocity can be produced through elastic recoil rather than fiber contraction. The elastic recoil of collagenous tissues surrounding the muscle has a greater shortening velocity than the muscle itself. This can be difficult to visualize but, in a countermovement strategy, there will be two speeds of shortening: elastic tissue shortens quickly while muscle tissue contracts more slowly to minimize its own loss of force. The interplay between the two types of force (muscular and elastic) uses the best features of both tissue types, one for fine control (muscular) and the other for speed, efficiency, and increased force (elastic).

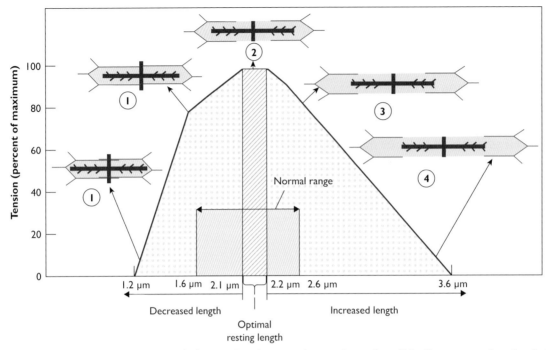

Figure 5.12. *Actin and myosin fibers have an ideal range of overlap to produce maximum force. If the fibers are too short (marked 1), there is less space available for further shortening. Too much length (marked 3 & 4) reduces the filament overlap and decreases the amount of pulling force. An optimal overlap between the two filaments provides maximum force potential (marked 2).*

Countermovement strategies take advantage of numerous tissue dynamics—elasticity, stiffness, tissue length, and velocity relationships. Sports-related literature commonly references countermovement (sometimes also referred to as a "stretch-shortening cycle" or "stretch-recoil cycle"), but it is much less talked about when considering normal movement. But whenever momentum acts across a joint, a blend of the benefits mentioned above assists the return movement.

Everyday movement may load less elastic energy than sports-related movement, but nonetheless the muscle fiber will stay quasi-isometric and the collagenous tissues will lengthen to some degree and therefore stiffen. The increased stiffness of the fascial tissue assists with the deceleration of the movement and creates a taut support around the contractile muscle tissue. Stiffening a muscle's fascial supporting structures gives the muscle a more responsive environment to transfer the force of its contraction.

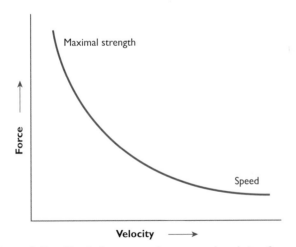

Figure 5.13. *Muscle force output decreases as the velocity of contraction increases. This means that a muscle recruited to contract quickly will, in effect, be weaker. The lengthening of the elastic tissues surrounding the muscle fiber means the MTU can shorten rapidly using elastic energy while the muscle fiber contracts more slowly, at a velocity suited to its optimal force output.*

Even in the relatively low-load stance phase of walking, there can be a 7 mm elongation of the Achilles tendon with a minimal lengthening of the muscle fibers (Fukunaga et al. 2001). Tendon recoil assists with toe-off and reduces muscle work, which is also reduced by the stiffening of the lengthened tendon. If the tendon had not lengthened, any ankle muscle that shortens during toe-off would first have to pull on the less stiff tendon before having any effect on the ankle.

To give an overly exaggerated image, picture the tendon as a very slender elastic band attached to a chair leg. Pulling on the elastic band will result in the band lengthening and no movement of the chair. Swap the elastic band for a piece of string, which is much less elastic and much stiffer. Pulling on the stiffer string will only lengthen the string a small amount and will move the chair. We know from the graph above that collagenous tissues alter their stiffness relative to length (fig. 5.11b), becoming more like strings and less like elastic bands as they are lengthened. A countermovement uses up the early portions of the strain curve—getting toward the mid-to-end range of joint position naturally stiffens the collagen tissues around the joint. This has two major benefits—some protection for the joint and more efficient transfer of force from the associated muscle fiber to control the joint movement. Control is needed both to decelerate the tissue lengthening and to create tissue shortening for the return. The muscles will then be better able to control the movement if their force is being transferred by "strings" rather than "slender elastic bands".

The roles a muscle can play during movement are directly influenced by its fiber arrangement. The force, length, and velocity relationships of fusiform muscles with their long parallel fibers differ considerably from those of pennate muscles with their short, angled fiber arrangement (fig. 5.14a). Working in parallel, and with fibers connecting directly between opposite ends of the muscle, allows fusiform fibers to contract quickly and act over a longer range. Shorter-fiber pennate muscles can only contract over short distances but do so with much greater power for the same volume of muscle (fig. 5.14b).

Once again, we must break down several factors to appreciate the relationships affecting

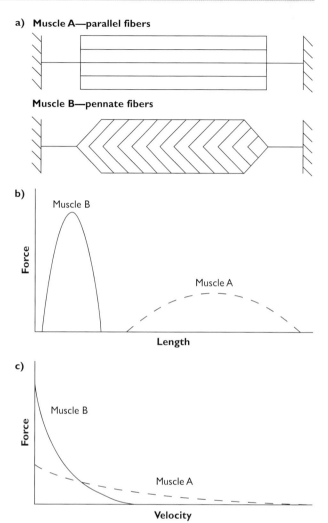

Figure 5.14.   *Muscle architecture, force, length, and velocity curves.* **a)** *Fusiform muscles (A) have long parallel fibers running from one end to the other of the MTU. Pennate muscles (B), in contrast, have angled fibers, like the barbs of a feather. Pennate fibers are therefore relatively shorter and can be arranged in unipennated, bipennated, or multipennated patterns.* **b)** *Differences in fiber lengths result in significant force/length differences. Pennate (B) muscles create more force but over shorter lengths than fusiform (A) muscles.* **c)** *Due to their greater shortening ability, fusiform (A) muscles create less force but over a wider range of velocity than pennated (B) muscles. (From Wilson & Lichtwark 2011.)*

performance. These include muscle volume (also known as anatomical cross-sectional area), the number of muscle fibers (measured by the physiological cross-sectional area), and the influence of fiber alignment (see fig. 5.15). Each feature has associated costs and benefits that affect the muscle's functional context and placement within the body. Some areas of the body will require more force, some may require faster contractions, some must deal with higher

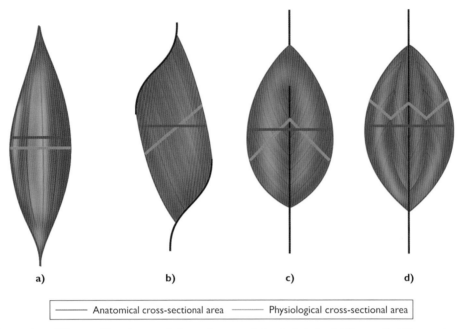

a)   b)   c)   d)

——— Anatomical cross-sectional area   ——— Physiological cross-sectional area

Figure 5.15.   The number of fibers making up a muscle has a direct correlation to its potential force output. The number of fibers can be estimated by calculating a muscle's cross-sectional area, which should bisect each fiber. A direct side-to-side line bisects each fiber of a fusiform muscle (a) but fails to measure each fiber of a pennated muscle. Angled sections must be made to bisect every pennated fiber (b, c, & d). Muscle volume, which affects its mass, is related to the cross-sectional area. There are therefore two important measurements that affect muscle performance—anatomical cross-sectional area, which relates to its volume, and physiological cross-sectional area, which relates to the number of fibers and a muscle's force output. Fusiform muscles will have the same measurement for both, but a pennate muscle will have a higher physiological cross-sectional area and therefore more, but shorter, muscle fibers.

forces from outside the body, while others are more involved with creating movement from within. Matching tissue architecture to the demands of each body area will increase overall efficiency of tissue development and growth, as well as reducing the cost of movement.

When walking or running, the distal end of each lower limb moves most relative to the rest of the body. As running shoe manufacturers have discovered, minimizing the weight at the end of the limbs can make significant energy savings over long distances. Our bodies also made the same discovery many years ago and packed our calves with pennate muscles. Using pennated architecture allows a muscle to bundle more muscle fibers into a smaller volume. Have a look at fig. 5.15, which compares anatomical and physiological cross-sectional areas. Each muscle shown has the same *anatomical cross-sectional area* (ACSA), meaning they take up the same volume within

the body and have the same weight but will differ in their potential force output.

Potential force output of a muscle depends heavily on the number of fibers it contains. The ACSA cuts through every fiber of the fusiform muscle but misses a considerable number of the pennated fibers. If we change the rules for the cross-sectional cut so that it must cut through every muscle fiber rather than directly across from side-to-side, the line does not change for the fusiform muscle but must be angled for the pennated. Angling the cross-section to include every fiber creates the *physiological cross-sectional area* (PCSA), which is a better measurement of potential force production of a muscle.

Fiber arrangement explains the difference in force potential and provides clues to the roles each muscle performs. Pennate muscles are positioned for production and, importantly, control of high forces imposed on the body through momentum. Fusiform muscles with an equivalent ACSA can manage relatively lower forces over a longer range of movement and with more velocity. Consider the difference in roles between the biceps brachii and the soleus muscles—crossing the elbow joint with its long range of motion but with relatively low loads, the biceps brachii consists of long parallel fibers, while the multi-pennate soleus muscle has high loads and a short range of motion.

Muscle architecture evolves according to demand. The biceps brachii is most commonly recruited to perform open-chain movements, helping guide the hand toward its various destinations. The soleus is most repeatedly used in closed-chain movements, tensioning to control and decelerate dorsiflexion, particularly when landing from a jump or while running. The calf muscles are required to control up to six times our body weight when running and even more when we land from a jump. The multi-pennate arrangement of the muscle fibers of the soleus provides the strength and force required without taking up too much space or adding more weight to the distal limbs.

Not only have the calf muscles got angled fibers but they also have long, elastic tendons making them capable of recycling more kinetic energy. As we know from above, tendons have elastic properties and can strain to absorb some of the stress created during, for instance, landing, and the resultant lengthening is controlled by their associated muscle fibers. The muscle fibers may tension concentrically, eccentrically, or isometrically as the tendon lengthens, depending on the movement requirements as well the various tissue strengths, stiffnesses, and their ability to control the movement.

■ ON THE ASCENDING LIMB

Fascial tissue offers three main benefits to our locomotor processes: increased efficiency, power amplification, and damping. As we discuss these benefits, we must keep in mind

that these are not discrete functions operating independently. Each dynamic constantly overlaps with the others, even when one is called upon more because of current movement demands. As mentioned by Sawicki and Huijing, the proprioceptive system (mostly) unconsciously monitors the requirements and makes the necessary adjustments to muscle fiber's tone and length to fine-tune stiffness levels and force output.

As we saw above, the elastic property of the fascial tissues helps optimize muscle force and increase power output. The tendon lengthens rather than the muscle fiber and, because the muscle fiber is not changing length, it can stay within its optimal force-length relationship. The force-length relationship (see figs. 5.12 & 5.16) shows that there is a narrow range of length in which muscles can produce higher force, so staying within that range will improve any muscle's ability to control movement. However, a problem could arise if momentum pushes the muscle length over the peak of the curve.

Once over the force-length graph's peak, the muscle begins to lose force output (as shown in fig. 5.16a). Any further increases in length will effectively weaken the muscle by reducing its

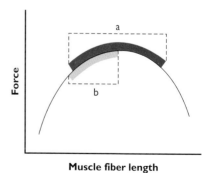

Figure 5.16. *Muscle fiber has an optimal force-length ratio (seen in fig. 5.12), but allowing muscle fiber to lengthen across the peak of the curve would result in decreased force output (as shown in red, a). Or, to put it simply, as the muscle lengthens beyond the peak of the curve it becomes relatively weaker and its ability to control movement decreases. Calibrating fiber length to operate within the ascending portion of the curve allows lengthening to increase force output (b). The result is that normal functional range remains within optimal force-length relationship.*

force production ability. Lengthening beyond the peak would become an issue for muscles designed to decelerate movement, momentum would constantly be edging the muscle into weakness when, in fact, the muscle requires more strength.

Thankfully, our muscle tissue has evolved an obvious solution by operating predominately on the ascending limb of the curve. Several researchers (Rubenson et al. 2012; Lieber and Ward 2011; Ishikawai et al. 2007) have found muscle fiber length remains on the ascending portion of the force-length curve (fig. 5.17). By starting from a relatively shorter position, the muscles only become stronger as they lengthen. If they were tuned to operate on either side of the peak, lengthening would first cause an increase in force followed by a rapid decrease as the ratio moves over the peak of the curve. Operating on the descending side of the curve would not make functional sense as more

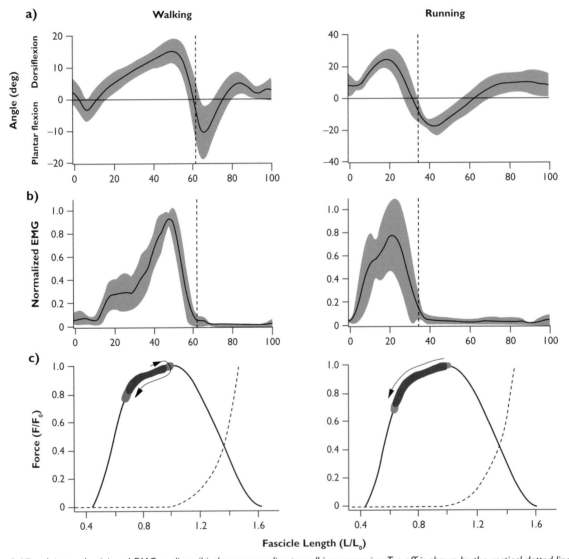

Figure 5.17.   Joint angles (a) and EMG readings (b) change according to walking or running. Toe-off is shown by the vertical dotted line at 62% for walking and 36% for running. Behavior of soleus fiber length in both walking (left) and running (right) occurs on the ascending portion of the force-length curve, allowing optimal force output for both activities. The arrow represents the direction of length change. (c) During both walking and running, the soleus fascicles operate on the ascending portion of the curve but only during early stance phase of walking do they lengthen before shortening. The fibers shorten during stance phase of running despite the increase in overall length of the musculotendinous unit during dorsiflexion indicating the muscle is working concentrically as the collagenous tissues lengthen. (Adapted from Rubenson et al. 2012.)

force is generally required to control movement as joints open and the lever-arms lengthen. Further, it makes sense to add protection to an area as it moves into end of range.

EMG and ankle position for walking and running shows soleus activity increases as the ankle moves further into dorsiflexion, then decreases with plantar flexion and the move toward toe-off. This pattern should remind us of Exercise 5.1 (p. 115), where heel lift and plantar flexion are provided by the body's momentum in concert with the position and associated tissue tension of the other joints through the rest of the body.

> The plantar flexors could be said to be "lifting" the body, but they are also preventing the foot from collapsing under the body. The next chapter will reveal much of the indirect work of the so-called plantar flexors, as they provide much of the "force support" to the foot's structure during supination in preparation for toe-off. The plantar flexors help stiffen the overall structure of the foot while also controlling the forward force from momentum.

Direction of muscle fiber length change in fig. 5.17c shows the different reaction to high loads. Fibers lengthen slightly before shortening during walking, a low-load activity. This contrasts with the fiber activity during running, and the associated higher impact forces that drive the ankle into dorsiflexion. Although we see the ankle being driven further into dorsiflexion during the short stance phase of running, the muscle fibers only actively shorten. The overall tissue lengthening during running to allow dorsiflexion must come from the associated tendon and surrounding fascial tissues—remember, the muscle fibers can shorten while the fascial tissues lengthen. The energy used to stretch the collagen-based tissues can then be recycled back into the system to drive ankle plantar flexion and help propel the body's forward momentum.

Recycling kinetic energy is only one metabolic benefit afforded by the fascial tissues. The whole system also benefits from the fascial tissues' ability to lengthen and thereby stiffen in response to momentum. The body's use of momentum to strain collagenous tissues changes the operating length range of muscle (Ishikawa et al. 2007; Rubenson et al. 2012). Rather than acting across the peak of the force-length curve, the strain and stiffening of fascial tissue moves the muscles' active range to the ascending portion of the force-length curve (fig. 5.17c).

If muscles were tuned to operate either side of the peak of their force-length curve, they would move onto the descending portion when trying to decelerate momentum. This would result in them becoming weaker as their associated joints open and, potentially, move toward their end of range. The ability to operate on the ascending side of the curve increases the relative strength of the muscle as it moves toward the end of normal joint range. Working on the ascending curve gives a protective mechanism as the tuning of fascicle length helps guard against over-lengthening of tissues across a joint.

■ FORCE CONTROL— DECELERATION AND DAMPING

Along with improving efficiency and enhancing power output, a third dynamic of collagenous fascial tissue is to assist damping of force. Damping[3] (or attenuation, fig. 5.18c) is the controlled deceleration to stop movement and dissipate the energy temporarily stored in the elastic tissues after they lengthen. Roberts and Azizi (2011) show that lengthening of tendons on landing allows high forces to be applied rapidly into the musculotendinous

---

[3]It can be important for one's "street cred" to be familiar with damping versus dampening. The former means to dissipate force and the latter is the application of liquid.

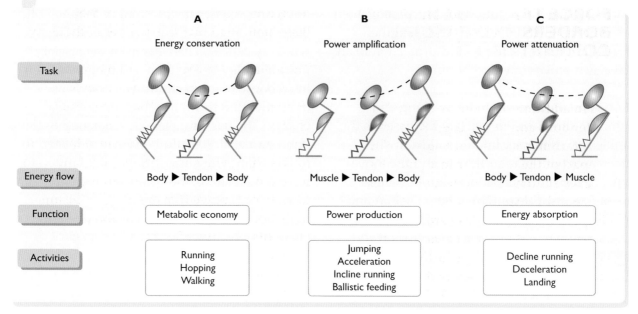

Figure 5.18. Attenuation or damping (C) is the last of three mechanisms described by Roberts and Azizi in their review paper on the role of springs. Landing often requires control of high force as the tissues lengthen. Muscle fiber produces less force as the velocity increases, and is therefore less able to eccentrically contract immediately following impact. To compensate for its loss of force during rapid lengthening, the muscle remains close to isometric (within its optimal force range) on landing and the collagenous tissues lengthen to control impact forces. This allows the muscle to eccentrically contract at a slower rate (and therefore with more force) to dampen the elastic energy captured within the collagen. The other mechanisms have been explored above—energy conservation, economy (A) is enhanced by the muscle fibers staying close to their ideal length while momentum is used to load elastic energy. Power production is amplified (B) by first pretensioning the tissues (we will see the benefits of this in the next two chapters). (Adapted from Roberts & Azizi 2011.)

system. Such forces are difficult and dangerous for muscles and often a source of injury. By first re-routing the impact force into the collagenous tissues, the muscle fiber can then react with a slower eccentric contraction to attenuate the energy—remember, the faster a muscle contracts, the less force it can produce. Roberts and Azizi point out that just as tendons allow a muscle to produce more force, they also enable the damping of higher forces than the muscles would otherwise be capable of controlling.

Impact forces enter the body rapidly with no respect for muscle fiber's ability to contract quickly enough and with enough force to control the reaction following impact. Muscles struggle to produce high force with rapid contraction (see figs. 5.13 & 5.14), so re-routing impact forces first into the fascial tissues, while the muscle contracts "quasi-isometrically",

allows the muscle fiber to lengthen at a slower velocity and maintain control.

Damping of force is particularly important for the foot and ankle as they receive most of the body's impact forces daily. Whether one mid-foot strikes while running, skipping, or jumping down from a height, there is likely to be rapid ankle dorsiflexion. The knee and hip, the other major joints involved in these movements, both have large and strong muscles to control any flexion, but the calf consists of a range of relatively small and mostly slender muscles. Thankfully, each of these muscles has a pennate arrangement leading into long tendons, with each muscle contained within its own epimysium, and the muscles are grouped together within fascial compartments, so there is a range of fascial support in the management of forces.

FORCE TRANSFER BEYOND BORDERS AND FASCIAL COMPARTMENTS

In addition to the force exerted at tendons and other direct muscular attachments to bone, a substantial part of the muscular force may be exerted through connective tissues within a compartment. A likely important function of exerting force on compartment walls is to increase their stiffness and create, in addition to the bony skeleton, an extended rather stiff connective tissue "skeleton".

—Huijing et al. 2003

As with the musculoskeletal descriptions we have explored so far in this chapter, anatomy texts often condition us to highlight the longitudinal arrangement of musculoskeletal tissues. Longitudinal force transfer is only one part—albeit a significant one—of the story, as force can also transfer horizontally from one muscle to its neighbors and beyond. This relatively new area of investigation by researchers is revealing numerous benefits of the web-like continuity of the fascial tissues, as they appear to play roles in the transmission and amplification of force as well as enhancing proprioception.

Transfer of force beyond the "normal" boundary of a muscle is only surprising because of the separation of tissues we see in anatomy texts. The over-used but informative analogy of an orange gives a different image of anatomical arrangements—cutting across the hemisphere of the orange reveals its integrity and connectivity. Although the pattern reveals the position of orange segments and their "borders" it also shows the continuity of fiber from one segment to the next. Just as individual

orange segments are outcomes of their dissection, so too are the muscles of the body.

The ability to transfer force from beyond an MTU, referred to as *extramuscular force transmission*, relies on that same continuity of fiber. Different sections of tissue vary in function and their constituents are adjusted to fit accordingly, but the change from tendon to ligament and joint capsule, or from epimysium to loose connective tissue (see fig. 1.13), are transitions of interconnected cell types. Barring accidents and surgeries, there are no gaps or separations in the body.

Before venturing into force transfer across muscles we must first address a never-ending issue within anatomy—that of vocabulary. There is an inherent problem in empowering an appreciation of anatomical parts as it gives the impression they act as independent agents. How does one describe the form and function of a muscle without giving the impression of it being a discrete unit? To dissect and to name bestows the power of description from which understanding can come. However, that description simultaneously removes the unit from its environment and its many relationships beyond its apparent borders. As we are trying to emphasize the interaction of the body, especially during movement, we must acknowledge the limiting effect of vocabulary to first allow us to build a larger gestalt. So, while it may be true to say that orange segments do not exist within the orange but are an outcome of manual separation, for the sake of narrative clarity we must accept a descriptive necessity and break the anatomical whole into its functional components.

With the above caveat in mind, the leg can be divided into four compartments[4]—**anterior**

[4]These are just the major muscles for each compartment, we will refine the number of tissues in each compartment in the following chapter.

(tibialis anterior, extensor digitorum longus, and extensor hallucis longus), **lateral** (fibularis longus and fibularis brevis), **posterior** (gastrocnemius, soleus, and plantaris), and **deep posterior** (tibialis posterior, flexor digitorum longus, and flexor hallucis longus)—and the foot is also compartmentalized into four or nine sections, depending on one's choice of reference (for future reference we will use just four).

The body is all compartmentalized, it is not a unique feature of the lower limb, as there are many benefits for dividing functional units into "bagged" groups. Separation allows fascial compartments to glide past one another easily and inhibits the spread of infection or bleeding from one section to another. However, containment also comes with the potential danger of compartment syndromes, whereby increased intra-compartmental pressure begins to impinge on blood and/or nerve pathways, eventually requiring release of pressure by cutting the compartment bag, a procedure known as a *fasciotomy*.

Intra-compartmental pressure is not always a bad thing, like many aspects of our system it is a matter of degree. During normal movement function we benefit from increases in compartmental pressure, as it increases tissue stiffness to add another dimension to the body's efficiency mechanisms.

Intra- and intercompartmental force transmission was investigated by Prof. Huijing (see p. 131) who performed numerous investigations. There is much to unpick in Huijing's statement, but we have already explored most of the dynamics he is referring to—adjustment of tissue stiffness being the most important. In numerous experiments, Huijing demonstrated how stress and strain travel beyond individual muscles and into the surrounding tissue, and any breach in the connective tissue web would disrupt the transmission of force.

Performing fasciotomies of the anterior compartment of rats under experimental conditions sometimes increased force output of the muscles contained within the compartment, but was more likely to decrease it (Huijing et al. 2003). Breaking the integrity of the containing "bag" affected force transfer from the muscles. It seems that loss of compression given by the fascial compartment reduced the overall tissue stiffness and reduced its ability to transfer the force of contractions. The reduced pressure inside the compartment due to the fasciotomy resulted in decreased stiffness and potential force output.

There has not yet been enough exploration into fascial compartmentalization, but the implications of the story so far are that the compartments play important roles in stiffness adjustment. As we will see in the next chapter, muscles are compartmentalized according to functional groups. For example, tibialis anterior is a dorsiflexor and invertor of the ankle and is grouped with other ankle dorsiflexors— extensors digitorum longus and brevis—in the "anterior compartment". All the muscles crossing the ankle joints are then grouped within the crural fascia.

Joint control is rarely, if ever, a single muscle action, it requires the cooperation from numerous muscles to stabilize and mobilize a joint appropriately. Functionally, it makes sense that active tensioning of tibialis anterior will also stiffen the connective tissue around its synergistic neighbors. Working within a taut, stiff fascial bag increases force output and reduces muscle effort, and the favor is shared across to other compartments due to the extramuscular force transfer via the fascial web.

To appreciate the functional implications of the fascial web, it may be useful to draw a comparison between the bone trabeculae and the fascial tissue in terms of a functional hierarchy of tissues. The trabeculae provide a self-organized inner "micro-skeleton" to provide stiffness to the bones of the "macro-skeleton". This inner skeleton adapts to the repeated stresses and strains of life over months and years. Similarly, the adaptable soft tissues form another "soft tissue skeleton" external to the "macro-skeleton", one with contractile elements that can automatically and unconsciously fine-tune its stiffness in response to the strains traveling through the body. In the search for minimal effort and metabolic cost, this electrically sensitive muscle tissue can monitor and adjust its own tone to optimize its force transmission for marginal calorie use.

Design of each tissue level appears to balance cost of production, tissue strength, and weight of material by using some form of constant feedback loop. That feedback loop, as we saw in the earlier chapter on bone formation, uses mechanoreceptors to constantly sense the force within the tissue web.

FASCIAL PROPRIOCEPTION AND THE STIFFNESS ADJUSTING SYSTEM

The intercompartmental co-tensioning and stiffening dynamic is a communication of force, but that communication can also be the possible transfer of information. Another Dutch researcher, Jaap van der Wal (2009), noticed that mechanoreceptors are held in place by the collagenous, fascial tissue. Challenging the notion of discrete tissue layers, van der Wal demonstrated that muscle, tendon, ligament, and joint capsule are in-series with one another rather than the parallel arrangement too often presented in introductory anatomy texts.

It makes functional sense for the "perceivers" of mechanical force to be placed within a continuous web that is responsible for the transfer of force. Van der Wal emphasizes the interplay between the architectural design and placement of tissue type, the

tissue's functional role, and the placement of appropriate mechanoreceptors combine to assist proprioceptive feedback. Force transfer beyond individual tissues via collagenous tissues communicates local changes in tension and stiffness to neighboring areas. If working correctly, both at the levels of the collagen and nervous system tissues, the body appears able to adapt itself to an optimal degree of stiffness to manage the task at hand.

Myofascial force transmission beyond individual muscles (Huijing et al. 2003) and the continuity of fascial tissue and its mechanoreceptors (van der Wal 2009) provide the mechanism for Sawicki's "stiffness adjusting system" (Sawicki et al. 2009). Thinking of the musculoskeletal system as constantly tuning its stiffness to achieve the task at hand by creating or controlling the necessary forces is one of the most useful changes I have made to my perception of the anatomy of movement.

SUMMARY

Once more we see how tissue architecture and function are entwined. The relationship between tissues and function creates the struggle to describe the measurable benefits of tissue stress and strain, muscle fiber direction, and contractions in a way that does justice to each aspect without presenting them as isolated facts. We return to the ecology idea of the body as a connected, interdependent system.

No one aspect of describable anatomy exists in isolation, but we have to explore each part as such to measure its role and effect. Once we have an understanding of enough individual dynamics, we can start joining them together like pieces in a jigsaw puzzle to understand the full picture of functional anatomy.

Each MTU has its own architecture, with variables of fiber direction, fiber length, tendon length, and stiffness. Each MTU lives in an area of the body with its own unique force (gravity, GRF, and momentum) demands and so its architecture has evolved to suit those demands: whether it needs high length and low strength, high strength and elastic tendons, or some other variation.

Due to the nature of actin and myosin filaments, muscles tend to be strongest when operating in their mid-range, and the surrounding collagenous fascial tissue seems to help by taking some of the strain, allowing the muscles to stay close to the peak of their force-length relationship as well as perform at their optimum force/velocity. Muscle and collagen fibers cooperate with their complementary features to control movement, with muscle fibers working to produce,

decelerate, or control momentum, and doing so concentrically, eccentrically, or isometrically as needed.

Responding to mechanoreceptors, the musculotendinous elements are the fast-acting adjusters of stiffness and are constantly reacting to the demands of the situation. The mechanoreceptors within the fascial network monitor the tensional balance and signal for appropriate responses.

Gary Gray, the famous American physical therapist and so-called "Father of Function", says we should look for the "truth of movement". Any successful movement requires the control of forces to achieve the desired outcome, and the control of forces is simply the creation of appropriate stiffnesses.

6

EXTRINSIC MUSCLES

There is nothing of a haphazard nature in the pattern of the human foot. When, with the adoption of erect terrestrial bipedalism, the weight of the body became transferred entirely upon the prehuman foot, its bones did not become merely enlarged under the magnified stresses.

—Morton, *Human Locomotion and Body Form* (1952, page 28)

■ INTRODUCTION

Although the size and shape of the calcaneus changed over time, the overall size of the human foot did not increase much as it became responsible for carrying our extra bipedal load. In chapters 3 and 4, we saw how strain is reduced in the femur by the stabilizing action of muscle forces that surround the bone. No one muscle carries the entire responsibility for the support of the bones of the foot, nor the support of the body as it moves above it, they work together to enhance tensional stiffness and provide balance and movement control.

By approaching the foot from different angles and attaching to different points, the extrinsic muscles provide some of the force closure, the enhanced stiffness needed for the foot as it rises toward toe-off. It is the cooperative power of the muscles' coordination, and optimization of their tissue shape that allows the bones of the foot to be as gracile as they are.

This chapter will focus on the groups of long muscles that leave the foot and attach to the tibia, fibula, and femur, many of which are household names. In chapter 7, we will explore the shorter, foot-only muscles, but, in each chapter, it is important to keep in mind the multitasking, the functional overlapping constantly present in the soft tissues. Placing the fascial dynamics of the previous chapter alongside muscle actions is necessary to build the overall picture.

Much functional musculoskeletal anatomy is quite straightforward. Functional anatomy is basically about "which muscle goes where" and "what does it do"?, so we can be quite reductive: all we need to know is which joints a muscle crosses and at what angle. Knowing just those two things gives us almost all the information we need.

Of course, we do not just want to list that information we want to understand the "*why*"—why is the muscle shaped that way? Why is its tendon a particular length and shape? The appreciation of shape will bring us deeper into seeing tissue connections and interactions during movement.

The shape of any muscle only makes sense when we see its whole environment, including its movement requirements. In many respects, shape and function are the same things—function determines shape and shape determines function—so we cannot understand one without the other.

This chapter has a few important tips and tricks for working out muscle actions and properties and may also help you understand the previous chapters by giving you more context. If you struggled with some of the content in the previous chapters, read through chapters 6 and 7 and then return to chapters 3 to 5 again. It took me 30 years to piece it all together so do not pressure yourself to grasp it all in a few hours of reading.

Similarly, if the muscles are less familiar to you, have a quick read through these two chapters and then jump into the assessments and exercises of chapters 8 and 9. The assessments and exercises we have included are deliberately straightforward and will help you understand the musculature. There are all kinds of fancy orthopedic nuances that can be included, making this an encyclopedia of the foot, but that's not my interest. I would rather think of this book as a full reference.

■ WHAT'S IN A NAME?

One of the many frustrations with anatomy is that no one seems able to decide what parts should be called. We have come across this problem with the compound joints of the foot, named in some cases using the anatomical standard and in others paying homage to long-dead, saw-happy French surgeons. The choice often depends on which convention one is following or what the intended readership may be—for instance, the surgical community is more likely to use the names Lisfranc or Chopart joint rather than the unwieldy but anatomically informative tarsometatarsal and midtarsal joints.

Another conflict in terminology is which convention to use for naming muscles. Muscles can be described using three sources of nomenclature—position, function, or shape—and each of these is used for the musculature of the leg and foot. All three conventions offer some useful hints once the terminology is deciphered and their customs explained. The convention that gives us fewest clues on position and function is that of shape. For example, the familiar shoulder muscles, rhomboids and trapezius, tell us nothing about where they are or what they do. However, they give us strong clues about the muscle's capacity: we know that the square-like rhomboid muscle is likely to have only one direction of pull and is probably involved in stability in contrast to the wide-ranging fiber angles of the trapezius, which provide lots of mobility.

Muscles named for their position tell us roughly where they are. For example, tibialis anterior must be on the front of the tibia. And there is more that can be deduced from these two words, as muscles are often named in opposites. If there is a tibialis anterior, we can guess there must be a tibialis posterior (and it should be no surprise that there is!). This guideline is also followed for the functionally named muscles as well—if there are flexors (e.g., flexor hallucis longus), the chances are that we must have extensors (e.g., extensor hallucis longus), and for each adductor, an abductor, etc. This heuristic stands true for most of the muscles we will see below, but it falls apart slightly at the hip where we have an array of muscles named as adductors, but none named as abductors—the hip abductors are generally named by their position as gluteals (buttock).

While the anatomical name does not appear to provide much functional information and the functional name seems not to indicate position, position and function are fundamentally entwined. If a muscle crosses the front of the talar joint, for instance, it must be a dorsiflexor; if it crosses the back of the joint, it must be a plantar flexor. We could rewrite that sentence to say, if the muscle is a plantar flexor it must cross the back of the joint, and if it is a dorsiflexor it must cross the front.

The ability to infer structure from function and vice versa is just another expression of the interlacing relationship between the two dynamics (see fig. 3.3). As muscle function is determined by the angle at which it crosses a joint, using the naming conventions allows us to make the reasonable assumptions that

tibialis anterior crosses the front of the talar joint and therefore must be a dorsiflexor, and is opposed in this action by its neighbor, tibialis posterior, crossing the other side of the talar joint. It is a rule that the position of the muscle determines its action.

Using the same logic in reverse allows us to guess the position of functionally named muscles. For example, we can deduce that flexor hallucis longus must lie along the plantar surface of the foot and come to the back of the leg. We can deduce that it probably has an opposing muscle called extensor hallucis longus on the dorsal surface of the foot and leg—which it does. In the upper body, flexors cross the front and extensors cross the back of joints. This relationship reverses in the lower body because of the torsion of the limb bud during *in utero* development that brings the "front" of the lower limb to the back (fig. 6.1). Limb rotation is why the foot's dorsal surface

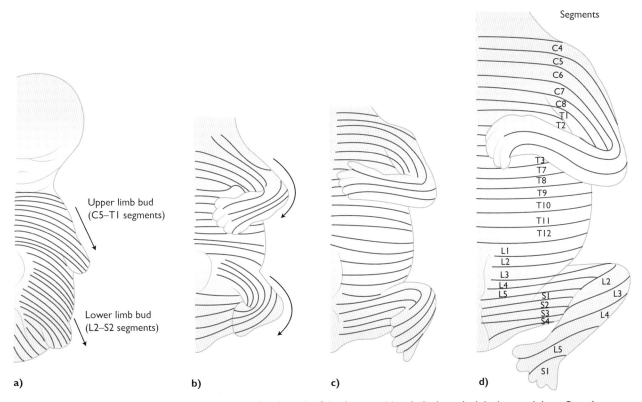

a)   b)   c)   d)

Figure 6.1.   The upper limb buds appear around the fourth week of development (a) with the lower limb buds a week later. Over the next two to three weeks, the distal ends flatten to form hand- and foot-like paddles as the proximal portions of the upper limb torsions laterally and the lower limb torsions medially (b & c). Below the knee, the lower limb continues to twist to bring the great toe to the medial aspect (d). The lines indicate the spinal segmentation of innervation to the skin (known as dermatomes) and are presented here for visual clarity of the torsions that occur during development.

is the top of the foot and gives us the term "dorsiflexion" to describe that surface moving toward the shin.[1]

Knowing the background to the conventions of nomenclature can help break the codes, as generally there is a reason and rationale for each name. Unless these rules are explained, learning muscles and actions just becomes an exercise is rote memorization. Scientific conventions take time to change, as we see with the fibularii muscles, which are still referred to as the peroneals in many papers, despite having their name changed some years ago. The two words come from different root languages—*peroneal* is from Greek and *fibularis* is derived from Latin. Both words refer to the pin-like fibula bone (apparently fibulas from various non-human species were used as pins) but there was a clash of language as Latin was used to name the fibula bone, while Greek had been used for its attaching muscles. There is consistency in the use of Latin to name both the tibia bone and its associated muscles, so it was suggested that the Latin form—*fibularii*—should replace the Greek name—*peroneals*—for the attaching muscles. Unfortunately, not everyone has made the change and you will still read scientific, peer-reviewed papers that refer to the peroneal muscles.

Another confusing anatomical standard exists around the use of the words abduction and adduction when describing actions of and within the foot. There are two conventions for the reference points from which the direction is described, either from the midline of the second toe (axial), or the midline of the body (mid-sagittal, fig. 6.2). We will see this in the next chapter when describing the actions of

the foot's intrinsic muscles, as they are named according to axial convention, which uses the second toe as its reference.[2]

The axial reference tends to describe motion of the toes relative to one another while the mid-sagittal convention describes the relationship through the foot as a whole. The switch back and forth between the conventions is usually obvious from the context in which they are being used. For example, spreading the toes would be an abduction from the midline of the second toe, while an abduction at the naviculocuneiform joint would be relative to the mid-sagittal plane.

MUSCLES, BAGS, AND PULLEYS

We saw three mechanisms of fascial efficiency in chapter 5: the spring-like role of tendons that allow muscles to remain close to isometric; the fascia's role in amplifying power output by enhancing the force-length and force-velocity ratios; and the tendon's role in attenuating or damping strain by allowing the muscle also to work eccentrically at lengths and velocities that optimize its force (fig. 5.18). A similar categorization can be made of the multifunctional capabilities of muscle tissues as they adjust their stiffness to act as gravity-resistant struts, controllers of elastic springs, motors to provide acceleration, or dampers of stored elastic energy (Farris & Raiteri 2017a&b).

Acting together as MTUs, muscle and fascia are constantly searching for the optimal degree of stiffness during movement. In this sense, even lack of movement, standing still for example, requires active tonus within certain muscles— the strut-like role of the MTUs. Most of the communication between our proprioceptive

---

[1]Think of the dorsal fin of a whale or shark on the top of the body, which is the strong and protected back. The ventral surface is considered to be the front and contains more delicate structures. This relationship is maintained in our torsioned lower limb where the dorsal surface (our front) is generally bulkier and more protected than the ventral surface (our back), which carries the delicate vessels to and from the feet.

[2]A similar problem exists in naming the movements of the hand and fingers, but the convention there is to use the third finger rather than the second.

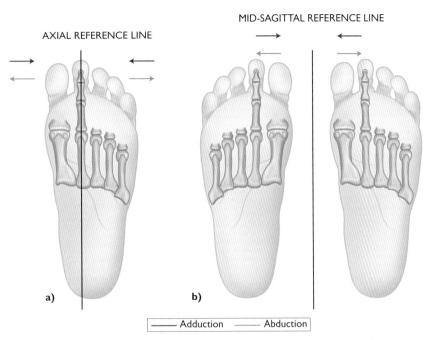

AXIAL REFERENCE LINE

MID-SAGITTAL REFERENCE LINE

a)   b)

——— Adduction ——— Abduction

Figure 6.2. Two conventions exist when referring to adduction and abduction of the foot and toes. The first, using a midline through the second toe (a), tends to refer to relationships and movement of the metatarsals and toes while the second uses the body's mid-sagittal line and usually refers to movement of and through the foot rather than the toes (b).

organs is preconscious, and a high percentage of the sensory input comes via the sole and tissues of the foot and ankle. Tissue health and the shoe environment for the foot is important, not just for the health of the foot but for balance and coordination of the rest of the body.[3]

As Morton repeatedly informed us, the feet must deal with a range of high forces, particularly that of gravity, and although he did not refer directly to momentum, he alluded to it in his writings when informing us of muscle action in creation and control of movement. Morton described the use of elasticity and the recycling of energy, describing it as a "deep-seated phenomenon that makes a direct contribution to the scheme of economic efficiency" (1952, page 250), but emphasized gravity over

momentum. Gravity is straightforward for us to understand, but the role of momentum and how it affects the soft tissues is a little more complex. Forward, downward, and rotational momentum lengthens tissues as they work to control the movement and this eccentric loading helps create the pretensioning and recoil dynamics described in the previous chapter.

Our relatively parallel feet provide the "rockers" (heel, ankle, forefoot, and toe) as we roll forward, and that forward momentum must be controlled and decelerated by soft tissues. Bone shape, joint alignment, and soft tissue angles all cooperate to create an efficient system that allows us to stack our tall, vertical skeleton on three main points of contact on either foot and then roll and swing ourselves forward. It is both remarkable and quite straightforward when reduced to basic elements.

The major keys to understanding the overall arrangement of the foot and ankle is the alignment of the two ankle joints and the

[3]Proprioceptive input is of significant value to full body function and is worthy of much more investigation than space allows. For further exploration I recommend the work of Dr. Emily Splichal and Naboso Technology.

angles at which the muscles cross from the leg to the foot (fig. 6.3). Seven major tendons cross behind the talar joint,[4] an indication of the importance of plantar flexion (when the muscles act as accelerators) and the degree of force involved in control of dorsiflexion (when the muscles act as decelerators and struts).

The two axes of the ankle joints feed into our ability to balance on just two feet. Our feet have more length in front than behind the ankle joints, making it easier to balance with a slight forward lean, and we have more muscle (in bulk and in numbers) placed behind the talar axis that contribute to the control of forward lean. But our slender feet only provide a narrow line of support left to right during movement. They are also inherently wobbly due to the offset between the calcaneus and talus along the subtalar axis (marked U-U[1], fig. 6.3b), and require muscles on either side of the ankle to control and balance side-to-side tilt.

As we saw in previous chapters, tilting of the calcaneus is one of the triggers for unlocking the foot into pronation, but the bony arrangement between the talus and calcaneus creates an area of high stress and instability. That instability is useful for shock absorption during impact, and the consequent pronation strains the supporting soft tissues with energy that can be recycled to re-form the supinated rigid lever in preparation for toe-off.

Once again, we see more tendons crossing on the side that requires more support, deceleration, and correction. The domed nature of the foot, the calcaneus-talus offset, and inward slant of the subtalar joint combine to create instability on the medial aspect. As we will see below, the seven major tendons that cross the inside of the subtalar joint[5] all have different angles

and attachments that use a range of strategies to correct pronation and support supination at different phase of movement.

Morton (1952) contrasted the strength of the calf with that of the upper limb, pointing out that even a child can bounce 50 lbs of their body weight on their feet while a full-grown man would struggle to bounce 50 lbs between his hands. Although Morton makes a somewhat unfair comparison as the calf muscles work almost directly under the center of gravity, in contrast to the bent elbows of the juggling man, there is still truth in the fact that although the upper and lower limbs share anatomical features, their relative strengths differ greatly. The leg and foot muscles have to control the body's momentum during acceleration (e.g., running and walking) and deceleration (attenuation on landing), often when the heel is lifted and the ball of the foot is in contact with the ground.

When the heel is raised, there is an offset between the point of support—the ball of the foot—and the body weight acting through the ankle complex. As we saw earlier, this "long lever" is made up of the many bones of the foot, in contrast to the bony levers of the femur and tibia. Support and compression are provided to the femur by its surrounding muscle and to the tibia by the attaching soft tissues and its triangular shape. The foot must produce a stable lever from a long line of oddly shaped bones. We saw the "form" closure created by the interlocking bones in chapter 4 and have mentioned the "force" closure of the soft tissues, which we can now explore in more detail.

The MTUs passing into the foot from the leg are an important part of the force closure mechanism of the foot, and are assisted by their architecture and by the tracks they take around the pulley system of the ankle (see also fig. 4.6). Tendons from three of the four leg compartments are behind the axis of

[4]Eight if you want to include the weak plantaris; the others are the soleus, gastrocnemius, fibularis longus and brevis, tibialis posterior, and flexors hallucis and digitorum brevis.
[5]The major tendons medial to the subtalar joint are the soleus, gastrocnemius, tibialis posterior, flexors hallucis and digitorum longus, tibialis anterior, and extensor hallucis longus.

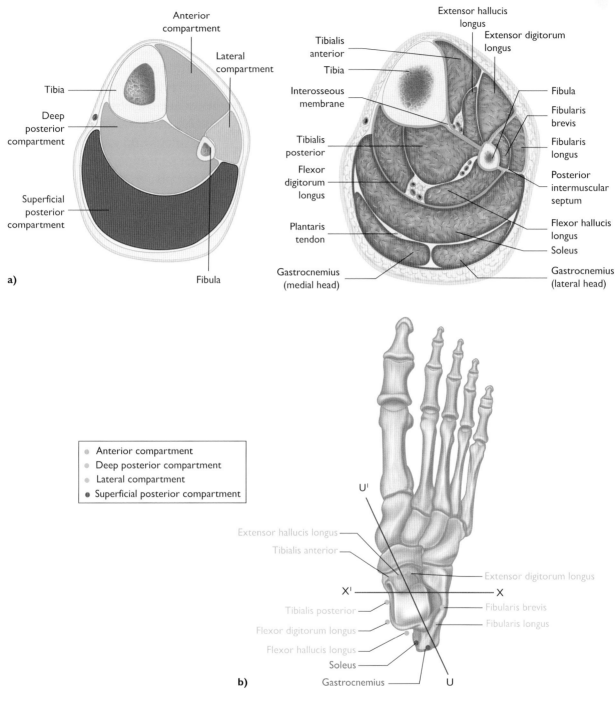

Figure 6.3.   a) Muscles from each compartment are associated with different aspects of the foot and cross the ankle joints in different quadrants. b) The two major joint axes require control from the extrinsic muscles. Plantar flexion/dorsiflexion of the talar joint occurs along the X-X¹ axis. All muscles crossing behind the axis of the talar joint will act as plantar flexors, those crossing in front of the axis are dorsiflexors. Inversion/eversion of the subtalar happens along the U-U¹ axis and muscles crossing medial to the subtalar joint provide inversion and those crossing on the lateral aspect will produce eversion. Functionally, we must reverse those "actions" to appreciate the muscles' common roles in gait. The muscles to the back of the talar joint will decelerate dorsiflexion—essential for controlled landings and to regulate dorsiflexion during the ankle rocker phase of gait. The muscles medial to the subtalar joint axis will decelerate eversion, part of the pronation response on contact with the ground, and they then assist with the foot's correction to inversion and supination prior to toe-off. (Adapted from Kapandji 2018.)

Retinacula – More than just tendon straps

As we have seen previously, anatomy suffers from the natural limitations of having to describe complex structures and their interactions. Named from the Latin *retinere*, to retain, the reputation and understanding of retinacula has suffered from this restricted nomenclature. Thankfully, a landmark paper from the Padua group led by Carla Stecco helped clarify and expand our appreciation of these important structures (Stecco et al. 2010).

By investigating 27 legs with a range of methods, they were able to confirm that the ankle retinacula are a continuation of the crural fascia, the deep fascia of the leg. Although being inseparable from the rest of the deep fascia layer, the retinacula are easily identified due to the thickening of the tissue.

Like the rest of the crural fascia, the retinacula comprise of three layers of parallel collagen fibers tissue that alternate in orientation and are separated by a thin layer of loose connective tissue. As suggested by their appearance, the collagen layers of the retinacula are more dense and their loose connective tissue layers thinner compared to the crural fascia. Although the retinacula are thickenings of the crural fascia, Stecco et al. propose they are not strong enough to play a significant part in a pulley-type system despite often being described that way.

Rather, their paper suggests that due to their continuity with various muscles, tendons, and bone they are sensitive to changes in position and tonus. Retinacula are rich in nerve fibers and proprioceptors which suggests they are therefore not passive stabilizers but fascial specializations for perception of ankle position and movement.

the talar joint, helping them support the foot as it lifts onto the ball of the foot,[6] and collectively they provide four times more force for plantar

flexion than is provided by the anterior compartment for dorsiflexion.

The largest and strongest of the plantar flexors, the soleus and gastrocnemius, attach only to the calcaneus, while the other tendons wrap around the malleoli and progress to the mid- and forefoot. The soleus and gastrocnemius are close to the foot's midline, while the muscles of the deep posterior compartment all pass medially, and those of the lateral compartment wrap laterally around the malleolus. Each compartment plays a different role in movement and balance of the foot, and having these strong muscles with long elastic tendons aids the many switches of roles the foot must make. The muscles need to produce power and absorb shock while expending minimal energy as they propel and balance us, and the constant adjustment of stiffness and direction of contraction requires information from the mechanical, tensional environment.

The long tendons of the lateral and deep posterior compartment muscles wrap around the talar pulley, through grooves in the various nooks and crannies offered by the bones and held in their tracks by strong thickenings of fascia, the retinacula (fig. 6.4). The retinacula form the superficial roofs for tendon grooves to prevent the tendons from bowstringing (imagine if the tibialis anterior tendon passed straight from mid-shin to the metatarsal rather than being guided around and held in place in the front of the ankle by the "strapping"). But retinacula are more than just supporting and guiding strappings— they also perform important roles for proprioception.

Far from being simple straps, retinacula contain specialized mechanoreceptors for sensing muscle tonus during pronation and supination (Adstrum et al. 2017). As retinacula are thickenings of the crural fascia, they are also connected to the fascia lata of the thigh, and this continuous layer of connective

---

[6] The plantar flexors also support the deceleration on landing from ball to heel.

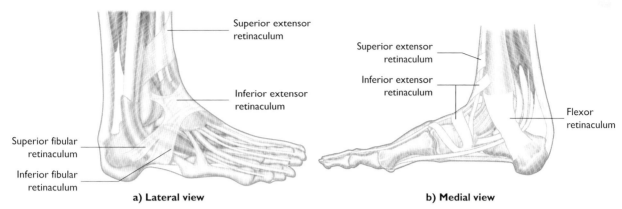

Figure 6.4. *As the tendons follow bony grooves around the malleoli, they are kept in place by the mechanoreceptive thickenings of the deep fascia. These thickenings, or retinacula, have regular fiber directions and play important mechanical and sensory roles. (Adapted from Wood Jones 1944.)*

tissue "may transfer anomalous traction to the retinacula, altering the proprioceptive system of the ankle" (Stecco et al. 2010, page 209).

Despite textbook appearances, the boundaries of the retinacula are arbitrary and vary with individual anatomy and patterns of use. Retinacula are sensitive to strain from the deeper tendons and, due to the continuity of tissue, to distal mechanics. In cases of challenged ankle stability and control, it can be useful to assess function and strain of hip and thigh tissues that can cause aberrant strain on these distal mechanoreceptive tissues.

CONNECTIVE TISSUE COMPARTMENTS

As we saw in the previous chapter, fascial compartments play a significant but undervalued role in force management. Although much work remains to be done for a fuller understanding of this dynamic, there are numerous areas where we see outer fascial wrappings providing mechanical advantages. The first of these was the formation of the retinacula around the ankle joint but, judging by the number of muscle attachments to these fascial planes, the compartments also act to stiffen and compress the deeper tissue.

The deep investing fascia that envelops the leg—the crural fascia—is a continuation of the fascia lata from the thigh, and it envelops and is therefore expanded by several muscles— including biceps femoris, sartorius, gracilis, semimembranosus, and semitendinosus (Standring, 2008). The crural fascia blends into the periosteum of the malleoli of the tibia and fibula and is particularly dense in the proximal and anterior portion, where it also receives attachments from the tibialis anterior and the extensor digitorum longus. As it receives fibers from contractile tissues of the thigh and leg, the crural fascia is stiffened by these muscle fibers as they work to control knee and ankle movements.

The deep investing fascia carries on into and around the other muscles of the leg to form the anterior and posterior septa—the fascial divisions between the inner compartments of the leg that we saw in fig. 6.3. The deep transverse fascia that runs between the posterior and deep posterior compartments wraps around the popliteus muscle and is continuous with semimembranosus. Even the interosseous membrane, the tissue between the tibia and fibula, blends with the tibialis posterior and carries into the interosseous ligament of the distal tibiofibular joint.

Although these compartmental bags are often presented and discussed as if they are separate, passive containers for the muscles, they are biomechanically active and responsive. These outer layers of tissue are connected to, and continuous with, deeper contractile muscles and are continuous to ligaments and joint capsules. Each fascial layer operates and cooperates as part of the body's mechanical and sensory system to help control and support movement.

Although we need to see the fascial tissues as continuous, anatomical descriptions are easier when we divide the body into sections. It comes down to the tension I have already mentioned in describing anatomy—does one follow an anatomical and "passive" convention, which eradicates the confusion of variables created during movement, or does one follow a functional convention which, while more enlightening and empowering for understanding the whole, requires the juggling of many factors at once and can be confusing at first sight? In this section, we will tread the line between the two by following the conventional four compartmental divisions, because it can provide a logical organization to the descriptions, while still analyzing the functional aspects.

▥ SUPERFICIAL POSTERIOR COMPARTMENT

The superficial posterior compartment consists of three muscles—gastrocnemius, soleus, and plantaris—and possibly the most famous of anatomical parts, the Achilles tendon (fig. 6.5). The Achilles tendon is formed by the triceps surae (Latin: *sura*, calf) which is a composite muscle made up of the gastrocnemius (Greek: *gaster*, stomach and *kneme*, leg) and the soleus (Latin: *solea*, pertaining to the fish of the same name and the common shape of both the fish, the muscle, and the sole of the foot).

The two main calf muscles combine to form the body's thickest and strongest tendon, and

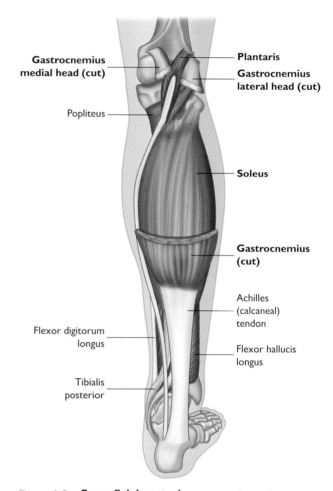

Figure 6.5. **Superficial posterior compartment.**

Soleus—*Proximal attachment*—*Soleal line, posterior surface of tibia, and posterior aspect of head of fibula. **Distal attachment**—Medial portion of top of calcaneus via the Achilles tendon. **Action**—Plantar flexion of the talar joint.*

Gastrocnemius—*Proximal attachment*—*Posterior surfaces of femoral condyles. **Distal attachment**—Lateral aspect of top of calcaneus via Achilles tendon. **Action**—Plantar flexion of the talar joint.*

Plantaris—*Proximal attachment*—*Lateral supracondylar line of femur. **Distal attachment**—Calcaneus via Achilles tendon. **Action**—Plantaris is considered a weak plantar flexor and weak knee flexor.*

together they carry around 93% of the force available for ankle plantar flexion, or more often, control and deceleration of dorsiflexion. The position and strength of the Achilles tendon makes sense when we see its role as a decelerator and appreciate how it can recycle energy during repeated rhythmical movements such as running, hopping, or walking.

Note on attachment and action listings. The listings are provided to give an extra layer of information, but these are available in almost every anatomy text. The listings may differ between sources due to anatomical variation and author preferences. As discussed in chapter 5, most references do not disclose that "actions" are the open-chain movements that would be seen if no resistance was given to a contraction of only the listed muscle i.e., an almost impossible scenario.

Through consistent usage, the muscles have become associated with their actions and are discussed as either "plantar flexors" or "invertors", and this is one source of the difficulties in learning the wider functional roles of the muscles. I urge you to remain flexible with how you visualize muscles and always keep in mind their role in controlling movement— often the opposite of their 'action'.

The source I have used for the listings is *Trail Guide to the Body* by Andrew Biel (fifth edition), which provides a comprehensive breakdown of surface and palpatory anatomy and is a wonderful resource for expanding the 3D representation of human anatomy.

The Achilles tendon has a spiral arrangement as the fibers from the soleus and gastrocnemius wrap around one another to allow the soleus to attach to the medial aspect of the calcaneus. The spiral helps add strength and elasticity to the tendon, which can increase its 15 cm[7] length by 4%. The tendinous strain takes advantage of the recoil capacity of the Achilles tendon's wavy and crimped fibers. Strains of more than 4% of its length will break the collagen cross-links within the Achilles tendon thereby moving it into the plastic phase, and straining beyond 8% leads to complete rupture, a too common injury during explosive movements.

Muscle power is not enough to produce the propulsion required for early phases of

a sprint (Lai et al. 2016). The system must take advantage of Achilles tendon strain to optimize the force-length and force-velocity relationships to produce extra power. The most common movement strategy to produce the required Achilles tendon strain is to "push" the heel down during the initial acceleration. The drop of the heel drives the ankle into dorsiflexion as one pushes the body forward and the countermovement strategy creates rapid lengthening of the tendon. The combination of speed of lengthening (which also causes the tendon to stiffen and therefore reduces its straining ability) and high force demand sometimes causes too much tendon strain and any spectators to the event witness an audible "gun-shot" as the Achilles tendon snaps.

Our use of the Achilles tendon as a spring is evidenced by having a tendon that is longer and twice as heavy as those of chimpanzees (Aiello & Dean 2002). The more connective tissue we have, the more strain energy it can carry, but that strain must be managed by the attaching muscles. A plot of the PCSA and fiber lengths of lower limb muscles shows soleus to have the greatest potential force output (see fig. 6.6). The number of fibers provided by the soleus can vary but the soleus often accounts for up to two-thirds of the Achilles tendon.

A study by Dalmau-Pastor et al. (2014), found that 52% of people had a higher proportion of soleus to gastrocnemius fibers forming the tendon. It makes sense that most people receive more fibers into the Achilles tendon from the powerful soleus to benefit from its ability to control high loads, particularly when we consider its attachment to the medial aspect of the calcaneus. Pronation causes, and is caused by, a medial tilt of the calcaneus, and, due to its position and strength, the soleus is perfectly adapted to help with shock absorption and assist with re-supination of the foot.

On looking at soleus' fiber length (fig. 6.6), one might consider it to have a limited functional

_____

[7] 15cm is an average length. Like everything else in our anatomy, it will vary from person to person.

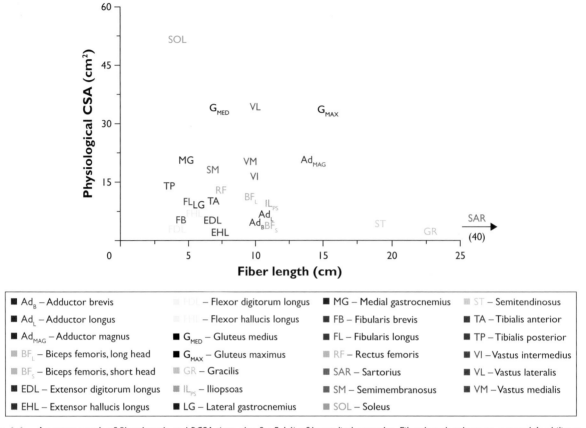

Figure 6.6. *A scatter graph of fiber length and PCSA, (see also fig. 5.14) of lower limb muscles. Fiber length relates to a muscle's ability to lengthen and shorten—longer fibers allow a wider range of movement—and PCSA indicates maximal force output. (Adapted from Lieber & Ward 2011.)*

range despite its important role in ankle movement. Soleus contrasts with gracilis and the semitendinosus, which have the longest fiber length of the lower limb muscles, allowing them to control movement over a wider range. The standard anatomy story is that we sacrifice length for strength when it comes to muscle architecture, as pennate muscles may pack more power into smaller volumes but their shorter fiber length reduces the muscles' operating length. This kind of cost-benefit analysis between length and strength is anchored in the anatomy-based story rather than the functional reality. A full cost-benefit analysis of tissue architecture must incorporate the fascial tissues into the equation as well, and the functional range of the combined tissues is affected by the length and stiffness of the tendons and is not limited to only muscle fiber length.

All the plantar flexors, but especially the soleus and gastrocnemius, have short muscle fibers but attach to long and elastic tendons that receive significant stresses due to their position during locomotion. The forces of impact on landing, walking, and running must be contained and controlled by strong muscles, which will benefit from the mechanical features associated with the collagenous tissues. The muscle fibers do not need to lengthen much because the elastic tendons can contribute to the functional range, facilitate movement, and contribute significant benefits to the force-length and force-velocity relationships of the muscle fibers. One must appreciate the role of these tissues in the regulation of the body's progress above the foot, whether it be during a sprint, hop, or a landing; the anatomical architecture only makes sense in terms of its functional environment.

The soleus differs from the gastrocnemius in only crossing the talar joint; the gastrocnemius also crosses the back of the knee. As each muscle attaches to a different aspect of the top of the calcaneus, it makes sense to give greater control of inversion/eversion to the stronger single-joint soleus muscle. As we have seen, the foot's half-dome arrangement with the in-set talus means the calcaneus tilts medially on impact and the bone's position is an important key to the mobile adaptor/rigid lever setting of the foot. Attaching the stronger single-joint soleus muscle to the inside of the calcaneus allows it to better control calcaneal tilt independent of knee flexion or extension.

Gastrocnemius length is affected by the position of the femur, which alters the muscle force-length relationship of the gastrocnemius' fibers. In contrast, the soleus fiber length is only affected by the positions of the ankle joints. Consider the natural joint reactions when one lands (see fig. 4.8c)—the ankle dorsiflexes, the knee and hip both flex as the foot pronates in response to the GRFs acting through the bone and joint alignments. Knee flexion shortens the gastrocnemius, reducing the muscle's ability to control the stresses at the foot and ankle. The force-length relationship of soleus is unaffected by knee flexion, and the lengthening of the soleus fibers assists the muscle's ability to decelerate both the dorsiflexion and the foot pronation to provide more local and independent control.

The hard-working soleus also acts as a peripheral vascular pump, helping push blood up the lower limb. As mentioned previously, the length of the human foot encourages a slight forward lean at the talar joint, bringing more body weight forward onto the forefoot. This relative dorsiflexion causes sustained tension in the soleus, which is formed of fatigue-resistant, type 1 muscle fibers. The consistent effort of this anti-gravity muscle helps it use its dense fascial encasement to encourage venous return.

The slow, steady, and strong soleus contrasts with the gastrocnemius, which consists of fast-twitch fibers that provide a little extra speed to the calf. The gastrocnemius is described as either a fusiform or a pennate muscle. This contradiction is indicative of its variable anatomy and its varied roles. Having more type II fast-twitch and fewer pennate fibers allows the gastrocnemius to transfer force more quickly than its shorter neighbor. Although its fibers might be less pennated than those of the soleus, gastrocnemius fibers are still relatively short and, like the soleus, the gastrocnemius MTU benefits from the added contributions of the long and thick Achilles tendon.

The final muscle of the posterior compartment is the *plantaris* (Latin: twig or shoot), which contains a high number of muscle spindles that help make it an "organ of proprioception" for control of plantar flexion/dorsiflexion and stiffness of the fascial compartment. Plantaris is a small fusiform muscle that is equivalent to the palmaris longus of the hand, which inserts into the palmar aponeurosis, but the plantaris, when present,[8] ends short of plantar aponeurosis. The plantaris' sensitivity and fascial connections make it more likely to be involved with overall tension of the surrounding fascial compartment than providing any direct assistance with plantar flexion, making it a common candidate for surgical harvesting and repositioning to replace other injured tendons.

LATERAL COMPARTMENT

The lateral compartment contains an interesting group of muscles that require flexibility in how we see and appreciate muscle action. As they pass lateral to the subtalar joint, the fibularii muscles are most often listed as evertors of the foot—which they are—and eversion is associated with foot pronation (see fig. 6.7). But the fibularii creating eversion at the ankle

[8]The plantaris is absent in 5–10% of the population.

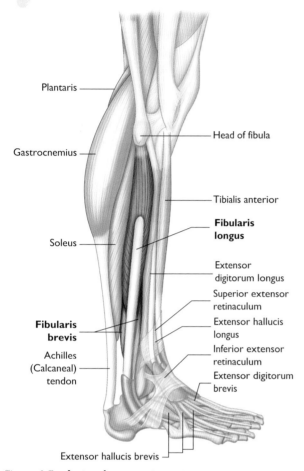

Plantaris

Gastrocnemius

Soleus

Head of fibula

Tibialis anterior

Fibularis longus

Extensor digitorum longus

Superior extensor retinaculum

Extensor hallucis longus

Fibularis brevis

Achilles (Calcaneal) tendon

Inferior extensor retinaculum

Extensor digitorum brevis

Extensor hallucis brevis

Figure 6.7.   **Lateral compartment.**

Fibularis longus—Proximal attachment—*Head of fibula and proximal two-thirds of lateral fibula.* ***Distal attachment—****Base of first metatarsal and medial cuneiform.* ***Action—****Eversion of subtalar joint and plantar flexion*

Fibularis brevis—Proximal attachment—*Distal two-thirds of fibula.* ***Distal attachment—****Styloid process of fifth metatarsal.* ***Action—****Eversion of subtalar joint and plantar flexion.*

important transverse portion of the half-dome, and their role is to support its integrity as the foot begins to supinate during gait.

The fibularii pass behind the lateral malleolus to assist plantar flexion (open-chain) and the control of dorsiflexion (closed-chain). The tendons are contained within a common synovial sheath that passes under a retinaculum and, as they separate, the tendons are guided along the lateral aspect of the calcaneus, passing on either side of the fibular trochlea on their way to their final destinations on either side of the foot (figs. 4.24b, 4.27a, & 6.10).

The fibularis longus crosses the sole of the foot in a groove between the bones and the long plantar ligament. Most commonly it has two slips, one that attaches to the lateral aspect of the base of first metatarsal, and a second that attaches to the lateral aspect of the medial cuneiform, adding to the stability of these two bones. An occasional third slip of tendon blends to the second cuneiform.

The attachment to the first metatarsal allows the fibularis longus tendon to pull the first ray toward the rest of the foot and, importantly, to plantar flex the first ray as the heel lifts and the toes begin to extend (see fig. 4.40a–d). Weakness of the fibularis longus can undermine the foot's stability in supination and its range into toe extension. Reduced function of fibularis longus can cause a potential double hit by reducing toe extension, which leads to less stiffness in the other plantar tissues that contribute to force closure.

As a strong, short, and pennate muscle, the fibularis brevis has several important functional roles. By drawing the styloid process of the fifth metatarsal proximally, the brevis maintains the space for the tendon for the longus to pass below the cuboid as well as supporting the overall dome of the foot (fig. 6.8). Both the fibularis tendons must make sharp turns behind the lateral malleolus, the

is an open-chain movement and we have to put the muscles into context by placing the foot on the ground and closing the mechanical chain. When describing the posterior compartment, it was easy to visualize the change between open- and closed-chain movement, but making the same flip can be more challenging when considering the fibularii.

The fibularis brevis attaches to the base of the fifth metatarsal and fibularis longus passes under the cuboid and across the foot to the base of the first metatarsal. The two muscles of this compartment therefore attach either side of the

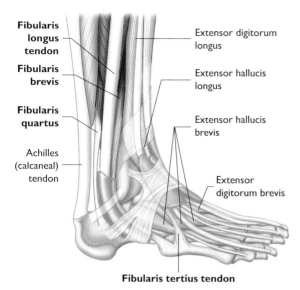

Fibularis longus tendon

Fibularis brevis

Fibularis quartus

Achilles (calcaneal) tendon

Extensor digitorum longus

Extensor hallucis longus

Extensor hallucis brevis

Extensor digitorum brevis

Fibularis tertius tendon

Figure 6.8.   The fibularii tendons passing under the retinacula are protected within a tenosynovial sheath, which can sometimes become inflamed as the tendons turn around the lateral malleolus. By pulling the fifth metatarsal posteriorly, the fibularis brevis helps maintain the cuboid arch for the fibularis longus as it makes its second turn to pass under the foot.

longus then has to make a second turn under the cuboid, making it more prone to injury (Hallinan et al. 2019). The superior fibular retinaculum is often unable to contain the tendons as they make the turn, allowing the tendons to come out of their bony groove. Jumping in and out of their groove gives the "snapping" feeling commonly felt at the ankle and affects the fibularii's mechanical advantage and mechanoreceptive input.

Fibularis brevis plays a crucial role in actively preventing lateral sprains because of its position on the lateral aspect of the ankle and is helped in this task by fibularis tertius (fig. 6.8). Fibularis tertius is unusual as, unlike the other "fibularis" muscles, it attaches to the top of the foot to act as a dorsiflexor (preventor of plantar flexion) and, because of its position and different innervation,[9] is officially part of the anterior compartment rather than the lateral.

Both the fibularis tertius and the fibularis quartus are sometimes suggested as recent adaptations for bipedal gait. These small and variable muscles are unique to humans but are only present in approximately 8% of the population[10] (Rios Nascimento et al. 2012). Incidence of the two muscles is suggested to be increasing, but this is probably due to greater awareness and improved imaging techniques rather than to any evolutionary dynamic.

The fibularis quartus often pops up in texts and, although it is associated with various symptoms, it is more likely to be asymptomatic. The correlation between the presence of the quartus muscle and dysfunction is probably because the muscle is more likely to be found on someone being investigated for ankle problems.

DEEP POSTERIOR COMPARTMENT

Often referred to as "**T**om, **D**ick, and **H**arry",[11] the tendons from the **t**ibialis posterior, flexor **d**igitorum longus, and flexor **h**allucis longus of the deep posterior compartment pass around the medial aspect of the ankle (see fig. 6.9). The deep posterior compartment helps counterbalance the lateral compartment and further supports the shock absorption and supination roles of the soleus. The deep posterior and lateral compartments act like the training stabilizers of a bike, helping to guide the foot's predominately sagittal progression but giving it some leeway to wobble from side-to-side. Together, the tendons from both compartments contribute the final 7% of plantar flexion power to the ankle complex, with most of that power coming from the fibularii but with tibialis posterior as the strongest of the five main muscles of the two groups.

---

[9]Fibularis tertius is innervated by the deep fibular nerve; the lateral compartment muscles are innervated by the superficial fibular nerve.

[10]References can vary from 8–26% (Rios Nascimento et al. 2012).
[11]The popular mnemonic uses a first letter from each of the names of the three muscles as shown in bold in the text.

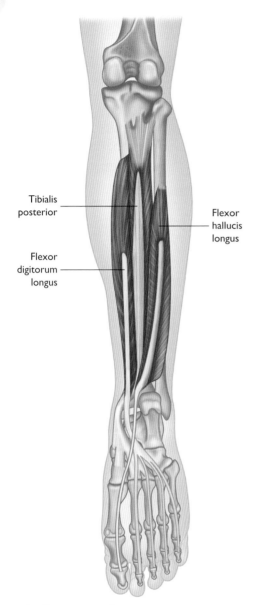

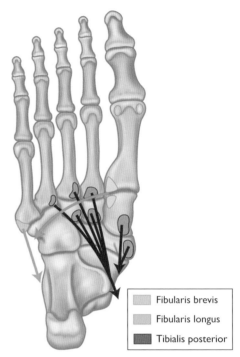

Figure 6.10.   *The tendon from tibialis posterior spreads out to attach to the base of most of the mid-foot bones. Tension from tibialis posterior will draw these pointed bones together and, assisted by the support from the two fibularii muscles on either side, help maintain the stabilizing transverse element of the foot's dome.*

Figure 6.9.   Deep posterior compartment.

***Tibialis posterior**—**Proximal attachment**—Proximal, posterior shafts of tibia and fibula; and interosseous membrane. **Distal attachment**—Plantar surface of navicular, all three cuneiforms, cuboid, and bases of metatarsals two to five. **Action**—Plantar flexion and inversion.*

***Flexor digitorum longus**—**Proximal attachment**—Middle, posterior surface of tibia. **Distal attachment**—Distal phalanges of second to fifth toes. **Action**—Flexion of toes (two to five), weak plantar flexion and inversion.*

***Flexor hallucis longus**—**Proximal attachment**—Middle half of posterior fibula. **Distal attachment**—Distal phalanx of first toe. **Action**—Flexion of first toe (MTJ and IPJ), weak plantar flexor and invertor.*

Due to its attachments on the mid-foot, tibialis posterior has several important functions to serve. After wrapping around the groove of the medial malleolus, the tendon splits into two main slips (fig. 6.10). Most of the larger tendon attaches to the navicular, while some fibers continue to the medial cuneiform and proximally to the tip of the sustentaculum tali. The smaller, second slip of tendon forms the attachment of the intrinsic muscles, the flexors hallucis and digitorum brevis, and attaches to the cuneiforms, the base of the four lateral metatarsals and the cuboid (where it often blends with fibularis brevis).[12]

Unlike the soleus, the tibialis posterior is quiet in standing despite its capacity to draw the foot into supination. Tibialis posterior's many attachments to the pointed inferior surfaces of the cuneiforms and metatarsals ideally position it to draw them together. But tibialis posterior's

---

[12]The attachments of tibialis posterior are variable, the list given here is the most common. A classification system has been suggested by Olewik 2019.

role is during movement. The muscle's pennate architecture, with short fibers and a long tendon, make it ideal for using the medial malleoli as a pulley as the ankle dorsiflexes. The dorsiflexion, even if only 10–15 degrees, tensions and stiffens the tendon to help force close the mid-foot and also supports the ankle syndesmosis (fig. 6.11).

Although tibialis posterior cannot compete with the soleus for strength, it is the third most powerful plantar flexor. To put this into context, the PCSA measurement (see fig. 6.6) shows tibialis posterior to have a larger potential force output than rectus femoris, iliopsoas, and biceps femoris, all large and strong muscles. Tibialis posterior's relatively

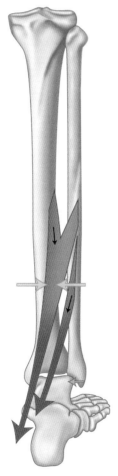

Figure 6.11. *The attachments of the tibialis posterior to the fibula, interosseous membrane, and the tibia allows the muscle to draw the two leg bones together as the ankle dorsiflexes. Pulling the fibula and tibia together during dorsiflexion supports the ankle syndesmosis when the wider, anterior portion of the talus must be accommodated between the two malleoli. (Adapted from Kapandji et al. 2019.)*

high PCSA but small excursion range (only 1–2 cm) makes it an ideal assistant for the soleus in creating stability during movement. The more powerful soleus controls the calcaneus, but tibialis posterior controls the inside of the foot, especially the navicular, giving active support and reinforcement to the spring ligament and the many other passive tissues around the height of the foot's dome.

Sadly, the tendon of tibialis posterior is commonly disrupted, and loss of this primary dynamic stabilizer can place extra strain on the spring ligament, the primary static stabilizer of the medial longitudinal arch. Loss of tibialis posterior strength, through overuse, underuse, or abuse can lead to "acquired flat foot",[13] which may limit a person's overall activity, and cause pain on the medial (ligamentous strain) or lateral (contact between the fibula and calcaneus) aspects of the foot. In the long term, acquired flat foot can lead to structural issues such as arthritis and bony spurs. (See chapter 8 & 9 for assessment and corrective exercise ideas.)

Tibialis posterior gains some extra support from its two compartmental associates, flexors hallucis and digitorum longus. The pathway taken by the flexor hallucis longus (FHL) tendon is particularly beneficial for supination as it passes directly under the sustentaculum tali on its way to the distal phalange of the big toe (see fig. 4.4). The long, rounded tendon can be easily palpated on the sole of the foot when the big toe is brought back into extension, an act that should also supinate the foot as it lifts the medial longitudinal arch and engages part of the windlass mechanism.

Extension of the big toe will stiffen much of the plantar tissue (explored in more detail in chapter 7), but it particularly helps the FHL tendon lift the sustentaculum tali to support the inside of the foot as the heel lifts in preparation for toe-off. Loss of toe extension therefore

---

[13] Also known as "adult acquired flat foot deformity" but "deformity" seems a bit harsh to me and so I prefer to drop it.

undermines this coupled relationship, as any reduction in extension will reduce the stiffness of the FHL tendon and challenge its ability to lift and support the sustentaculum tali.

The FHL is supported by the flexor digitorum longus (FDL), and the two muscles cross one another almost directly under the height of the dome at the so-called "knot of Henry" (fig. 6.12). Even though the digitorum longus supplies flexion ability to four toes, it is smaller and weaker than the long big toe flexor.

Like many of the muscles around the foot and ankle, it has variable attachments and slips, and the FDL may either provide tendinous slips to the FHL or receive slips from it. The FDL tendons fan out as they approach the toes and provide attachment for the lumbricals, short accessory toe flexors, and proximally, it receives an attachment from the quadratus plantae.

The common textbook story is that the quadratus plantae (the square muscle of the

plantar surface, figs. 6.12 & 7.10) attaches directly back toward the calcaneus and helps to straighten the pull of the FDL, which would be true if its primary function of the FDL was still to grasp and hold branches. But, thinking more functionally and bipedally, the quadratus plantae is aligned to the sagittal extension of the toes that will happen in gait and therefore helps the FDL control the direction of movement of the heel.

■ ANTERIOR COMPARTMENT

Each compartment of the leg can expand to some degree to facilitate fluid flow and muscle contraction, but the anterior compartment is the least expansile of the four (Standring 2008), which can cause problems when its contents increase in volume. Increases in compartmental volume can happen rapidly during trauma or occur over time, such as with changes to exercise levels. Symptoms of intra-compartmental pressure range from reduced blood flow and pain to numbness and reduced range of motion. In acute cases, surgical intervention is used to release the compartment, but with the more gradual onset cases, rest or activity changes may be enough to resolve the issue. Untreated compartment syndromes can threaten the health of the limb as loss of blood flow leads to tissue necrosis,[14] making surgical intervention essential. But, as we saw in chapter 5, the use of fasciotomies to release the pressure can reduce the potential power output of the muscles by up to 16% (Garfin et al. 1981).

Another potential weakness of the anterior compartment is the pathway of the common fibular nerve,[15] which wraps around the neck of the fibula. The nerve's position makes it vulnerable and prone to injury, which can cause flaccid paralysis of the only ankle

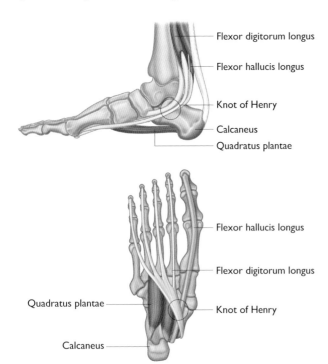

Flexor digitorum longus

Flexor hallucis longus

Knot of Henry

Calcaneus

Quadratus plantae

Flexor hallucis longus

Flexor digitorum longus

Quadratus plantae

Knot of Henry

Calcaneus

Figure 6.12.   Tendons of the FHL and FDL cross below the navicular bone and add some tensional support to the foot's dome. The two tendons are encased within tenosynovial sheaths to facilitate their movement but, being in an area of high stress, the structures are prone to tears and inflammation (Rajakulasingam et al. 2019).

[14]The tissue cells die due to loss of oxygen and nutrients.

[15]Also known as the common peroneal nerve, but we are trying to be consistent with the change to Latin.

dorsiflexors. The loss of dorsiflexion affects the walking pattern significantly as there are no other muscles that can directly compensate for the anterior compartment.

The anterior compartment consists of three main muscles—the tibialis anterior, and extensors hallucis and digitorum longus (fig. 6.13). Collectively they are responsible for drawing the foot up toward the front of the tibia (a.k.a. dorsiflexion) and for controlling the foot's descent following heel strike during gait (a.k.a. plantar flexion). Although they are weak and short (see fig. 6.6), the muscles of the anterior compartment are essential for foot clearance during swing phase of gait and deceleration following heel strike (see figs. 5.2 & 6.14).

During the swing phase of gait, the anterior compartment dorsiflexes the ankle to lift the toes, and then provides a controlled descent for the foot after heel strike. If muscle power or control is lost from this compartment, the toes cannot lift as the leg swings, creating a trip hazard, and a foot slap is heard following heel strike, as the foot is not decelerated effectively during the rapid plantar flexion. Common compensation patterns for deficits in the anterior compartment are: 1. a waddling gait, where the foot is lifting by leaning across to the opposite side; 2. a swing-out gait, when the foot is artificially lifted by abducting the hip on the swing side; and 3. A high-stepping gait, when the foot is lifted by increasing hip flexion on the same side.

The tendons from the anterior compartment travel to the foot under the strong extensor retinacula. The superior portion of the retinaculum runs between the tibia and fibula, and the Y-shaped inferior retinaculum runs from the lateral calcaneus to the medial malleolus and around the instep to blend with the deep fascia on the sole of the foot (Aeillo & Dean 2002).

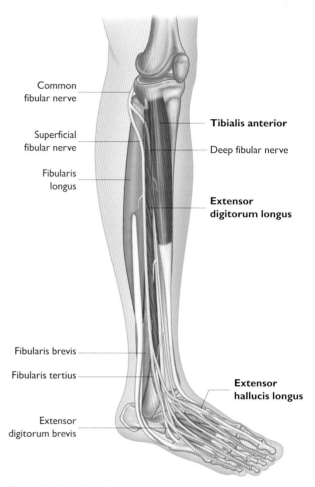

Figure 6.13.   Anterior compartment.

*Tibialis anterior—**Proximal attachment**—Lateral condyle of tibia; proximal, anterior shaft of fibula and interosseous membrane. **Distal attachment**—Medial cuneiform and base of first metatarsal. **Action**—Dorsiflexion and inversion of the subtalar joint.*

*Extensor digitorum longus—**Proximal attachment**—Lateral condyle of tibia, proximal, anterior shaft of fibula and interosseous membrane. **Distal attachment**—Middle and distal phalanges of second to fifth toes. **Action**—Extension of metatarsophalangeal and interphalangeal joints of toes two to five; dorsiflexion; eversion.*

*Extensor hallucis longus—**Proximal attachment**—Middle, anterior surface of fibula and interosseous membrane. **Distal attachment**—Distal phalanx of first toe. **Action**—Extension of first toe; dorsiflexion; inversion.*

The tibialis anterior passes under both retinacula to the medial aspect of the first metatarsal and the medial cuneiform,[16] acting

---

[16]Tibialis anterior attachments vary from equal to unevenly split divisions into the medial cuneiform and first metatarsal, having a second band to the first metatarsal, or, just a single tendon attaching to the medial cuneiform (Olewnik et al. 2019).

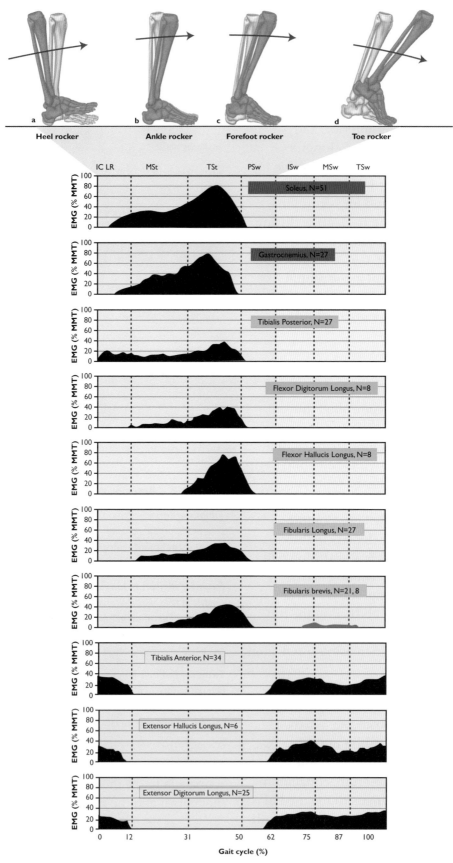

Figure 6.14. *EMG readings for the leg muscles during gait. Note the difference in timings between the anterior compartment and the other three as they alternate between increased activity through swing phase (anterior compartment) and stance (the other three compartments). (Adapted from Perry and Burnfield 2010.)*

not only as an antagonist with tibialis posterior for control of the talar joint's plantar flexion/dorsiflexion axis but also as a synergist with it for inversion of the subtalar joint (see fig. 6.3). The ability of tibialis anterior to invert the foot means the muscle supports supination of the foot in preparation for dealing with impact forces at heel strike—as the leg swings forward and the anterior compartment draws the foot into dorsiflexion, tensioning of tibialis anterior creates some supination during swing phase (see fig. 6.14).

The two long toe extensors also pass under the retinacula and oppose the two long flexors of the deep posterior compartment. Just as the tendons of FDL provide attachments for the lumbricals, the extensor digitorum brevis muscles attach to the tendons of its longer counterpart. Many of the long and short toe flexors and extensors merge into a complex arrangement of connective tissue surrounding the toe joints, which we will explore in the next chapter when looking at the intrinsic muscles in more detail.

The tendons of extensor digitorum longus form the extensor expansion which covers the proximal phalanges and divides into two lateral and one central band. The central band attaches to the middle phalange, the lateral bands converge again and attach to the base of the distal phalange.

As mentioned above, a common extra muscle in the anterior compartment is the fibularis tertius. This uniquely human muscle appears to be an additional head of the extensor digitorum longus but, unlike FDL, it fails to reach all the way to any phalange and attaches to the fifth metatarsal. As it crosses the ankle complex, fibularis tertius may play an important proprioceptive role in sensing sudden inversion, to protect the anterior tibiofibular ligament (our most frequently sprained ligament).

■ EXTRINSIC MUSCLES THROUGH THE GAIT CYCLE

There are a few caveats we need to point out before venturing into some analysis of the gait cycle. The first, and perhaps most important, is to realize that almost all gait analysis is performed on a flat surface[17] and at the walker's preferred speed. Any normal walk would have variations in speed and terrain. The idealized information presented on the gait cycle is to assist our visualization of what the muscles are doing when certain movements are performed and to help our interpretation of "real-life movement".

There is also debate over the accuracy of EMG readings, as the results can vary between individuals and be dependent on a number of variables such as sensor placement and sensitivity. But, as with the disclaimer above, we are using the EMG readings to create a general picture of muscle timing; the nuances are of less concern here. The black areas in the graph (see fig. 6.14) show when the muscle is firing, with the height relating to the strength of the contraction. One difficulty in reading EMG charts is that they do not show the type of contraction—whether the muscle is working eccentrically, concentrically, or isometrically—so we must assume the type of contraction based on what we know is happening in the foot and ankle. Hopefully this will make sense as we go through the readings below to tie many strings together from the previous chapters.

Gait cycle terminology can be frustrating, but we do not need to go into too much detail for our purposes. We will just look at the two main phases (see fig. 6.14): stance phase (when the foot is on the ground, colored green),

---

[17]This is most commonly a treadmill, which provokes another argument over the transference of the information as walking on a treadmill with the surface constantly moving below you is not the same as real-life walking. You don't have to be a scientist to know they are not the same, yet scientific convention seems to insist on doing it this way.

and swing phase (when the foot is swinging forward, colored purple). These phases are separated by two functional events—toe-off, which is when the foot leaves the ground, and heel strike, which is when it lands again. For ease of communication, the whole cycle, tracking one foot, is divided into percentages from 0% to 100% and, because walking is a cyclical activity, both 0% and 100% are the same event—the heel strike at the end of swing phase is the beginning of a new stance phase and the cycle keeps repeating itself.

The dividing point between stance and swing is toe-off, which is placed at 62% of the cycle, meaning that we have our foot on the ground for 62% of the time and it is swinging through the air 48% of the time. Many references will use the term *push-off* to denote this transition point, but I prefer to use *toe-off* as the push-off implies an active contraction—pushing forward with concentric muscular activity—which might not necessarily be the case, especially in a rhythmical walk on flat ground.

The first thing to notice in fig. 6.14 is the division between the three plantar flexor compartments (posterior, deep posterior, and lateral) and the dorsiflexion compartment (anterior). The three plantar flexor compartments are only active during stance phase, in contrast to the anterior compartment which switches on just prior to toe-off and stays active through swing phase and during the early portion of stance.

The activity of the anterior compartment only makes sense if we can see the readings in the context of function. As mentioned above, the dorsiflexors are responsible for foot clearance during swing phase and will concentrically contract to create dorsiflexion. On heel strike[18] (0% on the chart), they must control the rapid plantar flexion created by

the heel rocker with an eccentric contraction i.e., they shorten during swing then lengthen on heel strike to decelerate plantar flexion and provide a controlled landing for the foot (from 0 to 12%). This is why one must be careful when interpreting EMG activity—the charts do not tell us whether the muscle is working concentrically, eccentrically, or isometrically, and so we must infer some of that from what is happening across the joints during function.

Of the plantar flexors, only tibialis posterior gets excited in that early portion of stance phase and it remains active through to approximately 50%, which is when most of the other plantar flexors also reduce their activity. Although tibialis posterior does not tension anywhere close to its potential maximum, it has a double peak pattern on its charts. The early peak immediately follows heel strike when tibialis posterior's activation helps to support the inside of the foot's half-dome, i.e., its attachment to the navicular, in preparation for landing the whole foot and controlling the pronation response to the impact and the series of offset forces.

Once the forefoot fully lands, the body's momentum carries the leg over the foot on the ankle rocker between the talus and the tibia from 12%. The ankle joint moves from plantar flexion toward dorsiflexion and requires deceleration by the plantar flexor group, and this is when we see the rest of the posterior muscles switch on. The one muscle that joins tibialis posterior early in that process is the soleus, which may be stimulated by the medial tilt of the calcaneus at heel strike.

The knee is slightly bent following heel strike, and it straightens as the ankle dorsiflexes. This is because of the plantar flexors decelerating the tibia and fibula as they pass over the talus while the pelvis moves forward over the foot. The two large plantar flexors, soleus and gastrocnemius, contract to decelerate the ankle rocker progression (which aids the knee extension) but soleus starts earlier in the

---

[18]Heel strike is sometimes also referred to as "initial contact" as this allows discussion and comparison with running mechanics which do not always use a heel strike.

cycle while gastrocnemius builds up tension more gradually as the knee extends and as, eventually, the heel lifts.

In this controlled scenario, the heel lifts as a result of the hip, knee, and ankle joints reaching their normal limits. The body's momentum is driving the body forward and, if we consider only the trajectory of the pelvis for a moment, the hip passes into extension as the pelvis moves forward over the foot. Once the hip ligaments are strained during the naturally limited range of hip extension, the only place able to contribute to stride length will be the foot rockers. First the forefoot rocker and then the toe rockers will let the pelvis move further forward, and as the rockers provide extra motion, the heel of the foot must lift and the toes start to extend (we experienced this dynamic in Exercise 5.1).

As the heel lifts at around 31%, the foot requires extra force support to maintain integrity. By this time, the knee has also extended to strain the two-joint gastrocnemius, which helps it provide extra support to the one-joint soleus, which was doing more of the work while the knee was bent. This two-muscle, one- and two-joint arrangement allows the soleus to not only support the foot when the knee is flexed, but also to use the body's natural movement into knee extension to recruit the force from gastrocnemius when it is needed most.

As the foot progresses toward the toe rocker stage, we reach an almost maximal contraction of both soleus and gastrocnemius, two of the body's strongest muscles. Their gradual ascent ends at a sharp peak, and they switch off quite quickly. The two long toe flexors (FHL and FDL) only engage during the latter stages of stance, and remain active slightly later than the two main calf muscles.

The firing pattern of FHL and FDL reflects that of the two fibularii muscles, which, although they contract with a lower percentage of their maximum, also build up toward a peak as

the toes begin to extend. This is an important reminder that the fibularii are not just plantar flexors and evertors of the ankle but also play vital roles in the stabilization of the foot and, in the case of fibularis longus, in plantar flexion of the first metatarsal to assist with extension of the big toe (see fig. 4.40).

Appreciating the functional requirements aids our understanding of the force support provided by the soft tissue as the foot comes into its rigid lever position.

The movement context explains the timing for muscle firing, and we can better see the direction of contraction and, importantly, the eccentric work that is done to control momentum.

■ SUMMARY

In this chapter we have continued the exploration of form and function and added further context to muscle architecture, muscle position, and the angles at which their tendons cross joints. By dividing the leg into its four compartments, and the ankle complex into two axes, we have hopefully clarified the actions of each muscle.

Muscles crossing the front of the talar joint are classed as dorsiflexors and are opposed by the larger number of plantar flexor muscles that cross behind the talar joint. The greater number and strength of the plantar flexors is due to their role in decelerating rapid dorsiflexion; their force is further enhanced by their pennate fibers and long, stiff tendons, especially the twisted Achilles tendon.

The invertors and evertors cross medial and lateral to the subtalar joint to provide side-to-side stability for the narrow foot. Most of them are also plantar flexors and are therefore tensioned by the high forces commonly involved with dorsiflexion during movement. As these muscles attach to the mid-foot, they also force close and supinate the foot—in particular, tibialis posterior and the fibularii.

The extrinsic muscles have three levels of connection—one group attaches to the top of the calcaneus, one group to the mid-foot, and another goes all the way to the toes and provides flexion and extension. The two long toe flexors are particularly important during gait at toe-off position because of their relationship with the inside of the foot's dome.

In general, the important message of this chapter is that we must be fluid in how we see or speak of muscle action and we must be clear if the muscle is contracting concentrically (as in "actions") or if it is working to decelerate motion (often the opposite of their "action"). The forces acting through the body can be created internally when muscles act to produce force, or the forces can have an external source and require the muscles to prevent or decelerate movement.

Familiarity with musculotendinous pathways (such as the FHL) and common movement patterns (e.g., coming into toe extension) helps us build the four-dimensional picture of anatomy that is so difficult to gain from the two-dimensions of books.

7

INTRINSIC MUSCLES

The foot should not be studied as a
lone unit, because its form and function
have always been inseparable parts of
the complete human phenomenon of
human locomotion. Since acquiring
its human character, the foot has not
broken away from that association; its
physiology has merely been changed as
to deal with the work it now performs
in supporting and carrying our bodies
in the vertical position peculiar
to mankind.

—Morton 1935

■ INTRODUCTION

Our phylogenetic heritage and evolutionary
dynamics have provided us with feet that
resemble our hands—the overall genetic
blueprints for each structure are similar, and
the arrangement of bones and soft tissues could
be matched between the two by most non-
anatomists. The same is true for the features
of our feet and those of our primate cousins.
As we saw in chapter 2, the similarities are
not accidental—Darwin pointed out that
evolution is often a matter of repurposing

what has already been there. But therein lies
one potential roadblock along our journey
toward understanding the human foot. The
problem may not be initially obvious, but the
foot is often interpreted as if it is still a grasping
appendage. A problem that manifests, once
again, in the naming of the muscles.

One of our psychological traits is the ability
to recognize the consistency of form and
use of an object regardless of its orientation,
or size, or color. Generally, this perceptual
constancy, as it is called in the literature, is a
useful thing. It lets us jump into a rental car at
the airport and drive successfully even though
we have never been in that make or model,
nor driven on those roads before—the general
procedures are the same in most cars and
on most roads.

A problem with perceptual constancy arises
when we look at hands and feet and see their
very similar structures. We are incredibly
familiar with our hands and their grasping
abilities. The matching muscles on the human
hand and foot share a common genetic
heritage[1] and we give them similar names,

[1]Homologous is the technical term for structures of similar
genetic heritage.

following the same naming traditions. But having similar forms and similar genetic heritage should not imply that they have the same function. It is important to remember that, although structures might look the same and they might attach to similar places, they may—as Darwin warned us—have been repurposed.

Other primates might spend considerable time walking on their feet, but their feet are still recruited to grip and manipulate objects. In most humans, that is no longer the main function, or even a minor function, of our feet. Some of the naming traditions assume a functional constancy of muscle action, but that is not true—the soft tissues are functionally plastic and adapt their role depending on the movement needs. That is especially true of tissues within the feet.

Writing back in the early 1940s, anatomist F. Wood Jones warned us about the "actions" of muscles being only of academic interest because most texts insist on treating the foot as if it is a hand. (As Wood Jones describes it, the foot is a weight-bearing and propulsive structure that must resist the impulse to explode on impact with the ground and provide a stable platform to release significant ballistic force as the rest of the body moves over the top of it.) With that in mind, Wood Jones provides us with a few helpful suggestions for gaining a functional understanding of the foot's musculature.

Wood Jones' first target was the stupidity of the "actions" as they all assume an open-chain and unrestricted movement—which certainly does not match the roles described above—and therefore should only interest those in need of passing exams. The next target for his wrath was the idea of "origin" and "insertion" with the latter generally moving toward the former. Although we have dealt with this earlier in this text, it is interesting to point out that the naming of "actions" still usually follows the same tradition of "insertion" moving toward "origin" and that is proving difficult to

eradicate.[2] For example, while the flexors might still flex the big toe while sipping cocktails by the pool, they are more likely to anchor the toe to the ground as our body moves over the top toward toe-off position—thereby moving the "origin" away from the "insertion", just as we saw with the plantar flexors in chapter 6.

Our natural instinct for perceptual constancy can inhibit a more functional understanding of the foot. As we learn the approved names of muscles, those names can lead us along certain blind alleys. This is the case for the flexors and extensors of the toes which one would naturally consider to be antagonists to one another. However, in the complex world of the foot, they act in concert to coordinate the multi-joint arrangement of the phalanges and their extensor hood.

To truly understand a muscle, it is not its name or its actions that you need to know (although working familiarity with both does help![3]), but its position. Where do the muscles attach? Which joints do they cross? And what forces are those joints having to deal with during normal movement?

When it comes to the foot, the major roles for the muscles are to prevent it from exploding on impact—no-one wants an exploding foot!—and to bring the bones back together again for supination. Therefore, a major requirement for the tissues running between the foot bones is to manage the bones' integrity and keep them together. The muscles' first task is to provide stability, as opposed to movement—in most cases, movement is provided by sources beyond the foot, whether it is the momentum

_____

[2] I do realise the irony that I am also following the tradition by providing the same list of "actions" within this text. The other option is to provide you with every functional alternative and create a longer, more confusing text.
[3] Especially with exams! Unless you have thoroughly discussed the ideas in this text or had this text referenced during your classes, be careful with your answers to any test set by a traditional academic institute.

already present in the rest of the body or from the larger muscles further up the limb that have better mechanical advantage. Most often, the foot is reacting to movements in the body above it, constantly changing and adapting its form and tone to provide a base on which those movements can occur.

An adaptive foot has fine unconscious control over its many parts, and its musculature is able to fine-tune the stiffness of the foot. Much of that responsiveness is provided by intrinsic muscles that have been referred to as the "core of the foot" (McKeon et al. 2014). As we will explore, the intrinsic foot muscles have had increased attention recently. This is mostly due to the revival of interest in minimal footwear and a greater appreciation of the foot as our main point of interaction with the ground as we walk—without the prop of a stiff-soled shoe, the foot is better able to adapt to the contour of the ground. Each change in surface is a stimulation to the foot and therefore to the intrinsic muscles that must stabilize each of the small bones.

Recruitment of the intrinsic muscles is particularly high as we approach toe-off. Stiff-soled shoes will provide external reinforcement as the heel rises and the toes extend, but minimal shoes provide less buttressing and encourage the intrinsic muscles to support the rigid lever from inside the foot. It therefore makes sense that producing a reactive, intelligent, and strong foot should be a cornerstone of any training program.

As we will see in chapter 9, a functional appreciation of the foot can improve our approach to exercising it. Where hand physiotherapy can use various squeezing tools (most often, encouraging "insertion" toward "origin"), the foot requires load, to be challenged with much greater forces, and to learn to respond to changes in balance and position of the rest of the body (most commonly, "origin" away from "insertion"!). Working the foot muscles in isolation with

gripping movements will only have limited effects—limited in terms of strength but also in proprioception and motor control.

As mediators between the ground and the movement of the rest of the body, our feet must perceive changes in pressure and angle. Feet are incredibly sensitive, yet they are capable of handling forces many times greater than our body weight. We stand, walk, skip, bounce, and run on them all day while they are often squeezed into the restricted little boxes, which we call shoes, yet they still manage to provide proprioception through the skin and muscle. Any movement between the bones of the foot not only stretches and strains its intrinsic muscles to provide benefits of pretensioning but also stimulates the muscle spindles. And the mechanoreceptive muscle spindles are only one source of information; the ticklish layer of sweaty skin[4] is loaded with mechanoreceptive cells that are ready and willing to fire when called on.

This final chapter on the anatomy of the foot will show some of the ways in which the foot achieves the seemingly contradictory roles of absorbing high forces and acting as a sensor. This chapter will draw together many of the functional themes laid out previously— particularly the role of the fascial tissues for force enhancement. Then, in the following couple of chapters, we will lay out tools to assess the foot's functional abilities and suggest some strategies for improvement.

▪ DORSAL VERSUS PLANTAR— A SENSITIVE SOLE

Earlier we discussed the twist undergone by the lower limb while *in utero* that brings the "front" of the body to the back and vice versa (see fig. 6.1). In keeping with the general dorsal/ plantar arrangement of protection, the upper,

---

[4]Technically described as glabrous skin, the skin on the sole has a high density of nerve endings and sweat glands.

dorsal aspect of the foot is primarily bony, with thin layers of skin and fascia coverings. Most of the foot's soft tissue is located on the hairless plantar aspect and has several strategies to help it cope with the stresses and strains of daily locomotion.

The skin on the plantar surface of the foot is thick, with many sweat glands and, as we all know from any protracted summer holiday by the beach, the skin and its deeper layers can thicken and adapt to any increased exposure to stress. Just as manual labor will harden the skin on the palm of the hand, going barefoot will thicken the skin on the sole of the foot and, despite the added thickness, loses none of its tactile sensitivity (Holowka et al. 2019).

For extra shock absorption, the area of skin below the calcaneus also contains a thick layer of dense fat which helps with shock absorption and is divided into sectioned compartments to hold it in place (fig. 7.1). The fat pad under the heel is approximately 18 mm thick and is formed of U-shaped columns reinforced with elastic fibers that intersect the tissue at various angles. Tissues around the heel are arranged to receive impact forces—the fat pad at the heel differs from the fat pad under the metatarsal heads, which must deal with the compression

and shear forces associated with toe-off (Standring 2008).

Shearing forces are common in the foot as contact and friction with the ground (sock or shoe) temporarily anchors that area of skin while the inner, deeper structures of the foot still has some momentum. Strong ligaments run between each layer of the skin and the adipose layers to protect their relationship—like a rope between a boat and its anchor. These vertical ligaments are referred to as retinacula cutis (Latin: *retinere* = retain; *cutis* = skin), and they manage the amount of glide between the skin, the underlying fat pad, the deeper muscles, and the bones of the foot.

Without the retinacula cutis, the bones of the foot would be gliding around inside the skin, making it difficult to control movement. The retinacula cutis varies in length and number throughout the body, and gives the characteristic mobility to the skin that is common in the face, the knee, and across the low back (Nash et al. 2004). Try comparing the mobility of the skin on the top of your foot with that of the sole—there is much more freedom on the dorsal aspect. Having shorter, stronger tethering between the plantar layers allows more direct communication of force between the layers and reduces friction—the kind of friction you might remember from wearing ill-fitting socks in a pair of wellington boots on an unexpectedly long walk.[5]

It is relatively common for the fat to lose some of its integrity around the heel, especially during middle age. Atrophy of the fat pad can be caused by reduced elasticity of the collagen and a changed percentage of collagen fiber type, which is a natural part of aging. This is especially associated with female menopause, when lower levels of estrogen cause decreased production of the elastic type III collagen fibers

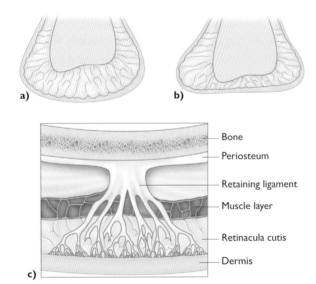

a)   b)

c)

Bone

Periosteum

Retaining ligament

Muscle layer

Retinacula cutis

Dermis

Figure 7.1.   The calcaneus receives extra protection from impact forces from a layer of thick, dense fat cells. The cells are arranged in U-shaped columns (a & b) that are supported and held in place by strong and tight retinacula cutis (c).

_____

[5]It was probably raining too and the novelty of splashing through puddles had long worn off—it was a thoroughly miserable experience as the friction blisters developed.

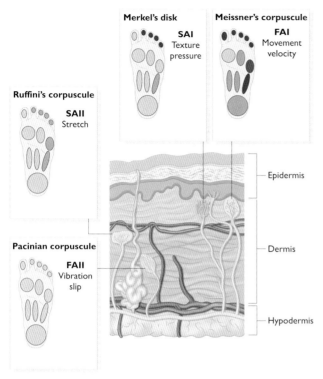

Figure 7.2.   Four types of mechanoreceptors lie within the dermal layer of the sole of the foot, providing afferent information to the central nervous system. Each receptor type is associated with a different sensation, as illustrated. Distribution density is indicated by the shading patterns from black (high density) to light gray (low density). Nerve endings are sensitive to stimuli for different periods of time and are referred to as either slow- or fast-, adapting depending on the length of time it takes for each to stop signaling in the presence of stimuli. (Adapted from Viseux 2020.)

The foot is the primary source of information regarding our body's center of gravity, its movement, and its position relative to the ground, therefore the foot is responsible for much of our proprioceptive control. Our sense of balance and ability to coordinate ourselves relies on several sources, including the semi-circular canals of the inner ear and their reflexes, the eyes, and the suboccipital muscles, but the feet are uniquely positioned to give feedback about our relationship to the ground. The foot manages this with a range of mechanoreceptors embedded within the dermal layer.

Those cutaneous nerve endings can then join forces with another mechanoreceptor type, the muscle spindles, that are sensitive to stretch and rate of stretch within muscle. Add to this the information from the mechanically sensitive retinacula around the ankle, and we see that the foot complex provides significant input for the control of posture using automatic reflexes as well as conscious control (Viseux 2020).

As postural control is organized at both a conscious and unconscious level, there are benefits from ensuring optimal receptor stimulation in combination with balance training exercises. One of the advantages of footwear with thin, flexible soles is the unimpeded mechanical information passing into the foot. Standard footwear has been shown to impair awareness of foot position (Holowka et al. 2019; Robbins et al. 1995).

Motor control and coordination are plastic skills that improve with training, a fact of particular importance to those with neurological issues such as Parkinson's disease (Olson et al. 2019). Exercise builds both skill and strength, and programs can be optimized to focus on one or the other. The best program for anyone with neurological challenges should include both weight-bearing exercise and balance challenges.

and increases in less elastic type I collagen fibers (Fede et al. 2019).

Aside from diminished shock absorption and protection, one of the dangers with reduced thickness and resilience of the plantar fat layer is that it can also affect mechanoreception. Postural control depends on a range of inputs and a large part of the local response for the lower limb comes from afferent input[6] originating in the sole of the foot. As with the palm of the hand, the foot's plantar surface is richly innervated with mechanoreceptors that respond to different stimuli such as vibration, stretch, and pressure (fig. 7.2, Viseux 2020).

---

[6]Afferent nerves send signals to the spinal cord, its response is carried by so-called *efferent* nerves.

COMPARTMENTS

Just as the fat cells must be held in place, so too do the muscles. It should be no surprise that the soft tissue of the foot is divided into compartments, since it is an arrangement used throughout the body (fig. 7.3). As we saw in the compartments of the leg, compartmentalization comes with its range of benefits and costs.

The costs associated with compartmentalization revolve around compartment syndromes where, mostly due to trauma, swelling starts to impinge on proper function. Compartment syndromes of the feet are less well known

because they are mostly only acute responses to accident, rather than the build-up of pressure that can occur in the soft tissues of the leg during changes in exercise.

It is possible that you might come across a compartment syndrome of the foot, especially as the concept of foot exercise is building momentum, so it is useful to be aware of them as a possible source of dysfunction. It is unlikely that you will ever need to assess one (and doing so is beyond the scope of manual and movement therapists anyway), which makes life easier for you and puts a little extra pressure on the surgeon who will have to decide how many compartments there are in

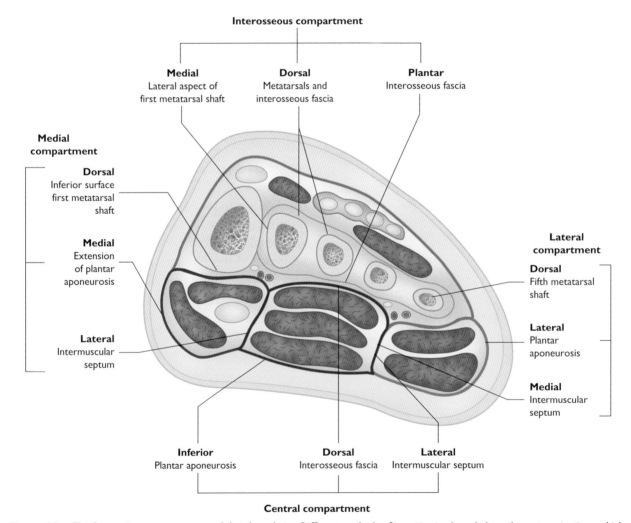

Figure 7.3.   The four major compartments and their boundaries. Different methods of investigation have led to other categorizations, which vary from three to ten compartments being listed (Reach et al. 2015).

the foot, how to measure their pressures, and, importantly, where to cut to release excessive pressure.

There is a lot of debate on the number of compartments in the foot, with the literature proposing 3, 4, 5, 8, 9, or 10 separate fascial compartments (Reach et al. 2007). The range seems to depend on when and how the investigations were done, but the most referenced texts divide the foot into four or nine divisions. For our purposes, we will use the most common listing of four compartments, which correlates to most of the texts you are likely to come across.

Our main goal is to appreciate that the foot's musculature is contained in a series of bags and, as we saw in chapter 5, these assist with force output. A study by Yamauchi and Koyama (2019) showed toe flexor strength increased when standing compared with sitting. When the test subjects stood, the foot deformation[7] caused enough pronation and therefore spreading of the foot to tension the fascial tissues. Working within a stiffened "bag" increased the toe flexor force output compared with when the toe flexor strength was measured with an unloaded foot.

In chapter 5 we introduced the concept of hydraulic amplification and how the correct intra-compartmental pressure enhances muscle force output. This concept is pertinent for the half-dome of the foot and how the intrinsic muscles could be imagined—like inflatable bags that act as both shock absorbers and elevators of the instep.

As one might expect, giving the intrinsic muscles more work to do will increase their size and strength. This simple argument is a strong part of "barefoot" thinking—that by reducing the damping roles of modern

footwear, the foot can do what it should always have been allowed to do, and the foot, along with the rest of the body, will benefit. Miller et al. (2014) investigated this by measuring the effect of a 12-week running program on the feet of healthy runners. After taking a range of measurements and dividing the 33 runners into random groups, the study found that those who ran in minimal shoes increased the cross-sectional area and volumes of flexor digitorum brevis and abductor digiti minimi, and significantly increased the stiffness of the longitudinal arch.

The results seem like a classic case of science being able to show us exactly what we should expect—letting the foot respond to the forces created when running increased their workload. Increasing the workload of any muscle, with an appropriate training schedule including rest and recovery, will cause it to develop. Although we most often feel the benefits of building biceps or quads by their increased ability to lift more weight, we might also be aware of how they "bulk up" and become more prominent. We even describe some bodybuilders as being "pneumatic" when they seem overly "pumped-up". Miller's study illustrates the direct benefit of that pumping to our arch support system, as the increased plantar muscle volume and cross-sectional area of the plantar intrinsic muscles was proven to directly relate to muscle strength (Kurihara et al. 2014).

For our purposes, we will use the most common listing of four compartments, which matches most of the texts you are likely to come across.

1. **Medial compartment.** Abductor hallucis, flexor hallucis brevis, tendon of flexor hallucis longus, and the medial plantar arteries, veins, and nerves.
2. **Central compartment.** This compartment is divided into three levels. The first level contains the adductor hallucis. The second

---

[7]"Deformation" might sound like a bad thing, but it just means the foot pronates and the bones spread a little.

level contains the quadratus plantae, lumbricals, flexor accessorius, adductor hallucis, and tendons of the FHL and FDL. The third level contains the flexor digitorum brevis.

3. **Lateral compartment.** Abductor digiti minimi, flexor digiti minimi brevis, opponens digiti minimi, and the branches of the lateral plantar artery, vein, and nerve.
4. **Interosseous compartment.** This compartment can also be divided into dorsal and plantar aspects. The dorsal contains the dorsal interossei muscles, and the plantar portion holds the plantar interossei, and plantar artery, vein, and nerve.

Another sheath of tendons passes above the dorsal interosseous compartment and contains the long and short extensor tendons, which could make a fifth compartment of the foot, a sixth if you want to divide the interosseous into two, eight if you like the idea of three sections in the central compartment, and a ninth is sometimes listed as a calcaneal portion of the central compartment to separate off the quadratus plantae. After a while, the discussion of how many compartments there are becomes quite academic, is heavily debated, and tempers rise quickly if one takes a particular stance on it. Be warned.

If you are concerned about the presence of a compartment syndrome, it is always best to refer for a full and proper assessment, but the general symptoms are easy to remember with the mnemonic of the five Ps—**P**ain, **P**allor, **P**aresthesia, **P**aralysis, and **P**ulselessness. Each of these is self-explanatory when you consider the effects of increased intra-compartmental pressure on the neurovascular bundles that pass through the compartments. Any compression of the vessels can affect neural conduction and blood flow to or from the area (**p**ain and **p**ulselessness). The swelling and tissue damage may cause pain and change of skin color (**p**allor), restrictions

to neural signaling may create painful pins and needles sensation (**p**aresthesia), reduce coordination, or cut it off completely (**p**aralysis).

FOUR MUSCLE LAYERS

As with the arrangement of the leg with its bulk of muscles in the calf, the foot has its soft tissue on the side that does most of the work, the plantar aspect. The plantar muscles are commonly described as being more developed in our prehensile primate cousins (Aiello & Dean 2002), but an argument could be made (as above!) that our relative foot weakness results from modern footwear and cultural inhibitions around bare feet. Morton and his contemporaries had all kinds of ideas of what was correct and proper, and the literature from the early to mid-twentieth century covering foot anatomy and health can make uncomfortable reading for today's more enlightened researcher. Sexism, racism, and downright snobbishness seemed to be the order of the day for many, and it is difficult to give them the excuse of being "products of their time", but they were. Today we know better than to judge a person by their footwear or its absence.[8]

Traditionally, four layers of muscle are presented in textbooks, and it is usual to list them from superficial to deep. Interestingly, the thick and strong "ligament" of the plantar fascia (also known as the plantar aponeurosis[9]) is not included within the listing and is usually considered a separate structure, but an argument could be made to include it as part of the first layer.

---

[8]Or do we?

[9]Naming of this structure is debated, with camps referring to the plantar "fascia" because it invests around muscles, or as the plantar "aponeurosis" because it joins a muscle with parts that it moves. Arguments can be made either way and I will interchange between plantar fascia and plantar aponeurosis to give variance to the reader.

As mentioned previously, anatomical description is rife with confusions between function and structure, partially driven by the need to separate and describe (anatomize), which is in competition with the desire to comprehend the functional whole. The plantar fascia has fallen victim to this tendency, despite its many relationships to the surrounding muscles having been understood for some time. For example, writing in 1944, Wood Jones described the relationship between the flexor digitorum brevis and the plantar fascia as "firmly bound at the heel" (page 163). However, as we will see below, the plantar fascia is continuous with many other contractile tissues as well. The plantar fascia is therefore in keeping with the work of van der Wal and his concept of "dynaments" in which he says we should not regard ligaments a purely passive structures that prevent joints from exploding, but also capable of stiffness adjustments via their continuity with surrounding muscles (van der Wal 2009).

The strong central portion of the plantar fascia is narrow posteriorly toward its calcaneal attachment and then branches out to each toe (fig. 7.4). The branches are tethered together by a series of transverse bands that prevent them, and therefore the toes, from spreading too much. The five branches and their interconnecting bands provide extra protection for the toes by providing anchor points for the fat pads that lie between the metatarsals, which, in turn, protect neurovascular vessels that pass between the bones. With so many important roles, it is vital that the aponeurosis can stay in place under pressure, and it achieves this through its connections to the skin via the retinacula cutis.

Laterally, the plantar aponeurosis wraps around the abductor digiti minimi muscle and forms part of the lateral band of plantar fascia that connects the outside of the calcaneus to the base of the fifth metatarsal. The fascia and the short abductor digiti minimi therefore span

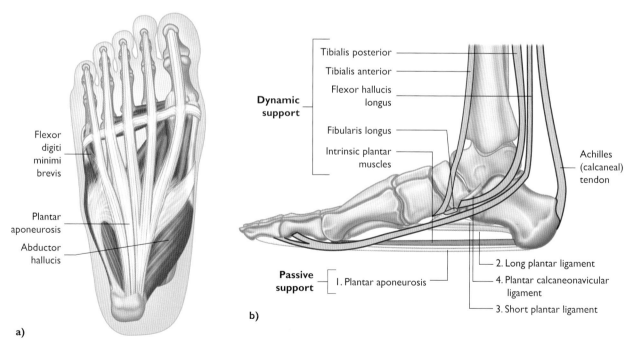

Figure 7.4.   *a) The inferior view of the plantar aponeurosis shows its strong proximal attachment to the calcaneus, and the divisions from the central band that reach to the ball of the foot where they are tethered together by transverse fibers. The aponeurosis extends laterally to encase the flexor digiti minimi brevis and medially to encase the abductor hallucis. b) This medial view presents the standard anatomical breakdown of the dynamic support from the extrinsic muscles we saw in the previous chapter, the three main layers of "passive" support provided by the plantar aponeurosis (a.k.a., the plantar fascia), and the long and short plantar ligaments. (Adapted from Wood Jones 1944.)*

the calcaneocuboid bridge, the passageway for the fibularis longus, an area that shortens during pronation and must lengthen again to allow supination. This is an area of interest to check in feet that seem reluctant or unable to form the rigid lever (we will explore this in the assessments in chapter 8.)

The human plantar aponeurosis has been considered unique in its form and degree of stiffness. The windlass mechanism was proposed by Hicks in a series of articles in the 1950s. Since then, the windlass mechanism has been a standard part of the story around how the human foot, unlike the feet of other primates, stiffens in preparation for toe-off. However, a recent comparative study of primate plantar fascia found several species also have well-developed central bands that, contrary to popular opinion, help stiffen their feet as part of a windlass mechanism (Sichting et al. 2020), see below.

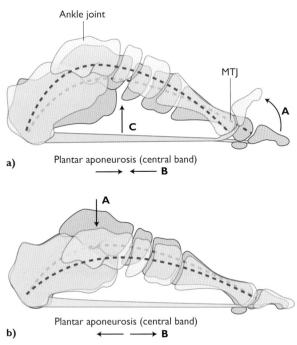

a)   Plantar aponeurosis (central band)

b)   Plantar aponeurosis (central band)

Figure 7.5. Since the work of Hicks (1955 & 1956) demonstrating the windlass mechanism, the plantar fascia has been considered an integral element for producing the rigid lever for toe-off (a). The plantar fascia also strains under load to capture elastic energy, which can contribute to locomotor efficiency (b). Sichting and colleagues suggest that these two roles are mutually exclusive as it is difficult to be both elastic and stiff. (Adapted from Sichting et al. 2020.)

The belief in the windlass mechanism as the prime "stiffener" of the human foot was recently challenged when a paper by Farris et al. (2020) questioned how the plantar aponeurosis could both act as a shock absorbing spring and be stiff enough to create a "rigid tie" between the heel and toes. Their work seems to indicate that the plantar intrinsic muscles are more important than the plantar fascia for stabilizing the foot as it rises into toe extension.

It appears that, rather than any one mechanism being solely responsible for creating and maintaining the rigid lever, there is a mixed strategy that blends the bony architecture (the midtarsal lock), the plantar fascia, the extrinsic, and the intrinsic muscles. Responsibility for creating and holding the rigid lever passes between each tissue during movement.

It is clear the plantar fascia is more than just a passive ligament, and it is tempting to conjecture about the effects of its continuity with the contractile tissues of the Achilles tendon, flexor digiti minimi brevis, and abductor hallucis (Stecco 2015), and flexor digitorum brevis (Wood Jones 1944). Due to its rich supply of mechanoreceptors and continuity to so many muscles, Stecco likens the plantar fascia to a "coachman guiding the muscles in the sole of the foot and helping coordinate all these structures during movement"—an image that further emphasizes the interactions between continuous tissues (fig. 7.6). It makes sense that roles and responsibilities are divided out among tissues and that they can cooperate with numerous levels of organization contributing to the same dynamic—especially when considering the high forces involved with supination and toe-off.

As Morton and Wood Jones warned us, the functional, moving body cannot be understood through textbook anatomy. The interactions and continuities are important and are only recently being investigated and appreciated

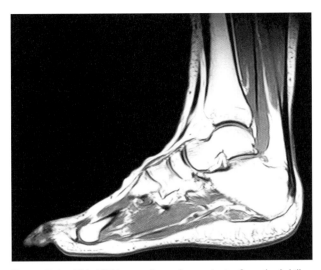

Figure 7.6. *This MRI image shows the continuity from the Achilles tendon around the calcaneus to the plantar fascia, allowing the triceps surae to tension the plantar fascia. The image also shows the flexor digitorum brevis lying on and connected to the deep aspect of the plantar fascia. As suggested by van der Wal, 2009, the ligamentous layer should be considered an active extension of the contractile tissues, as the intrinsic and extrinsic flexors can all adjust plantar fascia tension.*

Achilles Tendon, Calcaneus, and Plantar Fascia—A Functional Unit

The idea of tissue continuity between the plantar fascia and Achilles tendon has been with us for a while and was investigated back in 1995 (Snow et al.). Their study found a strong continuation between the two structures immediately following birth, but that it diminished with age which suggests that the continuity gradually ceases to be functionally significant.

However, two recent papers have added further clarity to the bone and soft tissue arrangement around the heel area. One paper showed the plantar fascia and Achilles tendon share morphological similarities in tissue thickness and cross-sectional areas either side of the calcaneus (Singh et al. 2021, fig. 7.6). The authors suggest that comparable measurements are indicative of a functional relationship between the two strong collagenous structures.

An earlier paper investigated the superficial bone tissue around the area of nine adult heels (aged 28 to 93, Zwirner et al 2020). The paper reports that alignment of the superficial trabeculae is oriented toward the two soft tissues at either end. This superoinferior trabecular arrangement contrasts to the obliquely fanning trabeculae pattern, both of which can be clearly seen in figure 7.6.

The superficial layer of bone around the posterior calcaneus was found to contain collagen fibers and adipocytes which suggests the previous continuity of soft tissues has part ossified but continues to act as a functional link between the Achilles tendon and plantar fascia. This functional connection supports the rationale of therapeutic strategies aimed at easing plantar fascia conditions through calf stretching and strengthening exercises.

from a holistic and functional approach. The paper by Sichting et al. (2020) illustrated this beautifully by mapping the major fiber directions of the plantar fascia of a range of primates (see fig. 7.7). Only the human plantar fascia was predominately aligned sagittally with both the central and lateral fibers oriented from posterior to anterior. Matching some of the gait patterns shown in fig. 1.8, other primates show a lateral to medial (see fig. 7.7b, c, & e) or medial to abducted big toe (see fig. 7.7a & e) transfer of force, that illustrates the overlap between locomotor patterns and tissue architecture.

The predominant fiber direction in the plantar aponeurosis matches the progression over the four rockers from heel to toe, and we see an interesting pattern when looking at the EMG readings of the extrinsic muscles in the previous chapter (see fig. 6.14). They all become less active after 50% of the gait cycle. Around that stage of the gait cycle, the heel is beginning to lift and the toes are extending—the work of the ankle stabilizers (the extrinsics)

is complete and the responsibility for the rigid lever moves to the four layers of intrinsic foot muscles (Farris et al. 2020; Zelik et al. 2014).

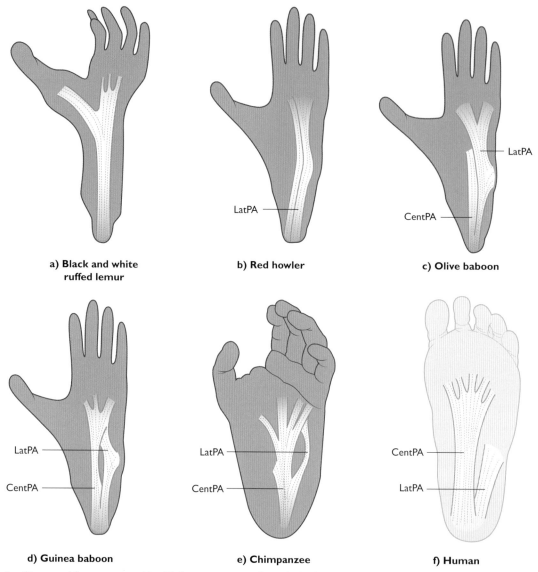

a) **Black and white ruffed lemur**

b) **Red howler**

c) **Olive baboon**

d) **Guinea baboon**

e) **Chimpanzee**

f) **Human**

Figure 7.7.   *Six general foot types were identified among primates but only the human foot showed consistent anterior to posterior alignment of the plantar aponeurosis (PA) tissue. Each of the others had varying degrees of deviation of the lateral (latPA) or central (centPA) portions of the aponeurosis. (Adapted from Sichting et al. 2020.)*

1. First Layer—Superficial

The three muscles of the first plantar layer fan out from the calcaneus to the toes almost like a deltoid (fig. 7.8). Although the flexor digitorum brevis (in the middle) is the only one named as a toe flexor, all three contribute to toe flexion (Mickle et al. 2012). Each muscle is therefore involved in deceleration and control of toe extension and, as all three span the half-dome of the foot, they will help draw the calcaneus toward the toes as the heel lifts and we come toward toe-off position. The functional position at toe-off, as we saw above, will stiffen the inside of the foot, and help maintain the rigid lever in preparation for toe-off.

Flexor digitorum brevis is one of the few "short" muscles that is superficial to a "long" muscle that crosses the same joints. The flexor digitorum longus comes from the back of the leg to the distal phalanges and is deep to the brevis as it crosses the sole of the foot. The tendons of the flexor digitorum brevis must split at the proximal phalanges to allow the long tendons to reach all the way out to the distal phalanges (see inset, fig. 7.8).

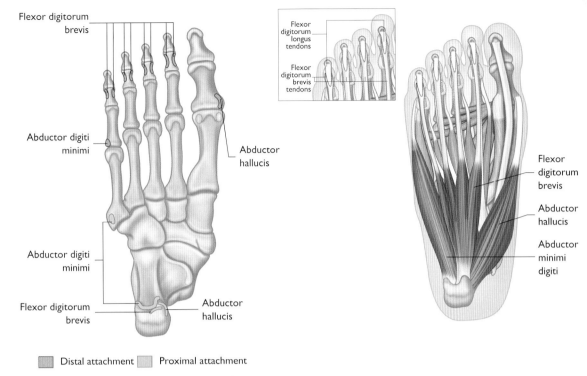

Distal attachment Proximal attachment

Figure 7.8. **First layer of intrinsic muscles.**

Flexor digitorum brevis—Proximal attachment—Medial process of calcaneus and plantar aponeurosis. Distal attachment—Middle phalanges of second to fifth toes. Action—Flexion of middle phalanges of second to fifth toes (proximal interphalangeal joints, a.k.a. PIPs).

Abductor hallucis—Proximal attachment—Medial process of calcaneus and plantar aponeurosis. Distal attachment—Proximal phalanx of first toe (MTJ). Action—Abduct the first toe. Flexion of the first MTJ.

Abductor digiti minimi—Proximal attachment—Lateral process of calcaneus and plantar aponeurosis. Distal attachment—Proximal phalanx of fifth toe. Action—Flexion of fifth toe (MTJ). Abduction of fifth toe (MTJ).

This is an unusual relationship as it is easier for tissues to arrange themselves with the longer muscles leapfrogging over the top of the deep tissues without the need to pass through them (see fig. 7.11). A similar arrangement occurs in the palm of the hand and allows the larger, stronger muscles to attach to the distal phalanges where more power is needed for grip and control.

Sequenced muscle attachments to each phalange provide fine control at each joint but mechanical advantage for grip reduces as one travels distally along the digits. To counteract the loss of mechanical advantage, the stronger muscle is allowed through to the distal phalange and the shorter intrinsic muscle controls the proximal interphalangeal joint, where it can assert more force.

Allowing the longer extrinsic muscles to pass the distal phalanges gives a range of benefits. The first is the increased force potential as outlined above and that also positions the larger, heavier muscle bellies more proximally to reduce the locomotor costs of moving heavy distal limbs. The increased length of muscle fibers that attach to the distal phalanges also provides a further advantage because of the direct relationship between fiber length and range of motion—the longer the muscle fiber the more it can shorten. Therefore, allowing longer muscles to attach to the bones that move furthest makes sense for both increased gripping force and increased range of motion.

As we saw above, several papers suggest that this first layer of intrinsic muscles has an intimate relationship with the plantar aponeurosis, and their blended attachment to

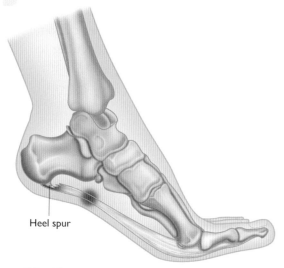

Heel spur

Figure 7.9.   The anterior process of the calcaneus is an area of high stress, making it susceptible to developing heel spurs, which sometimes lead to pain and discomfort (but, not always!). The attachment site for the plantar aponeurosis and the tissue of the first layer of intrinsic muscles can also develop a range of issues requiring expert differential diagnosis.

the anterior calcaneus creates a focal area of high stress. While most texts emphasize the muscles' actions at the toes, their anchoring at the heel focuses into a relatively narrow area. This is particularly true of the central portion of the arrangement, the middle section of the plantar aponeurosis, and the flexor digitorum brevis, as their fiber alignment matches the predominately sagittal progression of the foot as it comes up into the toe-off position. The proximity of their attachment and the tissue continuity between the flexor digitorum brevis and the plantar fascia fibers can make it difficult to differentiate between the source of pain that can develop in the area. Heel spurs, plantar fasciitis, and rupture, among many other conditions, can all occur in the area, and any pain in the area should be properly diagnosed to allow appropriate management (Yi et al. 2011), fig. 7.9.

2. Second Layer

The quadratus plantae is sometimes listed as the *flexor digitorum accessorius*[10] but I dislike

this latter name as I think it is a red herring, distracting us from the muscle's real function. The quadratus plantae is not present in other primate feet—remember those oblique angles of the plantar aponeurosis and the wobbly gait patterns of apes and monkeys? Humans have a straight plantar aponeurosis and a predominately straight walking pattern. A major function of quadratus plantae is therefore not to "accessorize" the long toe flexor as it flexes the toes, but to control the sagittal progression into toe extension. As we have been exploring all along—understanding function often requires us to reverse the commonly listed action. But most of the discussion around the angle and position of the quadratus plantae rarely, if ever, mentions the need for foot stability as the heel rises and we move toward toe-off.

As a toe flexor, it has been suggested that quadratus plantae is recruited for extra force during accelerated gait (Aiello & Dean 2002). Extra force production by the quadratus plantae might well occur when we need to increase walking speed, but can we be certain that the extra force production is to push us forward? Or is it the increased potential for instability of the foot that requires the quadratus plantae to increase its contribution to compensate? Once again, it may be an academic discussion as both dynamics occur simultaneously and both needs must be met. Does the answer have to be a binary one? Quadratus plantae's position will allow it to increase toe flexion for extra propulsion and, because it spans the plantar aspect, the extra force will also help stabilize the half-dome.

The sagittal plane progression over the rockers of the foot initially engages the plantar aponeurosis and the windlass mechanism

[10]Another occasional muscle is sometimes present, the *flexor digitorum accessorius longus*. Confusingly, some texts will mention its occasional presence while only referring to an other muscle as

the *quadratus plantae* rather than as the *flexor digitorum accessorius* in the rest of the text. If one does not know the quadratus plantae is sometimes called the *flexor digitorum accessorius*, futile hours could be spent looking for *the flexor digitorum accessorius brevis* which does not exist. Sometimes it almost seems like they want to confuse us.

for soft tissue support of the rigid lever, and then the deeper layers take over as the toes extend further. Where the first layer of intrinsic muscles is intimate with the plantar aponeurosis, this second layer, especially the quadratus plantae, is associated with another strong support for the foot called the long plantar ligament (fig. 7.10).

The quadratus plantae has two heads coming from the front of the calcaneus, with the long plantar ligament positioned between them. The medial head is the larger and longer of the two and the lateral head is flat and tendinous as it attaches to the lateral margin of FDL.

Like many muscles, it is variable between individuals: sometimes it is absent altogether or missing its lateral portion attaching to the fourth and fifth toe slips; and, in around 9% of cases, a third slip may be present (Pretterklieber 2018).

The lumbricals are another unusual group of small muscles as they arise from tendon and they produce both flexion and extension of the toes (though at different joints, fig. 7.10). This group of four small muscles originates from the tendon of flexor digitorum longus. The first lumbrical comes from the medial aspect of the tendon; the others all originate from within the

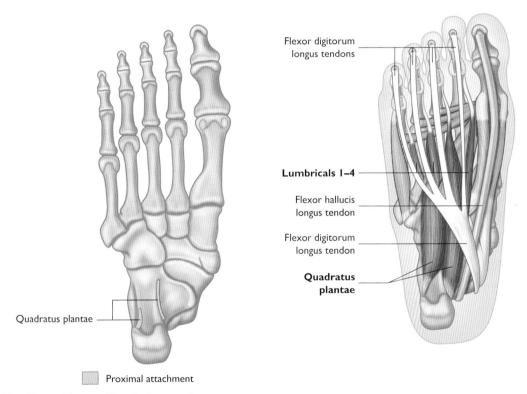

Flexor digitorum longus tendons

Lumbricals 1–4

Flexor hallucis longus tendon

Flexor digitorum longus tendon

Quadratus plantae

Quadratus plantae

▨ Proximal attachment

Figure 7.10. **Second layer of intrinsic muscles.**

Connected to the flexor digitorum longus tendon. The two heads of the quadratus plantae (also known as flexor digitorum accessorius) travel from the front of the calcaneus to the flexor digitorum longus tendon as it passes across the mid-foot. The flexor digitorum longus tendon divides into four slips to serve the lateral four toes and provides attachment for the lumbrical muscles that then attach distally to the bases of the second to fifth proximal phalanges.

*Quadratus plantae—**Proximal attachment**—Medial and lateral aspects of calcaneus. **Distal attachment**—Posterior, lateral aspect of flexor digitorum longus tendon. **Action**—Assists flexor digitorum longus to flex second to fifth toes. Is often suggested to straighten the line of pull of the flexor digitorum longus.*

*Lumbricals—**Proximal attachment**—Tendons of flexor digitorum longus. **Distal attachment**—Bases of proximal phalanges of second to fifth toes and extensor digitorum longus tendons (on dorsal surface of the toes)—part of the dorsal digital expansion. **Action**—Flexes the proximal phalanges of the second to fifth toes at the MTJ. Extends the middle and distal phalanges of the second to fifth toes at the interphalangeal joints.*

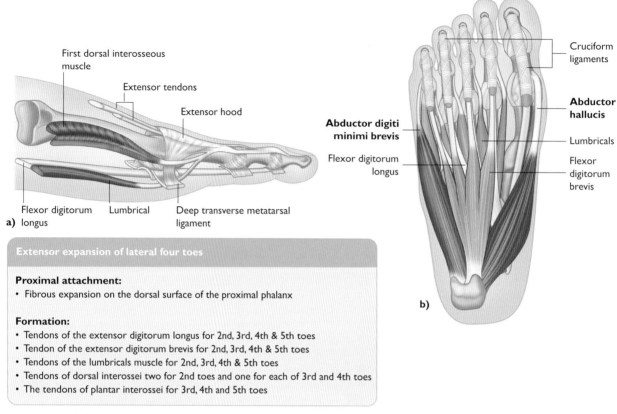

First dorsal interosseous muscle

Extensor tendons

Extensor hood

Cruciform ligaments

Abductor hallucis

Abductor digiti minimi brevis

Lumbricals

Flexor digitorum longus

Flexor digitorum brevis

Flexor digitorum longus   Lumbrical   Deep transverse metatarsal ligament

a)

b)

Extensor expansion of lateral four toes

Proximal attachment:
• Fibrous expansion on the dorsal surface of the proximal phalanx

Formation:
• Tendons of the extensor digitorum longus for 2nd, 3rd, 4th & 5th toes
• Tendon of the extensor digitorum brevis for 2nd, 3rd, 4th & 5th toes
• Tendons of the lumbricals muscle for 2nd, 3rd, 4th & 5th toes
• Tendons of dorsal interossei two for 2nd toes and one for each of 3rd and 4th toes
• The tendons of plantar interossei for 3rd, 4th and 5th toes

Figure 7.11.   a) As if it wasn't complicated enough, the extensor expansion is also known as the extensor hood, dorsal expansion, or hood, or as the dorsal aponeurosis. It is mostly formed from the continuity of tissues provided by the extensor tendons (hence its name) but it also provides anchor for the lumbricals and plantar interossei. b) The fascial wrapping of the digits is formed from the dorsal fascia, which receives tendons from the abductor hallucis and the abductor digiti minimi, as well as the extensors shown in a). Classed as hinge joints, the interphalangeal joints do not have any inherent bony support to prevent rotation, but they receive ligamentous support from the cruciform ligaments that prevent rotation between them.

angles of each tendon separation and therefore attach to two tendons each.

By contributing to a complex aponeurosis surrounding the toe joints, the lumbricals help the flexor digitorum longus and the toe extensors gain fine control of toe movement. Known as the extensor expansion, this aponeurosis provides various tendons with attachment sites as well as a retinaculum to help them alter their line of direction. We see that especially with the lumbricals as they drop below the deep transverse ligament and then rise again to the extensor hood over the middle and distal interphalangeal joints (fig. 7.11a).

3. Third Layer

This group of muscles is perfectly placed to provide a deep level of control to the tarsals and metatarsals during movement. As the first two superficial layers have taken up all the attachment sites on the calcaneus, there is no room left for the third layer of intrinsic muscles that span and support the mid- to forefoot. Instead, they attach to the midtarsal and metatarsal bones (fig. 7.12a). The distribution of their four fiber angles creates a box-like pattern on the sole of the foot, ensuring bony integrity from its range of angles.

We could consider three of the muscular heads (transverse and oblique portion of adductor

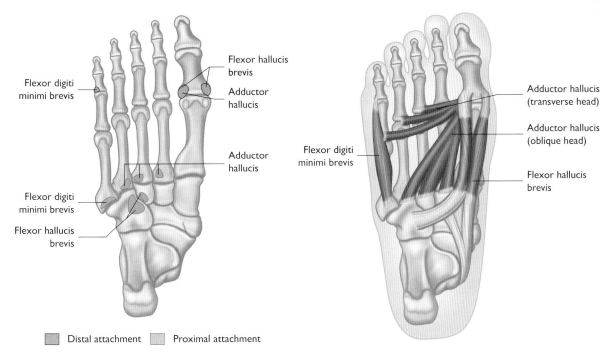

Distal attachment   Proximal attachment

Figure 7.12. **Third layer of intrinsic muscles.**

These muscles give movement and stability options as they traverse the foot from lateral to medial.

Flexor hallucis brevis—***Proximal attachment***—*Plantar surface of cuboid and lateral cuneiform.* ***Distal attachment***—*Medial and lateral surfaces of base of proximal phalanx of first toe.* ***Action***—*Flexion of first toe at the MTJ.*

Adductor hallucis—***Proximal attachment***—*Oblique head*—*bases of second to fourth metatarsals. Transverse head*—*Plantar ligament of third to fifth MTJs.* ***Distal attachment***—*Lateral surface of base of proximal phalanx of first toe.* ***Action***—*Adducts and flexes the first toe at the MTJ. Support and maintain the "transverse arch".*

Flexor digiti minimi brevis—***Proximal attachment***—*Base of fifth metatarsal.* ***Distal attachment***—*base of proximal phalanx of fifth toe.* ***Action***—*Flexion of fifth toe at the MTJ.*

hallucis and the flexor hallucis brevis) as another deltoid, that can either draw the foot into a cup-like shape to help with grip or provide a tether to the great toe from three different angles. The transverse head is best placed to adduct the toe and will also support the metatarsal heads and the ligaments running between them. The transverse head will strain during pronation, providing the muscle fiber with mechanoreceptive information and pretensioning its supporting fascial tissue to increase support for this distal arch. The other two heads of this deltoid, the flexor hallucis brevis and the oblique head of adductor hallucis, will assist the medial longitudinal arch. These two muscles share a tendon where they meet on the inside

of the proximal phalange, but they are differently innervated and can therefore act independently. However, the group is best considered together when all three heads will help support the half-dome—the same inverted shape created when they "cup" to help the foot grip or hold objects.

The flexor hallucis brevis divides as it approaches the great toe and the divisions receive tendons from the adductor hallucis medially and the abductor hallucis laterally. These large and strong tendons contain and manage the two sesamoid bones that create a tunnel for the flexor hallucis longus tendon (see fig. 7.13).

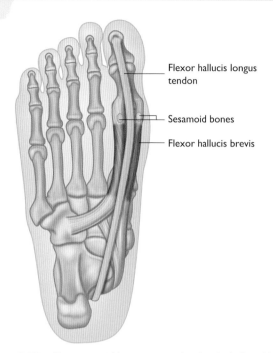

Flexor hallucis longus tendon

Sesamoid bones

Flexor hallucis brevis

Figure 7.13.   Two sesamoid bones exist within the divided tendon of the flexor hallucis brevis. They provide a track for the path of the flexor hallucis longus tendon but can be displaced through various foot deformities, most commonly hallux valgus, and become inflamed due to repeated strain.

The flexor digiti minimi brevis has a tendon that blends into the abductor digiti minimi. Overall, the blended tendons attaching to the toes from various sources provide stronger anchor points and though it might reduce individual control and range, the human foot requires more strength and stability than fine manipulation.

The tendons of the three muscles in this layer blend into the ligaments and joint capsules around the MTJs, and each muscle plays a part in maintaining the structural integrity and mobility of these joints. The metatarsal heads, and therefore their associated joints with the proximal phalanges, apply significant pressure to the ground as we progress into toe extension. The MTJ capsules respond by thickening their plantar tissue. These protective thickenings are referred to as *plantar plates* and are part of a strong and thick fascial network that has continuity with the deep portion of the plantar fascia (fig. 7.14).

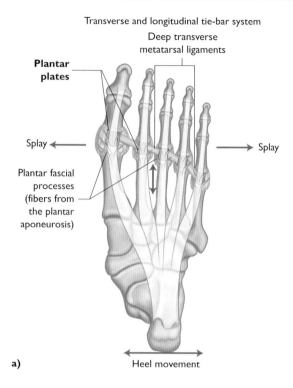

Transverse and longitudinal tie-bar system

Deep transverse metatarsal ligaments

Plantar plates

Splay

Splay

Plantar fascial processes (fibers from the plantar aponeurosis)

a)   Heel movement

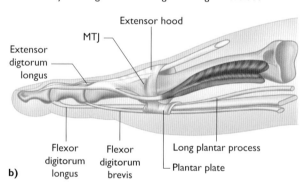

Both systems tighten when weight-bearing on forefoot

Extensor hood

MTJ

Extensor digtorum longus

Flexor digitorum longus

Flexor digitorum brevis

Long plantar process

Plantar plate

b)

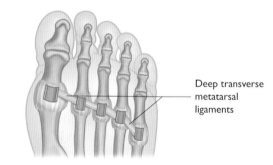

Deep transverse metatarsal ligaments

c)

Figure 7.14.   a) Weight-bearing causes the foot to splay as it pronates and the plantar tissues tension. Integrity is maintained through a series of tissue layers and directions. The plantar aponeurosis has fibers that travel to the MTJ capsules and support the plantar plates below the joints. b) The plantar plate provides shock absorption and glide for the metatarsal heads during locomotion and are held in place by the complex strapping of the extensor hood. c) The transverse ligament according to Morton (1922).

The metatarsal heads and associated plantar plates require a certain degree of mobility compared with the secure proximal joints between the metatarsal bases, the cuneiforms, and cuboid. The mobility/stability equation for the metatarsal heads is solved by the deep transverse ligament that spans between each head and encompasses each of the plantar plates. The deep transverse ligament and the plantar plates form the transverse tie-bar, an anatomical arrangement that prevents the forefoot from splaying and preserves the positioning of the plantar plates.

The continuity between the plantar aponeurosis, plantar plates, and the deep transverse ligament allows the foot to splay during pronation, which tensions the whole system. As the plantar aponeurosis is superficial and spans most of the foot, it will receive most of the stress during pronation. It therefore makes mechanical sense to let the superficial plantar aponeurosis tissue wrap around the deeper flexor tendons to reach the plantar plates and contribute to the pretensioning of the tie-bar mechanism.

The transverse head of adductor hallucis provides a contractile response to monitor and control the foot splay and has connections into the joint capsules for added support and security. Despite the tissue density and extra reinforcement, the plantar plates are prone to tearing and can sometimes allow the metatarsal to move within the capsular surround (Stainsby 1997).

Reduced integrity of the deep transverse ligament may contribute to the development of hallux valgus. In an early comparative anatomy paper, Morton (1922) suggested that the human transverse ligament is less established between the first and second toes compared with the connection between each of the other toes.

Morton blamed this fact on the need for wider mobility of the great toe for our arboreal ancestors, so we have been left with some of the anatomical pattern. It has since been suggested that the lack of tethering between the first and second metatarsals allows the first ray to migrate away from the second, a fact given some support by a cadaveric study that found reduced tensile support of the transverse ligament in feet with a halluxed toe (Abdalbary et al. 2016).

4. Fourth Layer

The two sets of interossei are not mirror images of one another. The plantar group only has one head per toe and covers only toes three to five. In contrast, the dorsal group is bipennate, with heads coming from adjacent metatarsals, and they include the second toe (see fig. 7.15).

Functionally, the coupling of flexion with adduction makes sense as the action of gripping requires a closing action. Releasing an object, whether it be a branch or tool, uses the opening movement of extension and abduction.

Although the flexor interossei only cover the third to fifth toes, they have the assistance of many other muscles within the plantar aspect. We require good control of flexion for gripping, and we require the force in the flexors to control the movement of extension.

Most human toe extension is produced either in response to our momentum as we progress over the forefoot and toe rockers, or with reduced resistance as we lift the toes during and immediately following toe-off. In either action, very little force is required, especially when compared to the shock absorption performed by the flexors.

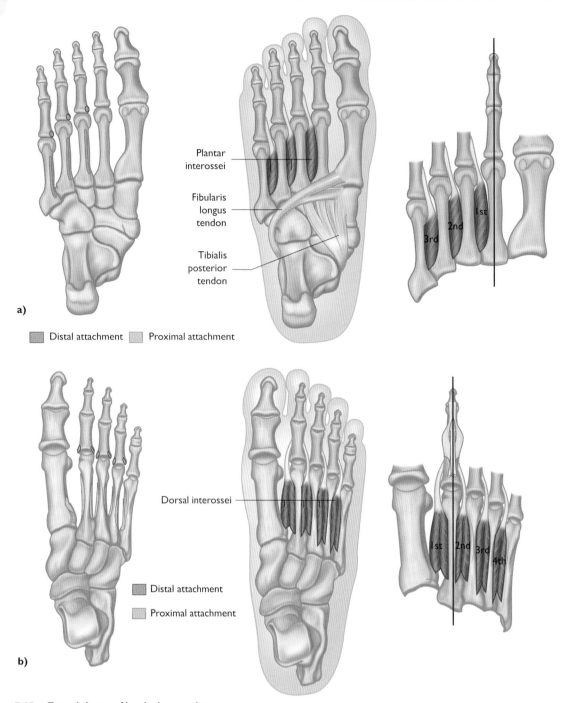

Plantar interossei

Fibularis longus tendon

Tibialis posterior tendon

a)

Distal attachment   Proximal attachment

Dorsal interossei

Distal attachment

Proximal attachment

b)

Figure 7.15. **Fourth layer of intrinsic muscles.**

a) The deepest layer of plantar tissues includes the tendons from tibialis posterior and fibularis longus (described in the previous chapter), along with the plantar and dorsal interossei. The short intereossei are often remembered by the mnemonic P-AD and D-AB—Plantar ADduction and Dorsal ABduction—but this is easily experienced by simply flexing and extending the toes to feel their natural inclination to adduct on flexion and abduct on extension. b) The dorsal view of the foot shows the dorsal interossei and the two extensors—extensor hallucis and extensor digitorum brevis.

Plantar interossei—**Proximal attachment**—*Medial surfaces of the third to fifth metatarsals.* **Distal attachment**—*Medial surfaces of proximal phalanges of third to fifth toes.* **Action**—*Flexion and adduction of third to fifth toes at the MTJ.*

Dorsal interossei—**Proximal attachment**—*Adjacent surfaces of all metatarsals.* **Distal attachment**—*First—proximal phalange of second toe. Second to fourth—Lateral surfaces of proximal phalanges of second to fourth toes.* **Action**—*Extension and abduction of second to fourth toes at the MTJ.*

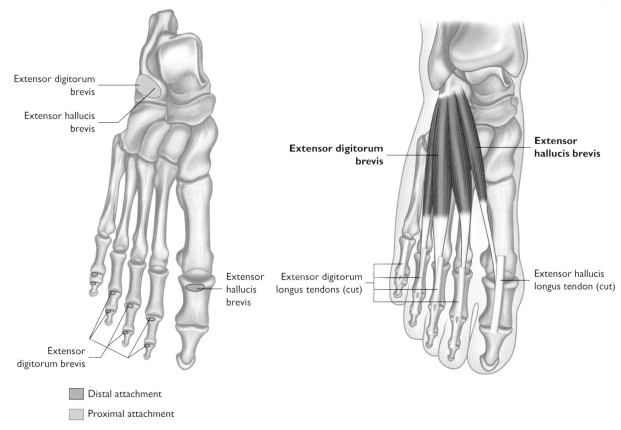

Extensor digitorum brevis

Extensor hallucis brevis

Extensor digitorum brevis

Extensor hallucis brevis

Extensor hallucis brevis

Extensor digitorum longus tendons (cut)

Extensor hallucis longus tendon (cut)

Extensor digitorum brevis

Distal attachment

Proximal attachment

Figure 7.16. **Dorsal extensors.**

*Extensor hallucis brevis—**Proximal attachment**—Dorsal surface of calcaneus. **Distal attachment**—Proximal phalange of first toe.*
Action—Extension of first toe at the MTJ.

*Extensor digitorum brevis—**Proximal attachment**—Dorsal surface of the calcaneus. **Distal attachment**—Proximal phalange of second to fourth toes. **Action**—Extension of first toe at the MTJ.*

TOE EXTENSORS

The short toe extensors are slender and variable muscles, they are sometimes considered as one muscle with four heads going to each of the first four toes (fig. 7.16). Many people are not even aware of their existence until they tie their shoelaces too tight and something begins to grumble underneath.

SUMMARY

The intrinsic muscles have a complex layering system, with some not quite adhering to the normal anatomical arrangements of superficial to deep, and long to short. The toe joints are encased in a sheath that receives tissues from a range of tendons, which creates passages for tendons to work their way either proximally or distally to provide fine control. This confusing arrangement provides extra control over the flexion and extension pattern through the toe joints and mirrors the similar arrangement in the hand.

Unlike the hand, the major role for the human foot is force management rather than fine manipulation. But along with the foot's many important roles in monitoring force transfer is its capacity for significant motor control to adapt to changes in posture and movement. A better understanding of these roles has created a resurgence of interest in the intrinsic muscles, much of which has been driven by research into the benefits of exercising barefoot and the use of minimal footwear.

Previously established ideas around foot support and the windlass mechanism for supination have been challenged and the significance of these smaller muscles has been highlighted. Most of the intrinsic muscles are oriented anterior to posterior and control our natural gait patterns—as reflected in the strengthening of the plantar fascia along the same vector and in contrast to other primates. Due to the natural shape of the foot, there is a triangular, deltoid nature to many of the muscular arrays, which makes functional as well as anatomical sense.

The foot is often seen as a tripod with its three common points of contact with the floor—the base of the fifth and first metatarsals, and the heel. We can view the musculature as either fanning out to the metatarsals from the calcaneus, or the reverse. When the heel is rising during locomotion and the metatarsals

are anchored on the ground, the medial and lateral muscles reach back and focus inward toward the heel. This viewpoint is particularly pertinent when we consider the requirement for stability as we move toward toe-off.

We have explored the natural bony mechanics that produce some degree of form closure for the foot during supination. In the previous chapter, we saw how the extrinsic muscles can assist with force closure, but they begin to reduce their activity prior to the last two rockers. The last two foot rockers are when the intrinsic muscles take over to provide the inner stability to the foot. They form what McKeon and his colleagues refer to as the "core of the foot." Sadly, this core has been undermined by modern life—either through lack of use or footwear.

In the next couple of chapters, we will go through some assessments to get an idea of the foot's performance, look at some exercise and mobility ideas, before finishing with an exploration of the role of footwear.

8

FUNCTION AND ASSESSMENT OF THE FOOT

With Mark Parfitt-Jones

▥ INTRODUCTION

Over the years I have found people approach chapters and workshop installments on assessment with a range of emotions. Those emotions range from excitement, as the answers to all the problems are about to be revealed, through to trepidation, because assessments are sometimes complex and difficult to interpret. This chapter aims to satisfy those at either end of that spectrum— with the caveat that to describe a full orthopedic assessment is beyond the scope of this text and probably beyond the scope of most readers' practices.

Key to applying assessments is understanding why you are using them. The text so far has aimed to arm you with an appreciation of each tissue's functional role. We zoomed in to the finer detail and out to the bigger picture as we moved from one chapter to the next; now we get to draw all the strands together with a review of the interactions between tissues and their function. A solid foundation of understanding the foot will allow you to apply the assessments and exercises with confidence.

The assessments included in this chapter will reinforce the information you have already read. Each test has been chosen for its usefulness in building a picture of what is or is not happening with a client's foot. That information then helps direct you to which exercises and stretches in chapter 9 are most suitable. The assessments are included here to encourage a deep understanding of what is happening within the foot, and why. This chapter is not a dry listing of every ligament and joint test for the foot.

Social media is driving a trend toward increased complexity of exercise and assessments. While many of them may be useful, there is the risk of falling into the professionally dangerous trap of over-complication while remaining under-informed. Spending time with this chapter will integrate the information you have read and put it in context. My promise at the beginning of the text was to encourage an understanding of the foot, not to provide a checklist of every anatomical landmark and every test for you to rote memorize—those are available in many other sources. Below, we will explore the "why", the "what", and the "how", all based on the evolutionary history, and the functional roles and capabilities of the foot provided by the bones and the soft tissues.

The assessments and subsequent exercises test and then support the main functions of the foot. A full orthopedic assessment is only valuable to those with complete management and treatment skill-sets—those complex, high-end skills should be taught hand-to-hand and preferably in person. Building competence in the tests below and working through the subsequent exercises will provide benefit to most feet, whilst allowing the practitioner to remain within their scope of practice.

The assessments included below are based around the question "can this tissue do what it should do"? And so, we begin our assessment by reiterating what the foot should be able to do: it should be able to manage shock absorption and force distribution; it should be mobile and adaptive; and it should be able to come together again to provide a rigid platform for propulsion.

As Lieberman points out (chapter 2), most discussion around the foot revolves around walking but the human foot has to perform many more tasks than just stepping forward. Our feet must help us walk, of course, but also run, jump, land, throw, fight, squat, rise, stand, pull and push, turn, twist, and dance. Each of these actions, and many more besides, placed some evolutionary pressure on the adaptability of the foot to make it into the form it is. Efficient gait might have been a major driving force to shape the foot, but if that was all it could do, our species would not have been as successful as we have.

Most functions of the foot can be split into four categories:

1. Shock Absorption.
2. Range of Motion.
3. Forming an Aligned Rigid Lever.
4. Propulsion and Force Output.

■ SHOCK ABSORPTION

The foot's shock absorption capabilities come from two main sources: the heel and its robust calcaneus that is partly protected by a thick fat pad; and the foot's ability to pronate, the unlocking of its many joints to distribute forces into the soft tissues. Pronation and the distribution of force feeds into many of the dynamics we saw in chapter 5—tissue strain helps increase muscle force output and loads elastic energy into the collagenous tissues.

Shock absorption can also be considered as force distribution. A healthy foot ensures no single tissue or tissue area needs to take all the impact strain. The foot achieves this through its series of bony alignments that oblige the foot to unlock and pronate. Whether one heel strikes while walking or lands on some part of the mid- to forefoot after a jump, leap, or running stride, the natural reaction of forces acting thorough the bones drives the foot into pronation. The interaction between bony architecture and gravity and ground reaction forces (chapter 4) ensures the soft tissues are recruited to control the shock.

A solid, immobile, supinated-type foot receives impact forces into its bones, not only causing distress to the bones, but also reducing proprioceptive information to the rest of the body. When working properly, the foot's role in force distribution ensures there is wider soft tissue involvement, and the forces received by any soft tissue is also a stimulation to the mechanoreceptors in that area. Force is therefore information, and the foot is our main distributor of that information upward to the rest of our body for overall proprioception and control.

Proprioceptive information is coming to us from the mechanoreceptor-rich sole of the foot, as well as the sensors within the soft tissues of the foot, leg, and hip. Much of that information is going upward to our central nervous system, but some mechanoreceptor stimulation is processed locally.

Local processing ensures rapid adjustment and fine-tuning of tissue stiffness levels (Sawicki et al. 2009). Speed of communication through spinal reflexes is too slow for the degree of tuning required by the foot and ankle as they navigate the constantly changing force environment. Ensuring clear pathways for force distribution therefore enhances our tone setting and efficiency. Blocking force distribution or channeling it into other tissues can be caused by joint and tissue limitations, and by the environment we put our feet into.

Footwear should be part of any assessment, as it can contribute to or limit the foot's function depending on the style of shoe or the abilities of the foot. We will explore footwear in chapter 10, but even a cursory glance at a client's shoe can provide some information on what their foot can and cannot do once you understand the essentials of the foot's mechanics. Investigating footwear and asking clients to move both barefoot and shod can all form part of a thorough assessment—and footwear can often provide an answer to a problem that is not obvious when assessing the unshod foot.

Although commonly advertised as providing comfort and shock absorption, any type of shoe can prevent or inhibit the foot's natural shock absorbing ability. That is not to say that shoes are bad—they serve many functions and can be very helpful in assisting a challenged foot. Despite what some social media posts might encourage us to think, few devices are either universally positive or universally negative, it depends on the context. Each device, whether it is a shoe or an orthotic, can alter force transfer, which may be a good or a bad thing. It is up to us to understand what those effects are and why they happen.

◼ RANGE OF MOTION

In my experience, many therapists struggle with the mismatch between what they see when a client moves in the real-world and the application of a specific range of motion tests. I find it useful to differentiate between long- and short-chain movement. Our normal, everyday movements are long-chain, complex actions, requiring contributions from many joints and tissues. But an important factor within that chain is that each joint and tissue should make an appropriate contribution. Unless I can investigate a particular area, it is nearly impossible for me to be sure where a problem within the long-chain might be or what type of issue is causing it.

All long-chain movements will require a contribution from each joint between the body's fixed point and the target of the movement being made—are you trying to get your hand to somewhere? Is one foot trying to kick something? Are you turning to look over your shoulder? If at least one foot is on the ground as you make any of these movements, the tissues of that foot will be asked to supply some contribution toward the overall range.

A common exercise in my workshops is to stand in neutral barefoot and to turn to your right as far as is comfortable for you, just as we did in the earlier chapters. This time, take note of how far you turn and feel the effect on your feet. If you turn to the right, your left foot should pronate, and your right foot should supinate. If not, check that you let your pelvis turn with you and, if you did, then you might have something interesting to note in the following assessments!

Now repeat the exercise without letting your left foot pronate (assuming it can do so).

Did you turn as far?

Can you try to get to your first range of movement?

How did that feel? Were you aware of any particular area, any strain, or any discomfort?

In the first exercise your feet contributed to your overall range of movement and, if you wish to repeat it, you might be aware of the mechanical chain through the rest of your body. In fact, almost every joint from your feet to your head had something to contribute. When we removed one (admittedly complex and multi-joint) range of motion—the pronation of your left foot—your overall range was reduced. However, we can compensate for that loss by asking other areas to contribute a little extra—those are likely to be the areas that complained a little.

When considering movement, it is useful to break it down into *range of movement* and *range of motion*. Each of our everyday activities, whether it is gait, cleaning, cooking, or sport, requires long-chain *ranges of movement*. We operate with the goal of getting our hands, nose, mouth, or feet from somewhere to somewhere else. Often, we do not care how we manage that, it just needs to happen, but successful *ranges of movement* require contribution from a series of individual *ranges of motion*.

There is a tendency to only check the range of motion of joints in areas that are complaining and maybe showing some pathology. But, as we have just seen, the areas that strained in your body during the exercise where we blocked the pronation of the foot were not the ones at fault, they were the areas trying to do a little more. It is important for us to acknowledge the interdependent relationships between ranges of motion along mechanical chains and, because of its position between the body and the ground, the ranges within the foot are of utmost importance. Each of the many joints in the foot has capacity for movement that not only allows them to contribute to the shock absorption and force distribution, but allows them to contribute to the foot's overall range of movement.

Our long stride evolved through a series of adaptations, especially to the heel, toes, spine, and pelvis. Each of these areas is reliant on the range of motion of the others during gait. If toe extension is reduced, it will either shorten the stride or cause the foot to rotate to compensate for the lack of range in the sagittal plane. Loss

of toe extension then changes the amount and the angle of forces passing up to the knee and to the hip, with consequences for movement efficiency.

Range of motion of the great toe, talar, knee, and hip joints are all interrelated and a deficit at one will have knock-on effects in the others. Reduced ranges will decrease the amount of tissue strain gained through momentum and result in increased work for the muscles (Sawicki et al. 2009; Whittington et al. 2008; Silder et al. 2007). You can feel this for yourself by taking a short walk and deliberately limiting your toe extension or ankle dorsiflexion and feeling the compensations that happen. The most likely compensations in this exercise are to increase muscle activity around the hip and pelvis.

The relationship between our hips and feet goes both ways, and restrictions at the hip could affect mechanics of the foot. For example, limited hip extension will affect the amount of ankle dorsiflexion and toe extension during gait.

Assessment for Pain or Increased Efficiency?

It is important not to fall into the trap of biomechanical determinism—the fixed idea that if a client has a mechanical deficit they are destined for pain and dysfunction. As we saw in chapters 3 and 5, our tissues adapt to repeated stress. Whether it is through Wolff's law (bone) or the equivalent concept for the soft tissue, Davis's law, it is always possible for a client's tissue to be perfectly adapted to their own unique alignment.

Our questions for assessments should focus on whether any client's discomfort might have a biomechanical element and whether there are areas that appear less efficient than they should be. By focusing our energy on improving efficiency, we remain within our appropriate scope of practice with the important secondary benefits of supporting psychological and emotional health through easier movement.

RIGID LEVER

As we have seen in the previous two chapters, one of the mechanisms to create the rigid lever is dependent on toe extension. Failure to properly extend the toe will reduce overall stiffness of the intrinsic and extrinsic tissues and therefore also reduce stiffness within the foot.

In chapter 3, we saw how the femur was stiffened by the surrounding muscles to form a rigid bone that supports movement between the hip and knee joints. If the bone were to bend when high forces are experienced, it would be less stable. On the other hand, if the femur were fixed and rigid it would be fragile and easily break when bending forces are applied. The body has created a best fit solution in producing a bone that is flexible with some safety margin[1] but that can become rigid when forces increase, with supporting muscles that react to and balance out the forces.

Imagine the difficulties we would have if the femur was a series of small bones rather than one long one—it would be incredibly difficult to stabilize them. Admittedly, we would increase our movement possibilities as more joints add to the ranges and directions of movement. But the new mobility possibilities would come at a cost to our stability and efficiency. Somehow our feet have evolved to balance out these conflicting demands and found a solution that allows a high degree of movement adaptability and yet provides the rigidity needed for a propulsive toe-off.

Human Exceptionalism

Although it is tempting to wax lyrical on the adaptive majesty of the human foot, it is no more specialized than that of any other animal. Can you imagine trying to take down a zebra with your front and back "claws", prancing along near-vertical cliff-sides, or leaping elegantly from branch to branch? Each mammal's foot has adapted to the ecology in which it is situated. The carnivore needs a large mobile foot armed with claws, the prancing goat requires long, slender, and precise hooves, while a leaping lemur benefits from protracted digits and an opposable big toe. It is only our tendency to human exceptionalism that supports the illusion that our mobile to rigid foot is somehow more evolved than the rest.

There are three mechanisms that help draw the bones of the foot together. The first is the form closure of the bones that we saw in chapter 4. The overlapping malleoli of the tibia and fibula create a coupling mechanism at the ankle joint that allows their rotation to transfer to the talus. From the talus, the lateral rotation passes forward through the bones of the foot, leading them to lock together and reform the half-dome. One of the keys to this "form closure" is the lateral rotation of the stance leg, which is driven by the forward swing of the other foot. If you are trying to solve a biomechanical issue in one foot, it is always worth paying attention to what is happening with the foot, hip, and knee of the other leg to be sure they can swing forward enough to drive lateral rotation into the other limb.

The second mechanism that draws the bones of the foot together is the force closure created by the extrinsic soft tissues. Ankle dorsiflexion of the stance leg during gait tensions all the plantar flexors. In chapter 5 we saw how the tendons crossing the back of the talar joint all assist form closure of the foot, drawing the bones together to support their close-packed

---

[1]The safety margin for the femur means that it is able to bend a little further than it is normally required to under everyday loads. Part of the balancing act the body manages in its housekeeping is to produce materials that are fit for purpose and still have a little in reserve.

condition. Supination is encouraged by the bias of tendon support crossing medial to the subtalar axis, with the soleus, tibialis posterior, and flexor hallucis longus being of particular importance. Soleus attaches to the medial calcaneus, tibialis posterior attaches to all the bones in the mid-foot region, while the flexor hallucis longus spans the medial longitudinal arch to go all the way to the big toe. These three muscles create a rearfoot, mid-foot, and forefoot anchorage that provides stability to an increasing number of joints.

The third mechanism that supports supination is the system of the intrinsic muscles. Chapter 6 explored these short muscles and how their various fascial relationships provide advantages through pretensioning of their collagenous tissues. The intrinsic muscles take responsibility for the rigid lever once the heel is lifted and the foot moves into toe extension. Along with the gastrocnemius, the soleus tensions the plantar fascia to support the intrinsic layers of muscle (see fig. 7.6). The intrinsic muscles are further assisted by the initial splaying of the foot as it spreads during stance phase, as the spreading of the bones and the movement into toe extension pretensions the layers of plantar fascia encasing the muscles. Although they are short and small, the positioning and pretensioning of the intrinsic muscles provides them with enough advantages to stabilize the foot during the toe rocker phase.

Almost regardless of what injury or discomfort a client presents with, these three mechanisms are all worthy of investigation, especially in cases of gradual or unexplained onset of symptoms:

1. Can the bones rotate enough?
2. Is there enough dorsiflexion to tension the plantar flexors?
3. Is there enough pretension reaching the intrinsic muscles, and are they strong enough?

An ideal toe-off position will load elastic energy into each of the tissues mentioned above, and then the plantar flexors and toe flexors will all have some degree of free energy to contribute to the swing of the leg once it is released from the ground. The human toe-off creates a catapult position in which elastic energy captured during the movement is then released to contribute to the next leg swing forward. However, a number of interdependent joint ranges have to cooperate to load the catapult as the knee and hip joints both affect movement at the foot.

Optimal load and release of elastic energy at each joint requires correct alignment between all the joints, as well as adequate range of motion at each one. In chapter 7, we saw the sagittal plane preference in our plantar fascia compared with that of our primate cousins, who all have some variation of medial-to-lateral force transfer. Humans track straight ahead into extension of the first and second MTJs, and that final position for toe-off should be aligned to the knee joint and anterior hip.

A quick experiment shows the effect at the hip of a laterally rotated foot at toe-off. Moving into a lunge with your feet in parallel should produce a stretch sensation at either your back calf or the front of the back hip. Moving into the same position with your back foot turned out will reduce the calf sensation and move the hip stretch to the medial tissue.

The tissue at the front of the hip is capable of dealing with high stress, more so than the tissue on the inside of the hip. But how the hip receives the strain is determined by the alignment of the foot and the stable base of the first and second metatarsals. Although the second metatarsal is generally longer than the first, there are two sesamoid bones lying below the first MTJ that balance out the length discrepancy for most of us. Occasionally there may be a structural or functional variance that creates issues with our ability to track through the big toe joint. These differences can be caused by variations in the structural lengths of the metatarsals, functional differences due to increased supination or pronation of the foot, or lack of stability of the first ray.

PROPULSION AND FORCE OUTPUT

Our evolutionary history has left us with the remnants of an opposable, grasping big toe, which means our first ray is less stable than the second and third. The first ray requires extra force closure from its surrounding muscles, as the joints and ligaments do not provide the same level of joint congruence and support as is present along the second ray. We should note that one of the main stabilizers for the base of the first metatarsal is the fibularis longus, which also plantar flexes the bone to provide more range of motion as the MTJ moves into extension. However, fibularis longus crosses the back of the talar joint and therefore requires adequate ankle dorsiflexion during gait to create tension through its fibers—and so we begin to see the interdependence between range of motion, force production, and stabilization.

Not only does the foot have to stabilize itself as it rises on the metatarsal heads, it must also deal with all the other activities that require it to produce, decelerate, and absorb high forces—jumping, landing, and running will push forces many times greater than our body weight through the foot. In most of those movements, the ankle will pass into dorsiflexion and recruit the extrinsic muscles, but many other movements requiring power and stability from the foot may be made from a more neutral ankle position. When that is the case, the joints and local muscles will have to step up and ensure enough mobility, stability, and force can be produced locally, since the strong plantar flexors will not be a position to assist as much.

The most common movement strategy for increasing force is to use a countermovement. By initially moving in the opposite direction, the target tissue is pretensioned and elastic energy is loaded into it in preparation for power production during the return movement. For example, to increase plantar flexor power, we use dorsiflexion; to increase intrinsic foot power, we use foot splay and toe extension.

Allowing the foot to spread and the joints to extend provides stiffness for the supportive fascial tissues and increases intra-compartmental pressure in the foot. Tissue stiffness is generally a neutral feature that, when properly tuned via movement range and muscle tone, can be used to optimize force. However, there is another interplay between joint range, muscle strength, and tissue stiffness: the joint must be capable of enough range to load the tissues; the muscles must be strong enough to control the countermovement and create its correction; and the fascial tissues must be resilient enough to carry the forces involved. Deficit in one either inhibits the whole system or places extra load onto one of the other areas.

ENOUGH AND NOT TOO MUCH

Getting the balance right is not easy. Each of the four dynamics (shock absorption, range of motion, creation of a rigid lever, and force production) require cooperation and coordination, as well as strength and mobility. These are all qualities that can be assessed and improved on. Any training program should incorporate a blend of challenges and, contrary to what you might see on social media, there is no one magical exercise, there are no "rubbish" ones that should be eradicated from the repertoire, and there are no perfect all-rounders.

There are, however, exercises that are incorrectly prescribed, incorrectly executed, and overdone. The cure for all these ills is to understand the reason and intent behind each movement. What does the movement require from the system? And what does the client's system require? Answer those two questions and you are on your way to creating a perfectly matched program.

Key to finding that match is good assessment and observation skills.

Having read through this text, you will be much more aware of the force transfers, the anatomical features, and the rationale for the assessments and exercises presented here. That previous information is the "why"—why are we doing these movements? Why is that assessment important? Why is the foot pointing that way?

What you are about to read is the "how".

▥ ASSESSMENT

I. Shock Absorption

Shock absorption requires the foot to pronate, which is a complex action of multiple joints and many soft tissues. For walking, the main question is whether the subtalar joint can evert or not; for running[2] and landing, shock absorption also requires dorsiflexion. There are numerous ways to assess the foot for its pronation ability and we will work through some of the visual cues first before checking them with passive and active movements.

---

[2]Running form is contested, variable, and, judging from on-line debates, for some an apparently emotive subject. My own preference, and that's all it is so please don't string me up, is for the foot to land below the hip joint with a relatively full contact so the ankle will dorsiflex to deceleration forces into the calf tissues. For more information, I recommend Benzie 2020 & Michaud 2021.

Visual Assessment

After a detailed consultation, it is natural to look at your client's feet. Literature varies on whether to observe gait before or after a static assessment; I think it is better to be flexible rather than follow any fixed rule. Gait assessment is difficult and can be as confusing as it is helpful, so it can make it easier to create a more controllable environment by removing variables. Conversely, sometimes postural assessments or orthopedic tests do not reveal much of interest that links to the clients' story, and having them walk can expose the hidden idiosyncrasies in their movement pattern.

The aim of any assessment is to establish a clear plan for any intervention, whether it is an exercise program or a manual therapy treatment. It is imperative to take your time and find a story that appears to match the client's needs. Work through each area methodically—it is better to spend longer doing a thorough assessment and coming to conclusions than to rush into a program without a clear plan.

With that in mind, there is no specific order to any of these assessment ideas. The order in which they are presented here is a reasonably good one to follow, certainly when first becoming familiar with them. But listing assessments for the format of a book that requires a certain order and unraveling of themes is not the same as being in an organic situation with a client.

During any session, in the assessment phase or not, I am always monitoring what the joints and tissues can do and where they are starting from. If I see a client with a high arched pattern, I do not actually have much information about the functionality of that foot. All I know is that they are starting from a relatively supinated position. They could have lots of range to move into pronation, they could have some pronation movement, or their foot could be stuck and rigid.

On the reverse, a low arch patterned foot might still be able to pronate and supinate, or only one, or neither. Visual assessment should not be a diagnosis, it is only the beginning of building a picture of the feet. But it can be a good anchor to get the therapist started as, unlike gait assessment, there are few confusing variables involved.

Our first question is—where is the foot along the pronation-to-supination scale? There are a number of visual cues to look for and the major indicators are (fig. 8.1):

- **The alignment of the calcaneus**—is it vertical, tilted medially, or tilted laterally? We are assessing the calcaneus because its sustentaculum tali is largely responsible for maintaining the position of the talus, which is often key to the pronation/supination relationship through the foot. This observation is sometimes referred to as the *relaxed calcaneal position*, and a deviation of more than 4° from vertical is sometimes considered an indicator of a pronated-type foot
- **The shape of the Achilles tendon**—is it curved? Often when the calcaneus is medially tilted, the tendon must correct itself to the alignment of the tibia
- **The shape of the forefoot when seen from the back**—are there "too many toes"? Because pronation causes the joints of the foot to rotate, more toes will be visible from the back when compared with a more neutral foot
- **The height of the navicular tuberosity from the floor** (we will assess this further below)

Finding Subtalar Neutral
It can be useful to assess where the talus is in relation to its neutral joint position. The visual indicators listed above will give you some clue, but it can be practical for other tests to find where the talus is and to observe what happens to the foot when the bone is moved into the center of its joints with tibia and fibula.

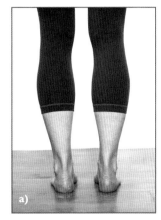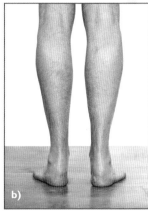

Figure 8.1   *a) The line of the posterior calcaneus should be relatively vertical. b) Medial tilts can be indicative of a pronated-type foot (as shown above). Lateral tilts (not shown) can indicate a supinated-type foot. As we can see in (b), if the calcaneus is tilted one way or the other, the Achilles tendon often bends to align with the soleus and gastrocnemius. The posterior view also allows the therapist to notice how much of the forefoot is visible from behind. More toes will be seen in a truly pronated foot because of the rotation caused by the pronation (as seen in a comparison of a and b). Less of the lateral foot will be visible in the supinated-type foot. A medial view can give some clues to the position of the navicular, which can also be measured by the navicular drop and drift tests below.*

To do this, find the talar head by palpating for the two hollows either side of it (see fig. 8.2), then rotate the leg (on a fixed foot) until the space between the talus and the two leg bones is equal. If the leg had to laterally rotate to find neutral, it is indicative of a pronated-type foot. If the leg had to medially rotate to find neutral, then it is probably supinated.

Navicular Drop
A visual assessment of the foot only provides some clues as to where to investigate further and should not be taken as indicative of any functional capacity. A commonly used metric to measure how much the foot adapts during weight acceptance is to measure the distance the navicular drops in response to weight-bearing.

The navicular tuberosity is a useful landmark because of its visibility and its position at the height of the medial longitudinal arch. As the foot pronates, the sustentaculum tali tilts and

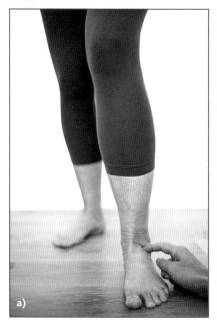
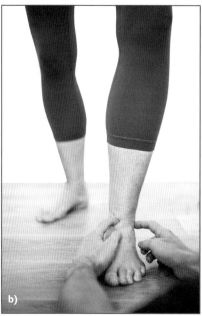
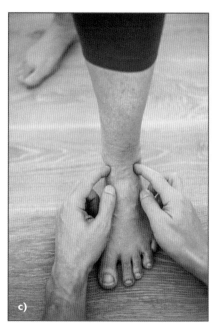

Figure 8.2 **Subtalar Neutral** *a) Take the foot into full pronation to find the fold of the lateral hollow, mark it if necessary. b) Take the foot into full supination to find the medial hollow. c) Place your finger and thumb into the hollows and turn the leg until the hollows feel even on both sides.*

the talus follows, the joint between the talus and the navicular opens, the spring ligament strains, and the navicular follows the talus downward. There should therefore be some movement of the navicular tuberosity during pronation, and it can be easily measured (fig. 8.3):

- Ask your client to sit or shift their bodyweight onto the other leg, place their foot and ankle into subtalar neutral (as above), palpate and mark the tuberosity, and measure the distance between it and the floor to obtain the base measurement

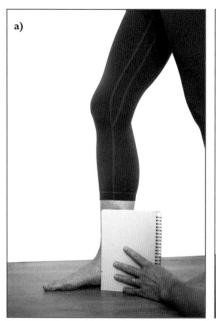
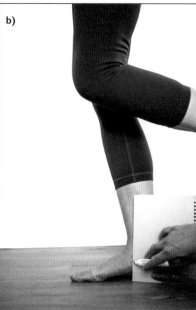
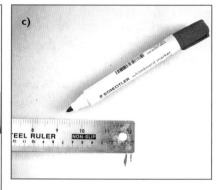

Figure 8.3 **Navicular Drop Test** *a) Have the client non-weightbearing and place their foot into subtalar neutral with a sheet of card under the medial aspect. Place a card along the medial aspect and mark the height of the navicular tuberosity. b) Have the client weight-bear and repeat the measurement, making a mark at the new location of the navicular. c) The card is removed and the distance between the two marks measured.*

- Have the client stand, or weight shift onto the assessed leg, and remeasure the distance between the navicular tuberosity and the floor
- The easiest method is to use a piece of card, as paper is usually too flimsy to control for an accurate reading
- Be sure to re-find the tuberosity for the second measurement as the bone will have moved under the marked skin

A general guideline is that a restricted foot will move less than 5 mm, "normal" is between 5 and 9 mm, and a foot with increased pronation is more than 9 mm (Navicular Drop Test 2020). These measurements are not absolute and need to be put in the context of the actual client. Things to consider are body weight, age, overall strength, and soft tissue health. A 6 mm drop might cause issues for an older person with fragile tissue but is easily managed by a younger person with reasonable muscle strength.

As with most orthopedic tests, there is variance in the published "acceptable ranges" and there is conflict over the reliability of this test. I do not recommend using navicular drop and navicular drift (below) to compare between clients; instead, it is useful to determine the program for a client and to measure their progress or change. As everyone's tissue sensitivity differs, a 6 mm drop will be insignificant to one and create discomfort for another—it will depend on their history.

Navicular Drift
A useful and quick add-on to the Navicular Drop Test is to measure how much the tuberosity "drifts" medially on weight-bearing (fig. 8.4).

To perform the test, start in subtalar neutral and use a card to measure how much the navicular tuberosity travels medially on weight-bearing.

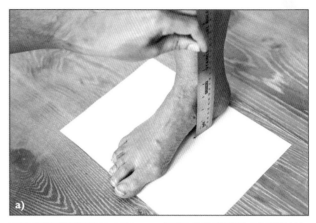

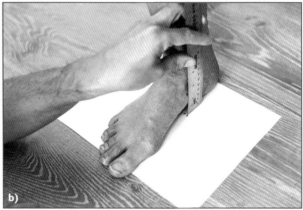

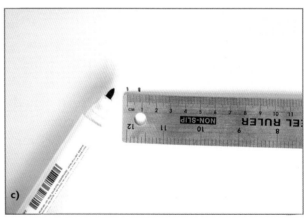

Figure 8.4 **Navicular Drift** *a) Have the client seated and place their foot into subtalar neutral with a sheet of card under the medial aspect. Drop a line directly downward from the navicular tuberosity and make a mark where it lands on the paper. b) Have the client weight-bear and repeat the measurement, making a mark at the new location of the navicular. c) The card is removed and the distance between the two marks measured.*

Measurements for the two tests (navicular drop and drift) can then be compared and, ideally, they should be relatively close to one another. The drop test measures the vertical movement of the navicular, the drift test measures the bone's rotational movement, and there should be a balance between the movement in the two planes.

There are some slight variations in these tests, and opinion is divided regarding their efficacy. They are useful in providing some guidelines and suggestions for exercise possibilities as they can indicate which tissues might be taking more force during shock absorption. Although increased movement of the navicular will strain the spring ligament, other tissues will then be recruited according to the navicular's predominant direction of movement.

For example, if the measurement for drift (transverse plane) is greater than the measurement for drop (sagittal plane), one might consider more rotational exercises to strengthen the decelerators of medial rotation of the bones. If the measurement for drop is the greater, one might consider strengthening both the intrinsic muscles and the muscles passing below the sustentaculum tali and navicular (FHL and tibialis posterior).

Findings that indicate an increased pronation tendency might suggest the presence of an "acquired flat foot". If that is the case, it would lead us to think about the strength of tibialis posterior and its associated plantar flexors, and we could apply the strengthening exercises from chapter 9. Reduced pronation and movement of the navicular would naturally lead us to consider the mobility exercises.

2. Range of Motion

There are three main ways to assess a joint's range—*actively, passively,* and *assisted.* These terms refer to the strategy used to get into position. If the client makes the movement themselves—for example, following an instruction such as "can you bring your toes off the floor"?—the motion is created by their own muscle action and is considered "active".

If the therapist makes the movement for the client—such as when the therapist uses their own fingers to lift the client's toes into extension—the motion is considered passive.

If the therapist helps the client make the movement and some effort is made by both parties, it is considered an assisted motion.

Each type of movement provides different information. An active range of motion test checks the client's ability to create, control, and achieve the range through an active contraction of the associated muscles. Inability to achieve full range during an active movement may not be due to limitations in the joint but caused by other factors, such as muscle weakness or reduced motor control ability. In that case, it might be useful to check their passive motion.

Using a passive test to move the joint allows the therapist to remove many of the variables associated with the client's strength and coordination. Active motion assessments test the muscle's strength and ability to shorten whereas passive motion assessments check the possible joint and tissue range.

If a passive test shows good range but less movement than an active test, it is a good idea to use an assisted movement to guide the client into the range. Assisted movements give both the therapist and client information, as the client's system receives some proprioceptive input from the therapist's guidance, which may help the client reactivate their motor control in that area.

Checking the range of motion at joints provides more information than just the angle through which the joint can move. Every joint has its own unique arrangement of soft and bony tissues and this will determine what happens when the joint reaches its natural end of range—its final "block". The feeling created by easing into that "block" is referred to as the joint's "end feel".

End feel can be assessed during a passive test when the therapist encourages the tissues into their final few degrees of motion. Each tissue type that limits joint range has a distinctive sensation when passively engaged during the assessment. Although categorizations might differ between references, there are five main types of end feel: bony, elastic, ropey, approximation, and empty.

- **Bony End Feel** occurs when two or more bones are brought into contact at the end of range and it will feel "definite", "solid", "absolute". Joints that have a natural bony end feel include knee and elbow extension, and subtalar eversion
- **Elastic End Feel** indicates that musculotendinous tissues are being stretched at the end of range and it will feel "springy", "bouncy", "elastic". Movement ranges that have natural elastic end feels include wrist extension, horizontal abduction of the shoulder complex, ankle dorsiflexion, and toe extension
- **Ropey End Feel** occurs when the passive soft tissues of the ligaments and the joint capsules limit the range. Examples of a natural ligamentous end feel are ulnar and radial deviation of the wrist, and subtalar inversion. These end feelings can be difficult to discriminate from bony end feel as they have a similar "definite" quality to them, but one can learn the subtle differences by comparing the end feel of knee extension (bony) with subtalar inversion (ropey)
- **Approximation End Feel** is when end range is not reached because other tissues get in the way. This happens with elbow and knee flexion, as the biceps of the arm and the calf of the leg get in the way before the joints have moved through their full possible range
- **Empty End Feel** is usually a bad sign as it means there is nothing limiting a bone's motion. This commonly happens in cases of ligament rupture, especially the cruciate ligaments of the knee, and is one of the diagnostic measures of a tear or rupture of the inner supporting structures of the joint.

Because each joint has a natural, normal limiting factor—soft tissue, bone, ligament, or approximation of tissues—any variation from the norm indicates the type of changes that are occurring at the joint. For example, if a joint would normally have a bony or ropey end feel, but an elastic one is felt on palpation, it is likely that the associated soft tissue has become hypertonic for some reason. Conversely, if there should be an elastic end feel but the joint feels as if it brings bones closer together for a solid, bony end feel, then there has been a loss of soft tissue integrity and there may be bony changes around the joint.

For most readers, it is likely that anything other than a normal soft tissue end feel would be beyond the scope of practice and the patient should be referred for a full assessment. An abnormal bony, ropey, approximation, or empty end feel can indicate joint changes, rupture of soft tissue, the presence of inflammation, and loss of joint integrity, respectively. Each of these is worthy of professional guidance.[3]

In the absence of pain, swelling or any other red flags such as recent injury, an elastic end feel is within scope of practice and appropriate mobilization and stretching can be used.

Ankle Dorsiflexion
Movement of the tibia over the talus is a vital part of shock absorption when landing from any kind of jump, leap, or skip. As the tibia moves into dorsiflexion it tensions the extrinsic muscles and recruits the very strong soleus and the Achilles tendon. Although the range (approx. 10° with straight knees and 20° when flexed) is not high, ankle dorsiflexion also plays an important role in supination by tensioning the soleus and deep posterior compartment muscles, lifting the heel, and locking the wider portion of the talus between the malleoli for extra control of the foot.

---
[3]A good resource to explore these topics more is https://www.massagetherapyreference.com/rom-end-feel/.

As the tibia and fibula pass over to the front of the talus (the trochlea/dome) during gait, they also rotate laterally due to the forward swing of the opposite leg. Increased joint congruence between the malleoli and the wider portion of the talus, coupled with tensioning of the plantar flexor tissues, gives form and force closure to the ankle and foot during the forefoot rocker phase.

Talocrural dorsiflexion is easily tested by having the client placed in a lunge-type position with the testing limb back and knee straight (fig. 8.5). It is often performed with a wall in front of the client for extra stability and support.

As the front knee bends forward the assessed (back) ankle should dorsiflex 10 to 15 degrees in response.

Execution of this assessment also gives information about knee and hip extension, and the stability of the rear foot. The client's knee should be able to straighten, and their hip should also extend by 10 to 15 degrees. Lack of range in either of these joints will change how the tissues are loaded during gait and generally lead to decreased efficiency of movement.[4]

As the client performs the test, the therapist can assess the foot's ability to stay in subtalar neutral. When dorsiflexion is limited, the subtalar or midtarsal joints are often recruited to provide some sagittal plane movement. If the subtalar joint is enlisted, the foot is likely to pronate because of the offset alignment of the subtalar joint. Dorsiflexion at the midtarsal joint line causes a midtarsal break. Either of these adaptations will place extra stress onto the passive tissues crossing the associated joints.

With the knee straight, the gastrocnemius will be lengthened, and this is part of the test. If the test is positive (i.e., dorsiflexion is limited),

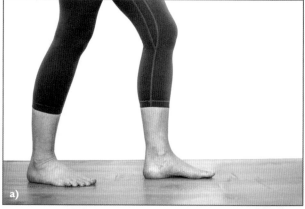

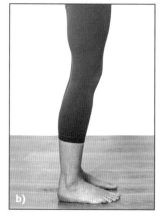
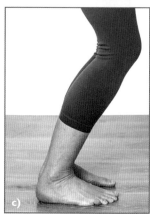

Figure 8.5 **Ankle Dorsiflexion** a) Standing lunge position using a wall for support. The client should be approximately 0.5 m away from the wall. The client bends the front knee slowly forward as the therapist either guides the foot and ankle to maintain subtalar neutral, or the client is cued to track the tibial tuberosity over the second metatarsal. A goniometer, rough visual check, or a postural assessment app can be used to measure the angle (approx. 10°). Note that the back foot should be straight ahead, parallel with the front foot – turning outward slightly, as shown, can be indicative of plantar flexor restriction. b) Repositioning the feet to neutral allows a differential test as the knees flex, c) and progress forward over the second metatarsal. Knee flexion reduces strain on gastrocnemius and should increase the dorsiflexion to approx. 20°.

we do not know which of the plantar flexors might be the limiting factor as it could be any combination of the muscles from the three posterior compartments. By repeating the test with the back knee flexed, we eliminate the two-joint gastrocnemius from the test.

If the test is now negative (i.e., dorsiflexion range is restored), we know to target gastrocnemius in a stretching routine. If knee flexion makes no difference to the test result, then gastrocnemius is less likely to be involved and most of the calf stretches can be

[4]For more detail, see *Born to Walk*, Earls 2020.

performed with a bent knee to target the other plantar flexors.

This test is often performed passively with the client seated or on a treatment table and is sometimes referred to as the Silfverskiöld test after the Swedish surgeon who developed it. The foot is held by the therapist to bring the ankle into dorsiflexion when the client's knee is bent and then dorsiflexion is repeated when the knee is straight. Although the information gleaned can be useful in building the picture of the client's overall functionality, the test has been found to have poor reliability (https://www.physio-pedia.com/Silfverskiold_Test).

Subtalar Inversion/Eversion
To review—talar movement is the relationship between the tibia (and, to a lesser extent, the fibula) and the talus for plantar flexion and dorsiflexion. The subtalar joint is the relationship between the talus and the calcaneus with its axis for inversion and eversion. The subtalar joint has movement in each plane, but least in the sagittal plane (which can be recruited to substitute for loss of dorsiflexion, as above), and the plane of most interest is the frontal.

Frontal plane movement in the subtalar joint allows the calcaneus to medially tilt (evert) on heel strike and revert to neutral again to help lock the foot in supination. Subtalar movement can be observed during long-chain movement, but its frontal plane range is best tested in isolation, with the client lying prone with the knee flexed to approximately 135 degrees (fig. 8.6). The therapist can cup the calcaneus and tilt it medially (eversion) and laterally (inversion). As described above in "end feel", subtalar inversion should have a ropey, ligamentous feel, while eversion should have a more solid, bony end feel caused by the calcaneus encroaching on the lateral malleolus. Although eversion is necessary for pronation to occur, it only has half the range that is available for inversion, partly due to the lower position of the lateral malleolus (Yates 2012).

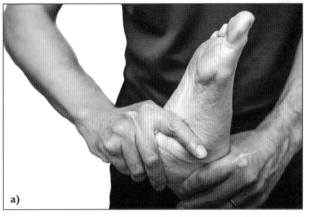
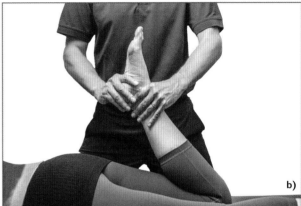
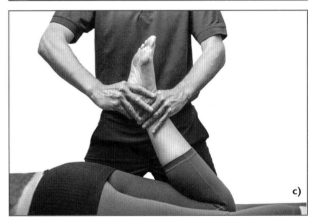

Figure 8.6   **Subtalar Eversion/Inversion** a) One of many assessments of frontal plane motion in the subtalar joint is to place the client prone with the knee bent to 135 degrees. b) The therapist can then cup the calcaneus and tilt it medially into eversion. A normal range is considered to be approx. 10° of eversion. c) A lateral tilt will assess inversion of the subtalar joint in the frontal plane. A normal range is considered to be approx. 20° of inversion.

Toe Extension
Toe extension is the important final position that prepares the foot, knee, and hip tissues for the release of energy for the forward swing of the leg during gait. The first MTJ is a commonly affected joint, and failing to achieve extension at this joint can have significant knock-on

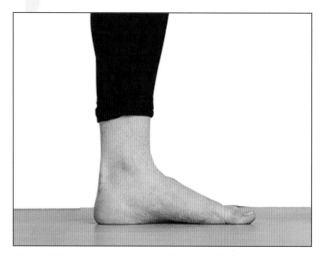

Figure 8.7. *Limited extension of the first MTJ often coincides with some degree of valgus of the big toe. Loss of extension at the MTJ can encourage extension to happen at the interphalangeal joint. We can see how the proximal and distal phalanges have adopted an extended position to create a compensatory "false toe extension", i.e., at the wrong joint. Rolling off the inside of the foot is often caused by reduced MTJ extension and places more stress on the skin along that aspect and the skin grows calluses to protect itself.*

effects along the mechanical chain, both in terms of force alignment as well as energy usage, as we have seen throughout this text.

A visual assessment often gives clues that the big toe joint is restricted, as the first toe may be adducted, its distal phalange might be pointing upward, or there may be callusing on the lateral aspect[5] of the toe (fig. 8.7). A bunion is often associated with limited toe extension, a relationship that might go either direction in terms of cause and effect. If toe extension reduces, the foot might turn outward to compensate, changing the angle of forces at the MTJ. Conversely, if a bunion begins to develop and the toe adducts, the MTJ loses its integrity and reduces its extension.

Reduced toe extension during exercise and gait is easy to spot as it either causes the foot to turn outward as the heel rises or the foot is lifted from the hip muscles to avoid rolling through the toe joints. The first MTJ receives a lot of stress and is one of our most challenged

joints and, as we mentioned above, it relates to other joints further along the chain. Therefore, checking toe extension with at least one form of passive test (fig. 8.8) should be an essential part of a client intake.

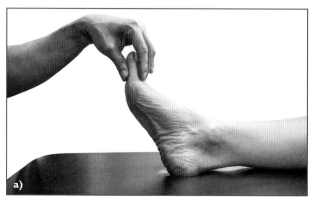

a)

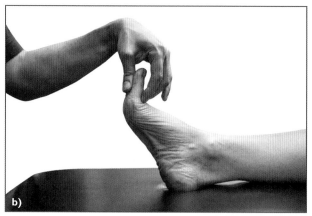

b)

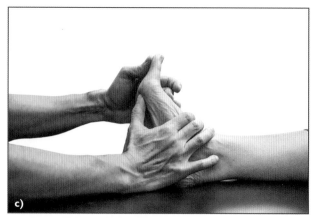

c)

Figure 8.8. **Passive Toe Extension** *a) With the client offloaded, take the proximal phalange between your finger and thumb, and draw it superiorly into extension. b) The MTJ should achieve 55 to 65 degrees of passive extension, and any restriction here exposes the end feel to provide information on the possible cause of the limitation. c) In a passive test, the full range is often accompanied by plantar flexion of the first metatarsal, which is impossible to achieve during gait. A loaded test is therefore necessary to check the joint's functional range.*

---

[5]Lateral to the midline of the foot, not lateral to the midline of the body.

Functionally, MTJ plantar flexion is of less significance and is rarely affected but, to be thorough, one could check that approximately 20 degrees of plantar flexion is available at the first MTJ.

It is tempting to prescribe toe extension exercises and stretches in these cases, but it is important to first rule out any joint and bone involvement. Loss of range can indicate changes in bone growth around the joint, which would contraindicate mobilizing the joint into extension. If osteophytes, or exotoses (see fig. 4.40d), have developed around the joint, they are likely to be further irritated during any forced extension which will stimulate further aberrant bone growth.

Thankfully, a differential passive range test is easy to perform to screen whether toe extension is appropriate for the client. Have your client relax as you draw their MTJ into extension passively. This will allow you to sense the end feel—if it is restricted and bony, do not prescribe stretches and mobilizations for them; if it feels elastic but limited, exercise and stretches will be fine.

The optimal range for first MTJ extension is 55 to 65 degrees, and many people appear to achieve this when performing the above passive test, but it is a false reading due to the drop of the first metatarsal (fig. 8.8a & c). Although the passive test does not mimic the joint's true mechanics during gait, use of this test is necessary to receive clear information regarding the bones.

A functional test is easily performed by having the client stand, and the tested foot in front with the knee bent (fig. 8.9). There should be some amount of body weight on the forward foot and the client may benefit from some balance support, such as a chair or wall. The therapist can then glide their thumb or finger under the distal phalange of the big toe and bring the toe upward, into extension.

This standing test for toe extension is variably referred to as Jack's test or Hubscher's maneuver, and it provides several findings. By placing the therapist's finger or thumb under the distal phalange, the interphalangeal joint is tested for extension, which should only be minimally present, if at all (fig. 8.7). As the MTJ is passively extended, the long and short flexors and plantar fascia tension and provoke

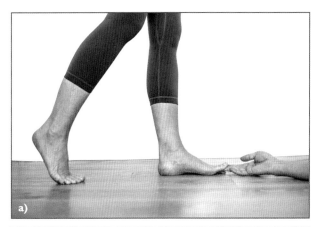

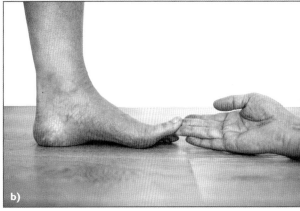

Figure 8.9.   ***Jack's (or Hubscher's) Test.*** *The MTJ of the first toe should be assessed in weight-bearing as well as unloaded. The passive unloaded test above can identify a hallux rigidus, where bone changes have occurred and extension is severely reduced. If unloaded passive range is within normal limits, a functional limit might still be present and requires the foot to be assessed in standing. Limited extension during Jack's test would indicate a hallux limitus, and exercise and stretching would be indicated. a) Have the client stand with the foot to be tested out in front. Provide a support for the client if they need one to aid their balance. b) The therapist slides a finger or thumb under the distal phalange and draws it upward to extend the joints. Adequate range (55 to 65 degrees) of MTJ extension helps engage the windlass mechanism to raise the medial longitudinal arch. Extension of the first MTJ can range up to 90 degrees, which is necessary for those wanting to wear high heels. Using the distal phalange to test the MTJ can expose compensatory extension at the interphalangeal joint (see fig. 8.7).*

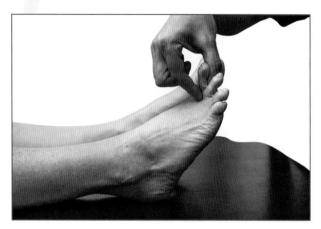

Figure 8.10.   *The other toes are less commonly affected by loss of range but should still be assessed for any abnormalities. The distal interphalangeal joints should each have 60 degrees of plantar flexion, and no dorsiflexion; the proximal interphalangeal joints should have 35 degrees of plantar flexion, and 30 degrees of dorsiflexion. The passive ranges are easily tested using the finger and thumb to control each phalange to isolate the appropriate joints.*

the windlass mechanism for supination of the foot.

While performing the test, the therapist therefore receives information on the integrity of both the interphalangeal and the MTJs, their level of resistance to extension, the quality of end feel at end of range, and the timing of the windlass.

3. Forming an Aligned Rigid Lever

Lack of propulsion during toe-off or walking with a toe-out gait can indicate an "unsupinated" foot. Each of the ranges measured above contribute to the foot's ability to supinate, and any reduction of range will reduce tissue stiffness through the plantar fascia, the posterior and deep posterior compartments, the intrinsic flexors, or some combination of each. Alignment of the foot must be close to the sagittal plane during the toe rocker for each joint and tissue to cooperate fully and create the solid platform needed for the release of energy at toe-off.

Reduced toe extension can lead to toeing out, but other factors can also be involved and require assessment. As we saw in fig. 4.36, the

parabola of the metatarsal heads is different in the human foot compared with other primates' feet and facilitates our sagittal progression in gait. However, there is some degree of normal variation in the lengths of the metatarsals between individuals. In an average array of metatarsals, the second is longer than the first, and then each subsequent metatarsal is gradually shorter as we work outward along the array.

Morton's Foot

The most important length relationship is between the first and second metatarsals, as their heads form the base for the last two points of contact during the toe rocker phase. If one is longer than the other, it will cause the foot to twist as it rises into toe extension (fig. 8.11). As we will see below, callus patterning on the foot can be a sign to check the relative positions of the two MTJ joints, as an imbalance causes uneven stress on the skin.

Morton (1935) was the first to seriously document the significance of altered metatarsal length, and devoted quite a few pages in both his books to the reasoning and assessment for what is now known as "Morton's foot". Some current references also refer to a longer second

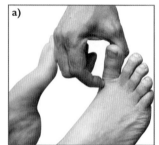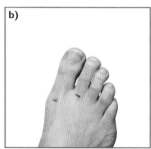

Figure 8.11.   *To check for the presence of Morton's foot, a) have the client relaxed and check for secondary signs of length differences and then, b) flex the joints to expose the position of the metatarsal heads. There should be a 1–2 mm difference between the ends of the two bones, as the shortness of the first metatarsal is compensated for by the two sesamoids lying below the joint. These two floating bones give a platform on which to rest the first metatarsal head and balance the lengths of the two metatarsal bones. A conservative treatment to alleviate any related dysfunction is to have a "Morton's extension" fitted by a podiatrist. The small pad of the extension is placed under the first MTJ and compensates for its lack of length, and evens out the imbalance between the adjacent joints.*

toe as "Morton's toe", but this is not something I have found in his writings. A longer second toe does not interfere with gait mechanics in the same way that a longer second metatarsal does. The important and defining feature of Morton's foot is the position of the MTJ, which is quite independent of the length of the phalanges.

A longer second toe is, however, an issue for shoe fitting. Most people size their shoes according to the space between the big toe and the end of the shoe and rarely check the available space for the second. Habitual wearing of ill-fitting footwear can lead to extra stress at the distal phalange, especially after walking downhill when the foot is pushed forward in the shoe, and can lead to deformity of the second toe joints. The cure for this is easy—buy shoes that fit the second toe, not just the first.

Mobility of the First Ray

The variation of tethering by the transverse ligament between the first and second rays was mentioned in the previous chapter. Possibly a hangover from our ancestral prehensile foot, the first ray has a tendency to lose much of its natural anchoring and become hypermobile. An unstable first ray has a similar effect as the Morton's foot above, and the two conditions often coincide.

Mobility along the MTJ should follow a predictable pattern that can be assessed by holding adjacent joints and moving them forward and back past one another. There should be considerable mobility between the fifth and fourth joint, less mobility between the fourth and third, and least mobility between the third and second. Mobility then increases again between the first and second joint, but it is only a matter of a few degrees of freedom. It is only by doing the test on a range of feet that one becomes familiar enough with the general feel of average mobility to be able to make the distinction between a hypermobile and normal ray without seeking supporting evidence such as the tests shown in figs. 8.11 & 8.12.

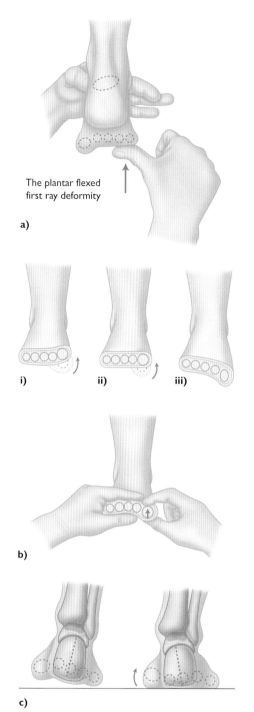

The plantar flexed first ray deformity

a)

i)   ii)   iii)

b)

c)

Figure 8.12. ***First Ray Mobility.*** *(a) When the foot is aligned in neutral and the first ray remains below the level of the others, it should be checked for mobility, (b) if it is hypermobile and rises above the level of the others (i–iii), it can create instability of the first ray and lead to pronation. If it is fixed, (c) the reverse will occur, and the foot will progress into supination as it is forced laterally. When the first metatarsal is only semi-mobile, coming into line with the others, impact forces will be transferred to the underlying sesamoids, creating inflammation that may lead to other compensations and limping. Resolution of these patterns may involve the fibularis longus, as well as manipulation of the joints, if they are restricted. (Adapted from Michaud 2011.)*

Callus Formation

The foot has evolved over many millions of years to transfer force effectively and efficiently. It has created many adaptive measures to allow a range of locomotor patterns that are reflected in the soft tissue and joint alignments. As we have emphasized throughout the book, the body adapts to the forces it is exposed to, and when the natural sequence goes awry, the foot can put defenses in place. The first and most common line of defense is the formation of calluses—hardening of the skin that is receiving more than its fair share of stress (fig. 8.13).

Similar patterns will be revealed on regularly worn shoes. At first sight, an expert reading of wear patterns can seem like reading tea leaves, but there is logic and rationale to the patterns of wear. The easiest callus pattern to explain is

that of Morton's foot, as the second metatarsal being longer than the first will create an area of high stress under its single point of contact during the toe rocker phase. The single point of support causes a line of callusing if the foot keeps going straight ahead, or a circular pattern if the foot rotates.

The pinch callus is a common formation on the side of the big toe, often around the interphalangeal line, and is associated with limited toe extension. The pinch is caused by the foot rolling over the side of the toe rather than extending straight ahead.

Each callus formation is a reliable indicator of how the repetitive forces of gait are traveling through the foot, as the skin has adapted to that force pattern for a reason. The callusing might not indicate the precise reason, but it does tell you where the forces are acting.

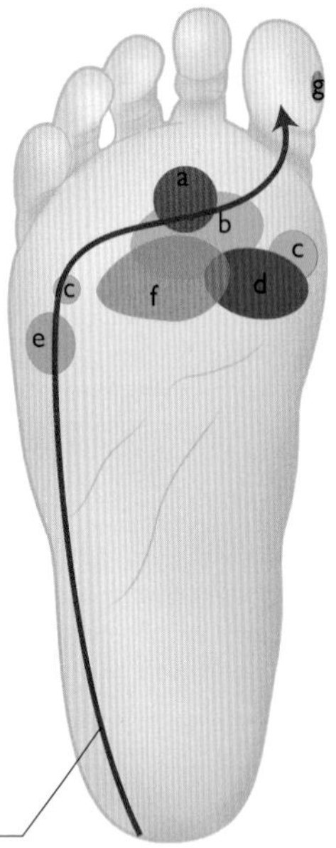

4. Propulsion and Force Output

Our movement is the outcome of interactions between the skeletal, fascial, and muscular systems, coordinated by the nervous system in response to forces. Achieving the rigid lever for toe-off requires coordinated input from each of those systems.

If the ligaments and joints allow a predominantly sagittal progression, we come onto the heads of the first and second metatarsals for what is considered a "high gear" toe-off, as all the flexor myofascia of the foot, knee, and hip can be recruited for forward propulsion. But if we deviate across onto the lateral metatarsal heads and into a "low gear" toe-off, fewer myofascial units can be used, and they will be recruited with less efficiency.

Tracking through each rocker therefore provides the foot-locking mechanisms, the tissue tensioning, and the aiming for release of energy at toe-off. To take advantage of

A – Under head of second metatarsal (linear or circular)—can be indicative of Morton's foot

B – Across the ball of the foot—check for hypermobility of the first ray

C – Under the fifth and first metatarsal heads—check for rigid and/or plantar flexed first ray

D – Under the first and second metatarsal heads—check for semi flexible first ray

E – Under the fifth metatarsal head— check for plantar flexed fifth ray

F – Across the ball of the foot—check for toe walking, restricted dorsiflexion, and tight calf muscles

G – Outer edge of the big toe—(pinch callus)—check for reduced toe extension

Line of force progression during stance phase (heel strike to toe-off)

Figure 8.13. **Callus Formation** *a) Morton's foot can cause linear or circular callusing under the second metatarsal head. b) An unstable first ray will also put more stress under the second metatarsal head or the wider area of the ball of the foot. A "pinch callus" on the outer edge of the great toe can be caused by loss of toe extension (see also fig. 8.7). c) Callusing under the first and fifth metatarsal heads may indicate a rigid plantar flexed first ray. d) Callusing around the ball of the foot and head of the first metatarsal can be caused by a semiflexible first ray. e) Pressure caused by a plantar flexed fifth ray can result in callusing under the head of the fifth metatarsal. f) Toe walking or overly tight plantar flexors places extra pressure across the whole of the forefoot.*

these benefits, we still must have the strength to control the foot through its various stages. As we have seen, different muscle groups are involved during the stance phase, initially it is the extrinsic plantar flexors and then responsibility passes to the intrinsic flexors.

An easy way to assess for overall strength and control is to have the client perform double- and then single-legged heel raises (fig. 8.14). This simple assessment will test the strength

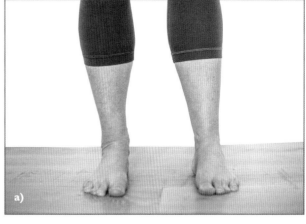

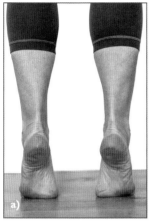 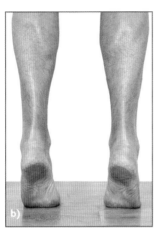
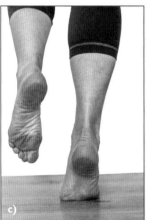 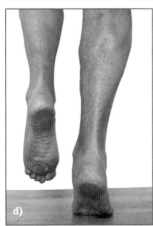

Figure 8.14. **Calf Rise.** *To assess plantar flexor strength, ask the client to raise their heels so they balance on their metatarsal heads. Relative strength of the muscle groups can be assessed by the number of repetitions that can be done with good form (see also chapter 9). a) From the back you can assess the tilt of the heel, the height of the rise, and the direction of toe extension. b) Here we see how both heels have laterally tilted – which may indicate the ability to supinate but we should also note how both feet have rolled outward to extend along the heads of metatarsals 2–5. c) A similar assessment can be made with a single heel rise. d) Placing more demand on the foot and ankle complex exposes the potential plantar flexor weakness.*

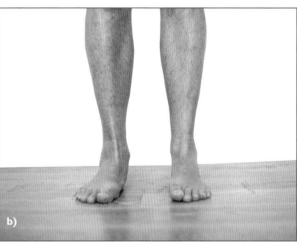

Figure 8.15. **Using Rotation to Assess Pronation & Supination.** *Standing in neutral and turning to the left should cause the right foot to pronate and the left foot to supinate, as the rotation of the pelvis causes the bones of the left leg to laterally rotate and the ones of the right leg to medially rotate. As we have discussed previously, the movement of the tibia and fibula is then coupled to the talus and into the foot because of the mortise and tenon relationship between the malleoli and the talus. The quality of the pronation and supination within each foot can be assessed using this movement but it is particularly useful to observe the ability of the lateral aspect of the supinating foot to open. The lateral band of the plantar fascia and the fibularis brevis span the gap between the calcaneus and styloid process of the fifth metatarsal. Any restriction in that area might benefit from the "figure-of-8" movements, foot wringing, and "knee-clock" exercises from chapter 9. In comparing the feet of (a) and (b), we can see how the pronation of the right foot causes a folding across the ankle in both but more drop can be seen on the medial aspect in (b)—the navicular drop test above could be used to give a starting baseline to measure changes from any prescribed exercises. The twist through the supinating left feet causes the calcaneus to move away from the styloid process and lifts the medial longitudinal arch for both (a) and (b). (a) shows less ability to pronate in the right foot but moving into supination appears significantly better (b), who also struggles to maintain floor contact with the great toe. Generally, the two samples shown here are indicative of the need for more mobility (a) and more stability (b).*

of both muscle groups and reveal information about joint tracking, while also providing immediate feedback to the client on their own strength and abilities.

As you assess the tilt of the calcaneus during the rise, remember the arrangement of the tendons crossing the subtalar joint in chapter 5. The deep posterior compartment and the soleus cross the inside of the joint and lift the sustentaculum tali to invert the heel; the fibularii cross on the opposite side and evert it. As the heel lifts, we want to see the heel invert—an indication of a strong and supportive tibialis posterior, FDL and FHL especially.

Rotation—Supination and Pronation

It is possible to have the strength for a heel raise but not possess the ligamentous length required for a supinated rigid lever. In chapter 2, we saw the lengthening required of the foot's lateral aspect as it evolved into our modern half-dome shape. During pronation, the inside of the foot lengthens as the joints open and the soft tissues absorb shock while the lateral aspect, especially the space between the calcaneus and the styloid process, shortens. To resupinate the foot, the reverse must happen as the joints, ligaments, and tendons allow the lateral aspect to lengthen again.

It is common for the lateral aspect of the foot to be restricted, and this can be assessed using a simple rotation (see fig. 8.15). Standing in neutral and turning the body one way will drive the feet into pronation on one foot and supination on the other. Since the movement starts from a neutral position, the tendons are not stretched and the movement is primarily testing the ability of the bones and ligaments to adapt.

■ SUMMARY

Having a clear idea of what is happening with the client's foot empowers the creation of a treatment plan. We should begin each session with a good understanding of which joints are restricted, which are safe and unsafe to stretch and mobilize, and which muscles might need extra strengthening.

Having an understanding of the general principles of assessment, how to do them, and knowing what kind of information can be gained through the different movements and end feels, arms the therapist with a vocabulary that can relate the limits, actions, and tracking deviations to the tissues. The assessments given above are far from comprehensive, the foot is a complex mechanical area and a lifetime of study is required to thoroughly appreciate it. But familiarizing yourself with the *principles* rather than the *mechanics* of each orthopedic test will position you for greater understanding when it comes to observing natural movement.

I recommend reading the above chapter at least once more, not necessarily to learn the assessment specifics but to follow the logic of what happens when movement is performed in certain ways and how the tissues—bone, ligament, or muscle—should react. The information is not a collection of arcane rules and regulations, just anatomical common sense. Grasping the common sense of the anatomical and functional arrangements will make further study of nuanced assessments much easier.

9

FOOT EXERCISES AND MOBILIZERS

Chapter authored by Lucy Wintle. See her biography on page 248.

> Wings are like dreams. Before each
> flight, a bird takes a small jump,
> a leap of faith, believing that its wings
> will work. That jump can only be made
> with rock solid feet.
>
> —J.R. Rim

> The intrinsic muscles are largely
> ignored by clinicians and researchers.
> As such, these muscles are seldom
> addressed in rehabilitation programs.
> Interventions for foot-related problems
> are more often directed at externally
> supporting the foot rather than
> training these muscles to function
> as they are designed.
>
> —McKeon et al. 2014

How many of us are guilty of neglecting our feet? Over the years we have been preoccupied with toning our glutes, sculpting our waists, working on our alignment and our posture, but until recently how many of us stopped to take notice of our feet and their relevance to everything we do in weight-bearing exercise? One thing we probably all agree on, having got this far in the book, is that this needs to change—while we might not want "rock solid feet" in the literal sense, we certainly want and need strong, adaptive feet that are capable of managing the stresses and strains of life.

I often think to myself, as I watch the myriad of "ever-more-challenging" exercises that we are bombarded with on a daily basis on social media "what is the point of that complexity if some of the simple tasks involved in standing, walking, and balancing cannot be achieved in the first place"?

Paying regular attention to correcting your foot patterns will pay significant dividends in the end, not only for your feet, but also for the rest of your body. It may take time to notice some of the changes, but a consistent approach will pay off in the long term. Some of the benefits you may notice, if you continue regular practice, are improved strength of your ankles, knees, and pelvis, better lumbo-pelvic stability, and better balance.

The exercises included in this chapter do not set out to be fancy or complicated, rather they are designed as a framework to point you in the right direction and lead you into enquiry.

Having read chapter 8 on assessment techniques, you should have a good idea of what your foot type is and therefore what your starting point is. Every foot will be starting from a different place and have its own story to tell. Fractures, sprains, shoe types, repetitive sports, and environment all contribute to the ecosystem of the foot. Do not forget that you are unique, and your foot might not tolerate what the person next to you finds easy!

I have divided the exercises into two basic categories: those that help strengthen the foot and those that aim to release—and a few of the exercises will do both.

As with all exercise that you undertake for the first time, it is essential to pay attention to your form, listen to your body, and not work through any pain. The number of repetitions quoted are a guideline and could prove too much as you begin your foot exercise journey. Always err on the side of caution and increase the repetitions as your awareness and strength build. It is better to do two or three of the exercises really well, rather than rushing through all of them.

Here is a list of the props required to complete all the exercises:

1. A small soft ball approximately the size of a squash ball.
2. A tennis ball or something of a similar size.
3. Length of elastic or resistance band.
4. A yoga brick or book with a depth of approximately 8 cm.
5. Although not essential, you might benefit from a small wedge if you have a particularly pronated or supinated foot— the type used as a doorstep will probably suffice.

Now you are set to go. Enjoy your voyage of foot discovery!

■ FOOT STABILIZATION EXERCISES

1. General Foot Awakening

This exercise is designed to bring awareness into the foot by stimulating the mechanoreceptors embedded within the skin on the sole, and to "open" the foot in preparation for further exercises. You may find that by working on the feet in this way, you are also bringing a sense of ease into other parts of your body. Maybe your pelvis or your lower back feels different? There is no right or wrong with this exercise…just what feels good!

Use a soft or hard ball of your choice, approximately the size of a squash ball, for this foot stimulation exercise. Standing on a hard surface will produce better results (fig. 9.1a).

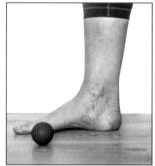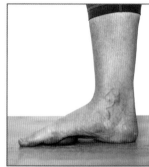

Figure 9.1a. Use your body weight to press down on the ball, applying appropriate pressure.

- Press and release the ball under the base of each toe (the head of each metatarsal)— starting with the big toe and moving out to the fifth toe (or vice versa). Move into the dome of the foot, still pressing and releasing, positioning the ball toward the lateral, then middle, then medial sides of the transverse arch. Repeat the process a few times.
- Now press into the ball and trace random patterns all over the sole of the foot, stopping at any places of "interest". Try to make these movements slow and methodical. Cover as much of the foot as you can in this exploration, bearing in mind that the lateral side of the foot has less soft tissue than the medial.

Once you have finished one foot, take a moment in standing to sense any difference between the two sides of your body. Do you feel more grounded on the foot you have stimulated? Maybe you have a better sense of connection to the floor with your toes, and you are more able to spread and lengthen them?

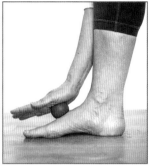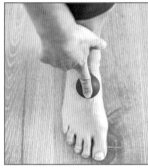

Figure 9.1b.   Trace a line between each metatarsal to gently spread the tissue between them.

- For the next stage, place the ball on the top of your foot. Choose a position that is comfortable for you to use your hand to work the ball between each metatarsal, such as a kneeling position with one foot out in front. Start at the ankle and gently press the ball from the ankle to the toes in between the metatarsals with a light pressure (fig. 9.1b). Repeat two or three times on each foot.

Your foot should now feel grounded, open, and released, providing you with a good sense of feedback from the surface on which you are standing.

2. Foot Clocks, Figure of 8, and Finding Your Tripod of Balance

By shifting where your weight is over your foot, this simple combination of movements will help you find a neutral or centered position in the foot. Taking the weight into different parts of the foot might highlight which movement is a challenge and what feels like familiar territory.

Foot Clocks
Begin with your pelvis in neutral and your feet hip-width apart. Keep both legs straight without locking your knees, and your torso lined up over your legs. Try not to let yourself be drawn into any side flexion or hip flexion.

- Shift your weight laterally to the right. Your right subtalar joint will evert and the left will invert. These are small movements. Keep your toes and metatarsal heads on the floor to encourage more subtalar movement.
- Now take your weight forward onto both sets of toes and metatarsal heads—your whole body is shifting anteriorly, and your ankles are slightly dorsiflexing (fig. 9.2a).
- Shift your weight to the left. Now your left foot is supinating, and your right is pronating (fig. 9.2b).
- Finally, shift posteriorly—sending your weight very slightly into the back of your heels.

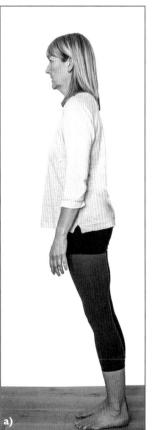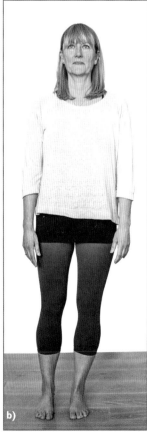

Figure 9.2a & b.   Use the feedback from the ground to sense how the shifts of weight travel into your pelvis.

Compare the range of movement and sense of support between the forward and back sway—our long forefoot provides much more range to shift our bodyweight forward than back.

Repeat the circle four times in each direction.

Figure of 8 and Tripod of Balance

• Using small shifting movements as above, draw a lateral figure of 8 (∞). Move laterally to one side, then forward, then medially back to the heel of the opposite foot, and out laterally again.

Repeat four times in one direction before you change and go the other way.

These movements are tiny (for me they are about the size of a golf ball). As you progress through the figure of 8, try to feel the shift of weight traveling into your pelvis and remember to keep your toes and metatarsal heads on the floor.

At the end of the circles and figure of 8, find a place of balance where your weight is evenly distributed underneath the base of your first and fifth metatarsals and the center of your heel. Feel how your right foot supports the right side of your body and your left foot supports the left side. We will refer to this weight distribution under the foot as the tripod of balance—your neutral and centered position. We will refer to the tripod as we progress through the following exercises. It should not feel like an effort to maintain a neutral foot position, rather you should have a sense of ease.

3. Toe Extension Exercise—Stepping Through
Prop—Small Soft Ball or Wedge

* Avoid this exercise if you know you have joint or bone limitations in your first MTJ (see chapter 8).

The ability to extend your first MTJ is vital to many functions of the foot. The movement in this exercise will help you assess the range and quality of movement in that joint. The exercise will also prepare the basic biomechanics of the foot for the exercises that follow.

Begin with your feet in a split stance i.e., one foot in front of the other, a natural hip distance apart.

• To extend the toes of the right foot, start with the right foot forward. Step forward with your left foot, leaving your right foot behind you and rising onto the toes of the right foot (fig. 9.3a). Try to keep the head of the first metatarsal on the floor to create extension of the MTJ at the base of the big toe.

Repeat several times before changing sides.

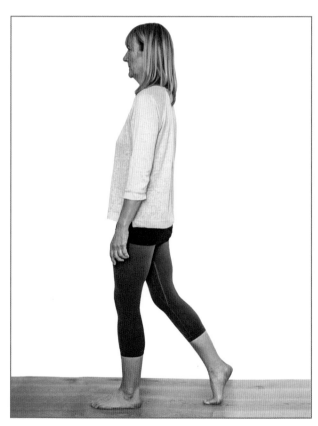

Figure 9.3a. Feel how hinging at the first MTJ tensions the plantar surface of the foot to assist with the windlass mechanism.

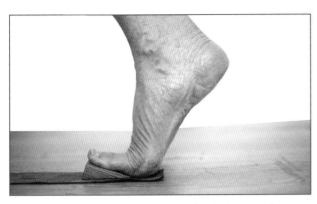

Figure 9.3b.   The addition of a prop under the big toe will create more toe extension at the MTJ.

- If you have the range of movement available in your first MTJ, you can advance this exercise by placing a prop underneath the pad of the big toe (not the metatarsal), see fig. 9.3b for placement. The prop can be either a small soft ball or a wedge that can slide under your toe with the thin end toward the first MTJ. Positioning the prop under your toe will increase the amount of dorsiflexion that occurs during the movement. Now repeat the above exercise, once again making sure the base of the metatarsal head stays in contact with the floor.

Repeat × 6 on each foot.

4. Bi-Lateral Heel Raises—Knees Extended

A straight leg heel raise will target the gastrocnemius muscle of the posterior compartment along with the long and short toe flexors. Keep your toes planted into the floor as you rise up and lower down.

- Find the tripod of balance for the feet with the feeling of even weight on all three points.
- Lengthen the toes to ensure they are not gripping or clawing on to the floor.
- You may opt to hold on lightly with one hand to a wall or other suitable prop at shoulder height. However,

resist the temptation to use this to lever yourself up.
- Now rise onto the heads of the metatarsals and maintain the position for a count of two seconds (fig. 9.4a).
- Slowly descend, keeping the toe pads in contact with the floor.

Repeat × 8

Note that it is better to hold on to something and achieve a full heel raise rather than to struggle with your balance!

To give a more full-body integration aspect to this exercise it can be helpful to initiate the movement by pressing the toe pads into the floor and lightly engaging the pelvic floor and deep abdominal muscles. This will give a sense of "internal" lift and may make the exercise easier for you. A comparison with and without pelvic floor/abdominal integration can help you decide if it is a valid inclusion or not.

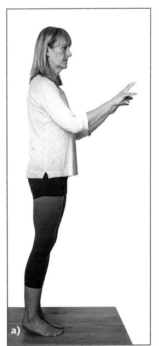
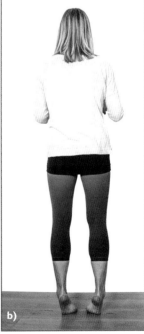

Figure 9.4.   (a) What is your starting point? If your weight is naturally more on your heels, you will feel more challenge as you lift off. If your weight is more forward, you may be more likely to fall forward slightly as you rise up. Hold on to a support if you cannot rise up. (b) If your foot supinates as shown, try to drive more weight onto the first MTJ and medial side of your foot.

Once you have completed the Short Foot exercise, 9.6 (this page), you may be able to feel how the pelvic floor can be integrated into exercises, using the feet as the point of initiation. While a whole book could be written on the pelvic floor, within the scope of this chapter we are simply concerned with how a subtle engagement of those muscles can help with exercises that require balance, lift, and control of the lumbo-pelvic area.

5. Bi-Lateral Heel Raises—Knees Flexed

Repeat the previous exercise with the knees slightly flexed. The bend of the knee makes this exercise target the soleus rather than the two-joint gastrocnemius. This exercise can be of particular benefit to anyone with an unstable, pronated type foot, as it can target the soleus, which attaches to, and can therefore support, the medial aspect of the calcaneus.

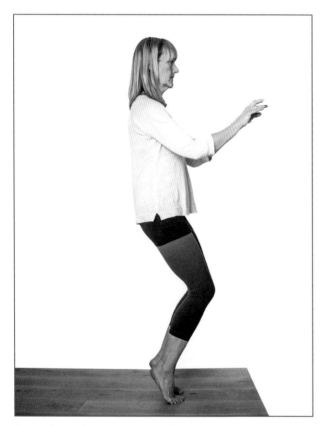

Figure 9.5. *Can you rise up and down slowly with control with your knees slightly bent?*

- Begin with the tripod of balance of each foot.
- Bend the knees then rise onto the metatarsal heads. Try not to straighten the legs as you rise (fig. 9.5).
- Slowly lower the heels back down onto the floor, keeping the knees bent.

Repeat × 8

Be mindful of your alignment as you do this. Keeping the tibial tuberosity lined up with the second toe helps to maintain ankle-joint centration and prevent the foot from pronating or supinating.

6. Short Foot—Stacking the Domes

The exercise known as "Short Foot" was originally described by Vladimir Janda (in Page et al. 2014). It got its name from the action of the foot doming up, which shortens the length and increases the height of the foot at the same time. A number of experiments have shown the Short Foot exercise to be useful in building strength of the intrinsic muscles and raising the half-dome of the foot (Hutchinson 2018; McKeon et al. 2014).

As we saw in chapter 7, increasing the tone of the plantar intrinsic muscles can help support the arches of the foot, increasing the height of the longitudinal arch, and the navicular. When the foot arch becomes stronger, it is better equipped to adapt to the loads and stresses placed upon it by activities of daily life and sports.

In the past, much emphasis has been placed on training the pelvic floor and deep abdominal muscles to improve lumbo-pelvic stability. Now we need to look at training the plantar intrinsic muscles to give the foot arches the stability they need and deserve.

The following exercise is subtle in its approach, encouraging you to isolate the muscles of the superficial group of the four foot layers—

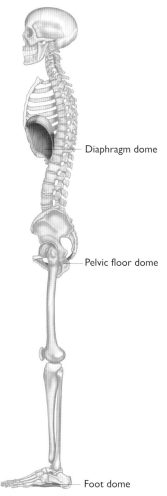

Figure 9.6.   *The body can be visualized as a series of domes—those of the foot, pelvic floor, and diaphragm.*

abductor hallucis longus, flexor digitorum brevis, and quadratus plantae. Similar exercises involve picking things up with your feet or scrunching a towel or band, but these tend to recruit flexor hallucis longus and flexor digitorum longus, which are extrinsic muscles. The Short Foot exercise is more intrinsically focused and subtle.

After some initial practice with this exercise, and you sense the intrinsic foot muscles engaging, you can incorporate that connection into further work to focus on strengthening the medial longitudinal arch of the foot. In this exercise, we are integrating the engagement of the intrinsic foot muscles, pelvic floor, and diaphragm.

Short Foot Starting Position
Stage 1—Foot Dome

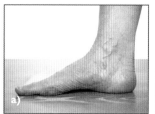 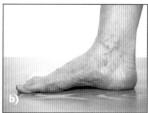

Figure 9.7.   *From its relaxed position (a), the longitudinal arch will gently lift as you engage your intrinsic muscles (b).*

- Find your tripod of balance.
- Gently press the pads of the toes down into the floor. Subtly draw the heel toward the metatarsal heads, and the metatarsals heads toward the heel, feeling the soft tissue in the arches of your feet doming up slightly (fig. 9.7b). Release and allow the arch of the foot to relax down. Try not to claw your toes or lock your knees. If you struggle to feel any activity in your feet, try visualizing the lift of the domes as you perform the exercise.

Repeat × 4

Stage 2—Pelvic Floor Dome
- As you lightly press the toes into the floor and lift the dome of the foot, pull up with the pelvic floor muscles. Visualize an up-doming of the sling of muscles that runs from the pubic bone to the tailbone and between the two sitting bones. An internal integration and, in some cases, a lift might be felt as the muscles engage.

Repeat × 4

Stage 3—Diaphragm Dome
- Breathe out as you lightly press the toes into the floor and lift the domes of the feet and the pelvic floor. Empty all the air out of your lungs and feel the diaphragm gently dome up. This will create a feeling of the cylinder around your torso shrinking slightly as the air is emptied out of the lungs. At the end of the out breath, all the domes are in their "up" position.

- Breathe in gently to relax the domes back down.

The key to success with this exercise is not to try too hard. Initially, it will be a challenge to achieve the three steps in a synchronized and integrated manner, unless you are used to this kind of "inner" work. Even then, this might be a different way of approaching the "core", especially when initiating the movement from the foot.

You can teach this exercise on its own initially, but as it becomes easier to synchronize the muscles of the foot with the muscles of the pelvic floor and abdominals, you can employ it as the basis of many other exercises, particularly those that require balance or power. For example, later in this chapter you will be challenging your balance by standing on one leg. Try to integrate your intrinsic foot muscles by engaging the Short Foot on the standing foot.

Movement practitioners may find that any poses that require balance on one leg (such as the Tree pose in yoga) will be enhanced by the integration of Short Foot. Any discipline which focuses on axial elongation will benefit, as will exercises where power is generated to move away from the floor, such as squats and lunges. Focusing on the foot will pay dividends.

This exercise can also be a nice way of focusing on postural alignment. For example, if either the pelvis or rib cage is displaced by a postural shift, the misalignment can affect the integration of the "domes". This can be a good exercise for feeling the internal connections that good alignment allows.

 Integration sequence

7. Bi-Lateral Heel Raises With Knees Extended and Ball Positioned at the Medial Calcaneus

The following exercise focuses on the tibialis posterior and the intrinsic muscles of the foot, both of which are extremely important for maintaining strength and height of the half-dome.

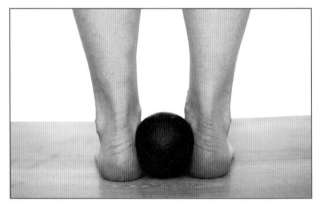

Figure 9.8a. *With your feet in parallel, place a ball behind the medial malleoli and hold it in place by squeezing the two heels together.*

- Place a tennis-sized ball on the floor, between your heels (fig. 9.8a).
- Find the foot's tripod of balance with the feeling of even weight on all three points.
- Lengthen the toes to ensure that there is no toe gripping or clawing on the floor.
- You may opt to hold on lightly with one hand to a wall or other suitable prop at shoulder height. However, resist the temptation to use this to lever yourself up.
- Rise up onto the heads of the metatarsals. As you do so, squeeze the ball between the heels, bringing the calcaneus into a lateral tilt and therefore encouraging the foot into supination and the "rigid lever" position (fig. 9.8b).

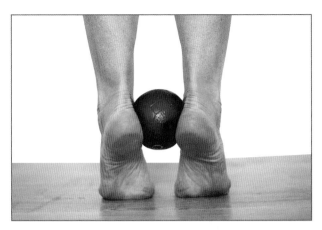

Figure 9.8b. *Actively drive the heels into the ball to create the "rigid lever".*

- Slowly descend, releasing the squeeze on the ball and letting the calcaneus return to its neutral position. The toes should not extend as you find your tripod of balance.

Repeat × 12

8. Single-Leg Stance—Transfer of Weight Onto One Foot

Standing on one leg is an essential part of walking successfully. The ability of your foot to adapt to the weight transfer and increased load of single-leg stance is vital, not just for the feet, but for strengthening your hips and lumbar muscles as well.

We can also examine two different strategies to explore balance—dynamic or static—and both can be equally beneficial. Initially, when one comes to single-leg balance exercises, the foot will feel unstable and will wobble quite a lot—that is normal and forms the initial stages of the strengthening and proprioceptive re-training. An aim might be to have a stable foot, but that would also require the rest of the body to stabilize above it. As the source of much proprioceptive input and the only contact between the ground and the body, the foot is continually reacting to changes in the body's center of gravity. Balance training creates a strong and intelligent foot by challenging the fine control of the intrinsic muscles.

Stage 1
- Begin standing with your feet a little less than hip-width apart, your hands either by your side, or, for more feedback from your pelvis, on your iliac crests.
- Find the tripod of balance of both feet.

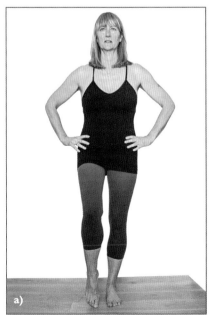 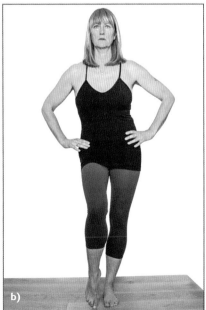 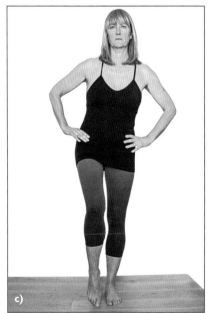

Figure 9.9. *a) As you hold the position, be mindful of how your pelvis balances on top of your standing leg. (b & c) Numerous compensations can occur around the hip joint that encourage the pelvis to drop or shift too much.*

- To lift the right foot from the floor, accept the weight into your left foot and hip. Engage the "Short Foot" dome under your left foot for stability and balance, and slowly peel your right foot up onto the tip of your big toe (bringing your right hip and knee into flexion). Rest the tip of your toe lightly on the floor (see fig. 9.9a).

Assess this position before going to the next stage. Can a neutral lumbo-pelvic position be maintained? How has your left foot adapted to the extra weight-bearing? Has your foot pronated and therefore the medial longitudinal arch collapsed? If this is the case, the height of your navicular will have dropped, and you can assess by how much as per the navicular drop and drift assessments in chapter 8. If that is the case, work on strengthening and stabilizing your foot more before moving on to the next stage.

Stage 2

- With the big toe of your right foot very lightly touching the floor, slowly lift your right knee, creating more flexion in the right hip and knee (fig. 9.9d). If you can successfully maintain your balance and height of the arch, add a further challenge by slowly lowering and lifting your right leg to lightly tap the floor with your big toe. Adding the movement of the free leg provides extra strength and motor control challenge to the exercise.

If you are having difficulty controlling the foot in the frontal plane and the calcaneus is excessively medially tilting (foot pronating), then providing a small prop like a thin door wedge or folded small cloth under the medial aspect of your calcaneus (fig. 9.9e) might help to bring your foot into a more stable position. Continue with the exercise and reassess the stability of your foot and the balance in your pelvis. Has the use of the prop enabled you to recruit your gluteus medius more successfully

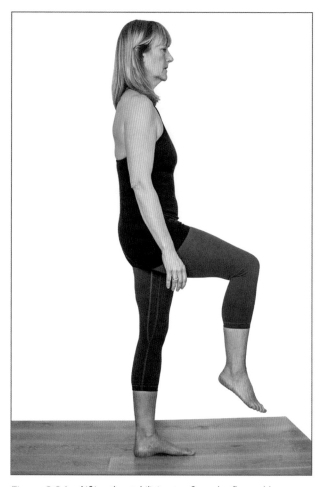

Figure 9.9d. *Lifting the stabilizing toe from the floor adds extra load to the supporting limb, so use the foot dome exercise under your standing foot for control and stability.*

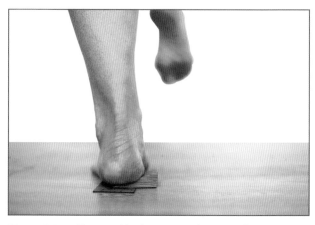

Figure 9.9e. *Extra workload can cause the stance foot to pronate. Loss of the arch can affect both knee and hip alignment. Careful placement of the prop will improve the alignment of your foot, knee, and hip.*

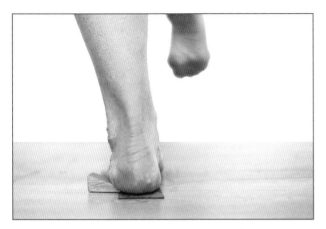

Figure 9.9f. *With the prop in place, can you weight-bear more effectively through the medial side of the foot?*

and helped you achieve improved pelvic alignment?

On the other hand, if your calcaneus is excessively laterally tilting (foot supinating), placing the prop laterally under your calcaneus (fig. 9.9f) might be of benefit, allowing you to bring more weight onto the plantar surface of the foot and therefore gain more contact with the floor. This will provide more feedback from your big toe into the medial aspect of your hip joint.

9. Single-Leg Heel Raises

Take the challenge a step further by rising onto the toes of one foot. This is a great way to work your plantar flexors, intrinsic muscles, and to train your balance. This exercise is more difficult than it looks—holding onto something can help get you started.

- Find your neutral foot position with your tripod of balance engaged.
- Lengthen the toes, ensuring that there is no toe gripping or clawing on the mat.
- Hold on lightly with one hand to help you balance. Resist the temptation to pull yourself up though!
- Lift the right foot off the floor behind you (i.e., knee flexion but not hip flexion).

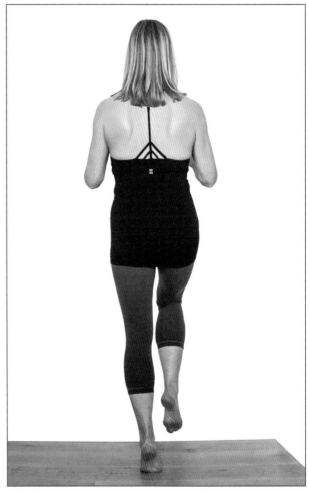

Figure 9.10. *In the rigid lever position, the calcaneus will laterally tilt.*

- Rise up onto the heads of the metatarsals of the left foot, bringing yourself into a supinated "rigid lever" position (fig. 9.10).
- Slowly descend with control, keeping the toe pads in contact with the floor.

Repeat × 6.

This exercise can be quite a challenge for those with unstable feet and weak plantar flexors, so moderate the repetitions as necessary. Those with an active lifestyle, especially runners, should gradually progress to at least 3 sets of 15 repetitions on each side, aiming for equal strength on both sides, as suggested in Michaud 2021.

10. Single-Leg Heel Raises With Lateral and Medial Resistance
Prop—Band

You can be selective with the following exercises to match the foot type. A weaker foot with a tendency to pronate will benefit from strengthening the deep posterior group (variation 1), while the more supinated foot, or one with an unstable first ray, will gain more from strengthening the lateral compartment (variation 2).

It is useful to have a chair in front of you, and hold on lightly.

Tie your band around something substantial and immobile. Now make a loop in the band (big enough to step into) and knot it. This can be a bit fiddly and a long length of band will make it easier. In my example, I have used a packet clip to adjust the length of the band to make life easier.

Variation 1
- Step into the loop with your right foot so that the band is just above your ankle joint.
- Create resistance by stepping away from the prop and bringing tension into the band, which will be pulling your leg laterally (fig. 9.11a).
- Balance on your right foot and rise onto the toes, keeping the foot and ankle stable—you are resisting the lateral pull of the band. This exercise will help to strengthen the tibialis posterior, flexor hallucis longus, and flexor digitorum longus muscles of the deep posterior compartment. The extra balance challenge will also encourage you to work the intrinsic muscles of your foot.
- As a practitioner, it can be helpful to assist and guide the client's calcaneus as they perform the exercise.

Repeat × 6–8. Do not change feet before proceeding with variation 2.

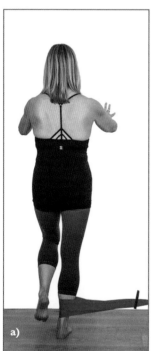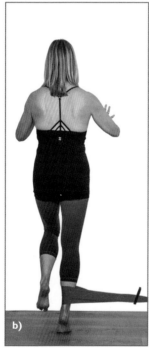

Figure 9.11.   a) Place the band around the leg and adjust the band or your starting position to increase or decrease the tension on the band. b) Start with gentle resistance and assess as you rise and lower down. Step further away for more resistance.

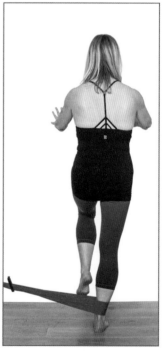

Figure 9.12.   Wrap the band around the leg to create a medial pull.

Variation 2

- Now turn around so that the band is still around your right leg. The pull is now from a medial direction.
- Come into a balance on the right leg and rise on to the toes again, resisting the medial pull of the band. This time you will be challenging the fibularii of the lateral compartment. The extra load on the fibularis longus should help it stabilize and plantar flex the first ray during the toe rocker phase of gait.

Repeat × 6–8.

Repeat both lateral and medial resistance exercises with the left foot in the band.

11. Small Knee Bends
Prop—Wedge

Quite often in movement and exercise classes there is a temptation to place a prop between the knees to correct the alignment of the legs in various exercises. If we think of the knee more as a "floating joint" that is at the top of the tibia and the bottom or the femur, it may highlight why making the correction either at the foot (as below) or from the pelvis (usually by engaging the abductors) can be more beneficial. It is also worth bearing in mind that one foot may have a different pattern to the other. For example, someone with a rotated pelvis may have one foot that is supinated and one that is pronated, and we can balance the feet through the appropriate use of wedges.

- Begin with your feet hip-width apart and with the tripod of balance for each foot.
- Bend your knees, keeping your back upright and lengthened. Feel your knees moving forward over your toes and your ankles moving into dorsiflexion. Do this a few times to feel the movement at the ankle joint and the lengthening of the soft tissue of the posterior compartment.
- Repeat the knee flexion and assess the tracking of your tibial tuberosities—you

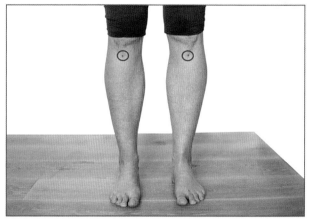

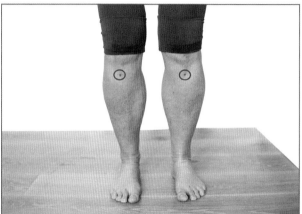

Figure 9.13a.   The tibial tuberosity is a useful and easily found bony landmark. It is the small rounded protuberance directly below the patella, and is the insertion of the quadriceps tendon. Performing the knee bend in front of a mirror can be useful for additional and immediate feedback.

will probably need to check this in a mirror. Do they pass neutrally over the second metatarsal, medially toward the big toe (pronation) or laterally toward the third toe (supination)? Do they do the same thing on both sides?

Repeat × 6

For many people, this exercise is challenging, not because of the tibial tuberosity position, but because of limited range of ankle motion. Tightness in both the posterior and lateral compartments of each leg can reduce the range of motion at the ankle in dorsiflexion. We will address this in our foot mobilization exercises later in this chapter.

- If your tibial tuberosity is passing medially over the big toe, place the prop under

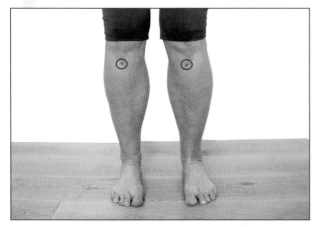

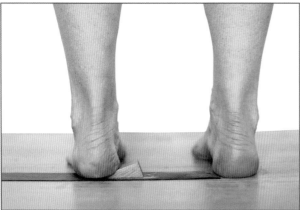

Figure 9.13b. A wedge positioned at the medial calcaneus of a pronated foot can help the knee track over the center of the foot.

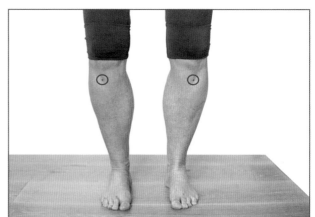

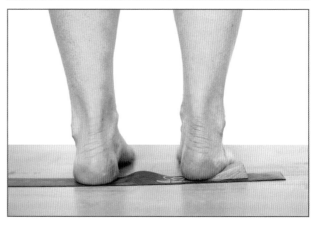

Figure 9.13c. Placing the wedge laterally on a supinated calcaneus can help unlock the foot and improve knee tracking.

the medial side of the rearfoot. This will bring the calcaneus into a more neutral, less medially tilted position. Now repeat the exercise and monitor the position of your tibial tuberosity as you go in to dorsiflexion. Has it changed? Is the tibial tuberosity able to stay in line with the second metatarsal and the foot retain a more neutral position?

Repeat × 6

• If your tibial tuberosity is passing laterally toward the third toe, place the prop on the lateral side of the rearfoot, attempting to bring the calcaneus into neutral from a laterally tilted position. Continue with the above knee bend, watching to see if the tibial tuberosity position has been corrected.

Repeat × 6

12. Abductor Hallucis—Big Toe Training
Prop—Short Ruler

Strengthening this muscle is a marathon not a sprint. You will need to practice regularly to gain some control. Initial mobilization using your forefinger may help to stimulate your sensory motor control. Many clients ask what they can do to stop their bunions getting any worse. Start with Short Foot (Exercise 9.6) alongside this exercise. Be prepared to do both exercises daily to see results.

It is useful to assess the active and passive range of movement of your big toe before you start this exercise. Refer to the passive assessment and end feel descriptions given in chapter 8.

This is a challenge for those with a weak foot and a well-formed bunion, but nonetheless a worthwhile exercise. Big toes that deviate medially might benefit from strengthening the abductor hallucis to prevent the hallux valgus progressing to the stage of compromising the stability of the foot.

Stage 1

- Starting with your right foot, place a short ruler (or piece of wood) along the medial side of your foot or use a line on the floor or floorboard.
- The measurement will give you a good idea of what is happening at the head of your first metatarsal. Does your big toe deviate away from the ruler to the right (fig. 9.14a), indicating a bunion?
- Using the intrinsic muscles, try to pick your big toe pad up and move it medially toward the ruler (fig. 9.14b). Hold it there for a count

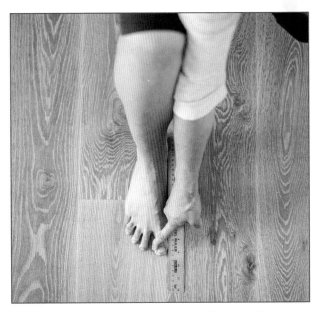

Figure 9.14c.   Using your hand to guide and train the big toe can help recruit the abductor hallucis.

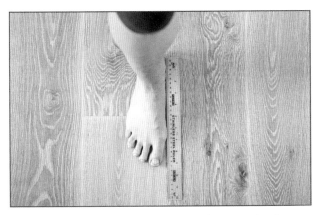

Figure 9.14a.   An example of big toe misalignment related to a bunion, this may be an indication that abductor hallucis is weak.

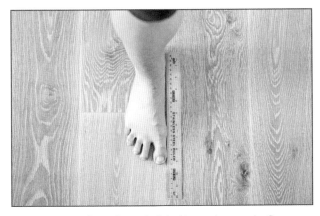

Figure 9.14b.   Press the pad of the big toe down to the floor to help engage abductor hallucis.

of 5 and release. The foot may make many devious compensations here. Keep your first metatarsal head in contact with the floor and do not let your foot supinate.

Repeat × 6–8

If the big toe does not move much, leave the ruler in position, and kneel down so your right foot is still in front. Use your right forefinger to gently move your big toe away from the second toe (fig. 9.14c). Hold it there for 5 seconds and let it move back naturally to its starting position.

Stage 2

If you are already able to move your big toe independently toward the ruler without your foot making compensations, try adding the next stage:

- Once the big toe is abducted, and with the toe pad pressing lightly into the floor, try to spread digits two to five laterally (without the big toe moving), see fig. 9.14d. It should feel as if your big toe is stuck in place and the other digits are moving and spreading laterally with a sense of the forefoot widening.

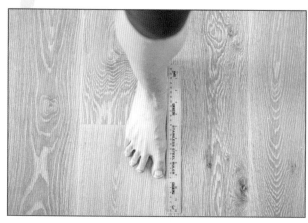

Figure 9.14d. Have you got the control to both keep the big toe in place and spread the other digits?

Repeat × 4–8

Physically holding the big toe in place while you do this is a good initial introduction to what can be a challenging movement in the digits. You are trying to abduct the toes. Do the toes separate and spread? Or do they go into a hammer or claw position.

Toe Spacers/Toe Correctors

There are many products available on the market that are designed to help you bring your toes into a more neutral position. Toes become misaligned for a variety of reasons and impede the proper function and stability of the foot. Claw toes, hammer toes, and bunions are all forms of toe misalignment which might benefit from Toe Spacers (fig. 9.14e). When you

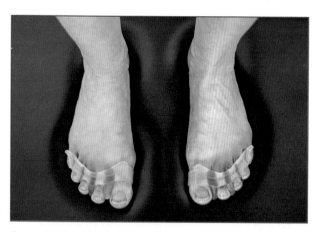

Figure 9.14e. Toe Spacers or Correctors slide in between each toe and can give you a sense of separation and stability.

start working on the toe exercises, if your toes simply stick together with no feeling of individuality, then working on your toe splay can help you to progress.

◎　◎　◎

■ FOOT MOBILIZATION EXERCISES

Soft tissue elasticity can only be used if the feet and ankles are adequately strong and mobile. The exercises above deal with many of the common weaknesses, so now we need to ensure there is adequate range of motion through the major joints.

We think of a high arch as being a good thing, but if your foot cannot move out of its supinated position and spread into a more open position, your soft tissues cannot absorb impact forces and your foot will struggle to establish an optimal interface with the ground. A tight, rigid foot which is closed or excessively supinated can be indicative of reduced mobility and adaptability.

Imagine if you jump off a step—when you land you want your foot to elastically open and the force of the impact to travel into the large muscles and fascia of your leg, thigh, pelvis, and beyond. The tensegrity of your body relies on the ability of your feet to start the body's sequenced reaction to the impact and below, we have outlined suggestions to increase mobility and improve ease of movement.

13. General Foot Release

Repeat Exercise 9.1. You will be able to find the sweet spots on the sole of each foot, and you can massage those in more detail with the ball.

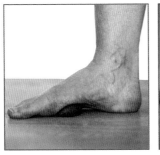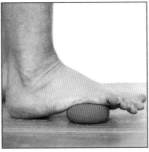

Figure 9.15a. *Those with high arches may find the insertions of tibialis posterior, and flexors digitorum longus and brevis give some informative feedback when pressure is applied to them.*

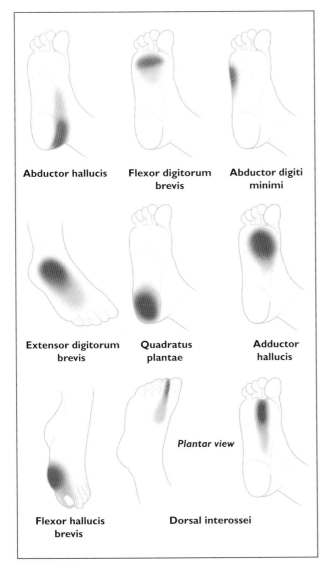

Abductor hallucis   **Flexor digitorum brevis**   **Abductor digiti minimi**

Extensor digitorum brevis   **Quadratus plantae**   **Adductor hallucis**

Plantar view

Flexor hallucis brevis   **Dorsal interossei**

Figure 9.15b. *Trigger points on the foot.*

14. Ankle Mobilization—Self Mobilization of the Foot

As you go around in the circular motion of this exercise, try to assess the quality of the

movement. Do you feel stiffness or ease of movement? What is the feeling in the bones and joints, muscles, and connective tissue as you circle? Are the bones held rigid and compressed, or do they feel as if they are floating within an elastic net? What are your restrictions? Can you feel a difference between soft tissue restriction and bony restrictions?

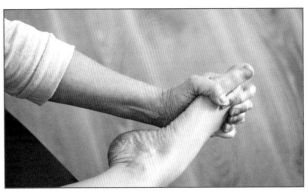

Figure 9.16. *Use your fingers to act as toe separators as you use the hand to mobilize the foot and ankle.*

With your right foot on your left thigh, place your left fingers between each toe. Start with your little finger between toes five and four and place a finger between each toe, working toward your big toe (fig. 9.16). Your thumb cups around the side of your first MTJ.

- Starting clockwise, begin to move the foot in circles initiating the movement with your ankle. Let the ankle drive the movement as the hand remains passive. Draw a nice full circle.

Repeat × 6 circles; then change to anti-clockwise

- Now initiate the movement with the left hand and let the ankle remain passive.

Repeat × 6 circles in each direction on each foot

15. Foot Wringing (Eversion and Inversion)—Self Mobilization of the Foot

This exercise will help you achieve a sense of the opposing movements in the forefoot and

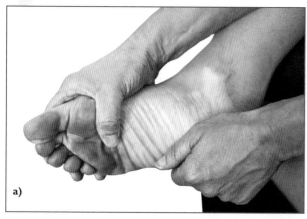

a)

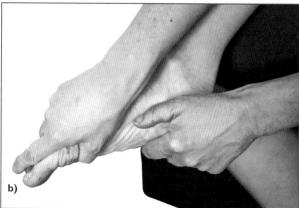

b)

Figure 9.17a & b.   Keep the right foot as passive as possible. Your right hand is guiding the forefoot and your left hand is guiding the rearfoot. Slightly alter the position of your right hand so each turn engages with a different section of the mid- and forefoot. Note the cupping of the hand around the calcaneus.

rearfoot, and gauge your general mobility (or lack of it). Is one direction easier than the other? Do you feel with one of those directions that you may have a blind spot or sensory motor amnesia (SMA)[1]?

Begin in a seated position with one leg crossed over the other. In this example, begin by crossing your right leg over your left thigh.

- Gently turn the calcaneus away from you (fig. 9.17a) toward the floor and draw the mid-foot and forefoot toward you, then reverse the movement in the opposite direction by drawing the calcaneus toward

you and turning the mid-foot away from you (fig. 9.17b).
- Change legs. Now your left hand is guiding your forefoot and mid-foot and the right hand is on the calcaneus. Continue as above.

Repeat the "wringing" movements on each foot.

Move the foot as if you are nurturing the bones gently beneath your hands creating fluidity and ease. Do not pull or push too hard, and note that to avoid irritating the nerves along the medial aspect, it is best to guide the calcaneus with the heel of your hand rather than pressing with your thumb.

16. Toe Extensor Lengthening and Anterior Compartment Release

The anterior compartment of the lower leg contains the muscles that produce ankle dorsiflexion, and of course, therefore, they resist plantar flexion. As they pass down the leg, they are held in position by the retinaculum (see chapter 6). Limited ankle range of movement can be partly attributed to this group of muscles and the associated retinaculum. This exercise aims to lengthen these muscles and promote glide under the cuff or strap of the retinaculum.

Stand in a split stance near the wall (to help with balance) with your right foot behind you in plantar flexion with the toes curled under (fig. 9.18a).

Stage 1
- Shift your weight forward, driving from the pelvis and ribs so you feel as if you have left the right foot behind. The right foot remains in place, and you should feel a stretch in the anterior compartment of the lower leg. To get a sense of the whole of the front of the right leg opening, keep your pelvis slightly posteriorly tilted as you draw your weight forward.

---

[1]SMA "is a memory loss of how certain muscle groups feel and how to control them. And because it occurs in the central nervous system, we are not aware of it, yet it affects us to our very core." Hannah (2004), *Somatics*.

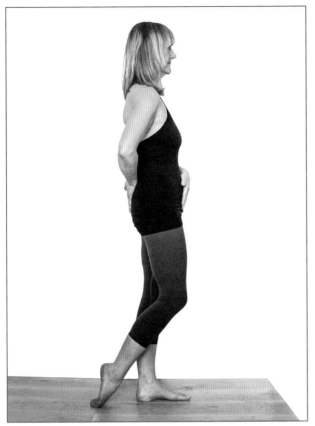

Figure 9.18a. Do not press your right toes directly down into the floor—try to be quite light on the right foot. Keeping your right hand behind your pelvis will remind you to initiate the movement by shifting the pelvis forward in a posterior tilt.

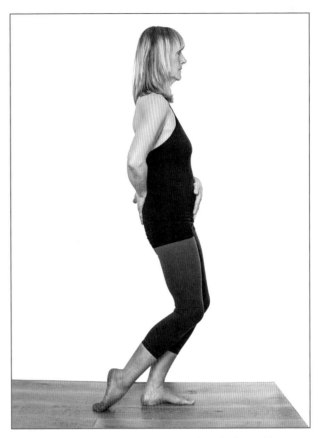

Figure 9.18b. Adding a small knee bend on the forward leg increases the balance challenge on the left side and gives you another opportunity to practice the Short Foot doming. Maintain the pelvic posterior tilt as you do the knee bend.

- Hold the forward position for a count of four, then release.

Repeat × 4 and step back down

- Continue with stages 2 and 3 before changing sides to stretch the left leg.

Stage 2
- Still in the above stance, with your right toes in plantar flexion and a sense of drawing the foot forward, slowly bend your left knee (fig. 9.18b). Keep your back upright and posteriorly tilt the pelvis. This can sometimes enhance the stretch. Hold on to the wall if necessary.
- Progress to stage 3 before swapping sides.

Stage 3
- Rise up from the last knee bend and lift your right foot off the floor and take your right hand around your forefoot (see fig. 9.18c). Get a sense of the space between your tibia and your foot. Drawing your hand into your foot as the foot opposes that action adds some post-isometric relaxation[2] into the stretch.
- You will be stretching the whole of your right anterior leg compartment.
- Hold for a count of 8 before releasing into a passive stretch.

Now change sides.

---

[2]A post-isometric relaxation occurs following a held contraction and is often used as a stretching technique for high tone areas.

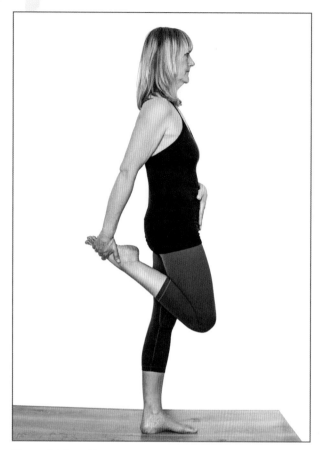

Figure 9.18c.   Maintain a posterior tilt of your pelvis (visualize a weight dropping from your tailbone) as you take hold of your right foot.

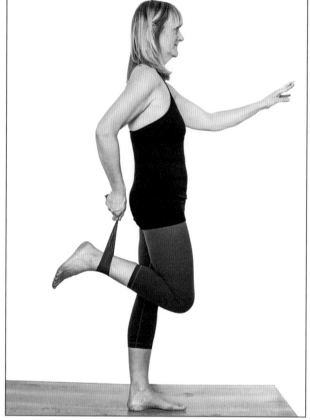

Figure 9.18d.   If you cannot reach the foot behind, use a band or yoga strap around your lower leg to facilitate the stretch.

17. Kneeling Ankle Dorsiflexion and Plantar Flexion

Take a kneeling position with your right leg in front of the left. You can place a pad under your back knee for comfort if necessary.

Make sure your right knee is directly over your ankle joint, so that the tibia is centered on the talus (fig. 9.19a). You can choose to put your hands on the floor either side of you or on a yoga brick for some support and balance.

- Shift your weight forward to bring you into a position of ankle dorsiflexion. Go as far as you can without the calcaneus lifting off the floor (fig. 9.19c). This movement tensions the plantar fascia and Achilles tendon to force close the foot.

Those with hypermobile tissues should ensure they do not travel into their "end range" bony

feeling at the knee joint and ankle joint. Those who are less mobile need to try and anchor the calcaneus to the floor.

- Now shift your pelvis backward, extending your right knee. Your ankle will move into plantar flexion. Keeping your toes on the floor as you move back will activate the intrinsic muscles and once again force close the foot but from a different tissue level than during the dorsiflexion movement above.
- Slowly repeat both movements backward and forward, paying attention to how the tibial tuberosity tracks over the ankle.

In a pronated foot type, the tibial tuberosity is more likely to track medially (i.e., toward the big toe) as you shift forward. In a supinated foot type, the movement is more likely to take the tibial tuberosity laterally toward toes three to five.

Interventions with a Prop
Pronated Foot Type

- Place the small prop (wedge or rolled up small cloth) under the medial side of the calcaneus. Repeat the shifts forward and back and see if you can direct your tibial tuberosity more over the second toe.

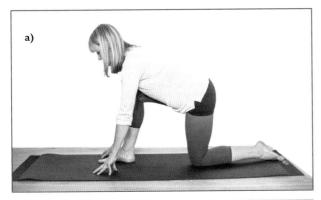

a)

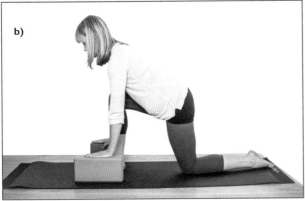

b)

Figure 9.19a & b. a) Begin with a 90/90 kneeling position, right leg in front of the left and your hands placed either side on the floor. b) Use yoga blocks for your hands to prevent over-reaching downward or allowing the rib cage to collapse.

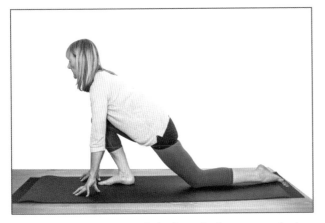

Figure 9.19c. Press your right heel into the floor as you take the front knee forward. You have gone too far if you feel the heel lift.

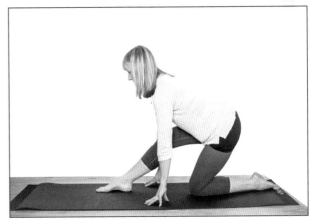

Figure 9.19d. Press your toes into the floor as you take the pelvis back and extend the forward knee. If the toes lift you have gone too far.

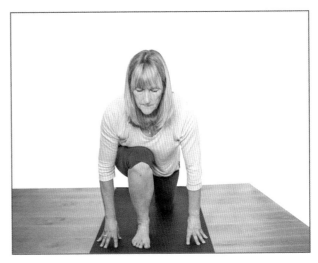

Figure 9.19e. Assess the position of the tibial tuberosity as you move into dorsiflexion—is it traveling into a neutral position over the second toe?

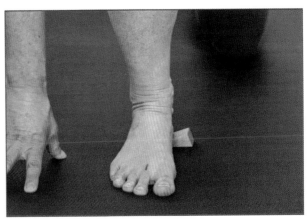

Figure 9.19f. Has your alignment improved with the prop in place under the medial calacaneus?

Supinated Foot Type

If your big toe gets pulled off the floor, place the prop under the lateral side of the calcaneus or the lateral side of the mid-foot to try and create more "opening" of the bones. Repeat the shifts and see if the foot can adapt more freely to the movement you are creating at the ankle.

We have already done this movement in Exercise 9.11, but this variation brings more range of movement into the tibia both posteriorly and anteriorly. It can be beneficial for you to watch the adaptation of the foot as the ankle dorsiflexes and plantar flexes.

18. Lengthening Off a Yoga Block

This exercise is relevant for both strengthening and mobilizing the foot and ankle complex. For a weak foot and ankle, focus on both the lift and lower phase of the movement with emphasis on squeezing the ball. Those in need of more length can spend a little more time in the stretches at the bottom of the movement.

Yoga bricks can vary in size. The depth of the yoga block here is approx. 8 cm/3".

Stand on the yoga brick and place the ball between your heels.

- Hold on to the wall initially as you assess your balance and slowly lower your heels toward the floor, keep your toes long and rooted to the brick. Keep the legs straight to focus on the posterior compartment gastrocnemius stretch. Hold for a slow count of 5.
- Rise up onto your toes, squeezing the ball as you go up (fig. 9.20b). This is a repeat of the heel raise we performed earlier. Release the "squeeze" as you return.
- Send the heels back toward the floor again. With your heels lowered, slightly bend your knee to relax the gastrocnemius and focus the stretch into the soleus. Hold for a count of 5 and rise back up.

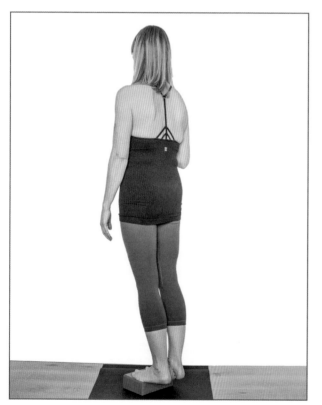
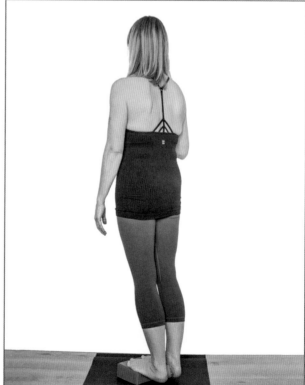

Figures 9.20a & b.   In this gastrocnemius stretch, keep your toes rooted to the brick.

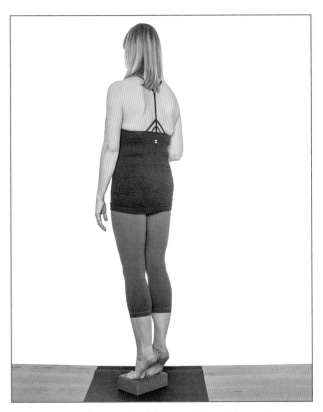

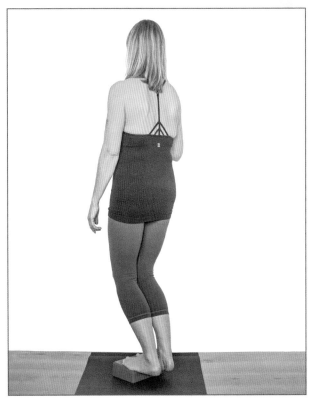

Figure 9.20c. *Drive the heels into the ball and rise back up onto the toes.*

Figure 9.20d. *Bend your knees and hold the soleus focused stretch.*

- Each time you lower your heels, alternate between straight legs for gastrocnemius and slightly bent knees for soleus.

Repeat × 8

19. Knee Clocks—Mobilizing the Subtalar Joint
Prop—Small Soft Ball

- Stand with your right foot forward and the ball directly under the subtalar joint.
- Looking down, draw a circle with your right knee around your right ankle joint. As the knee moves out to the 3 o'clock position, your subtalar joint will invert. Now move your knee to the 12 o'clock position and your ankle will move into dorsiflexion. Around toward 9 o'clock will bring your subtalar joint into eversion and finally back to the 6 o'clock position will move your subtalar joint into plantar flexion.

Move slowly and methodically, sensing the movement massaging the subtalar joint.

Repeat four times then reverse to clockwise. Sense the difference in the feet before you move on.

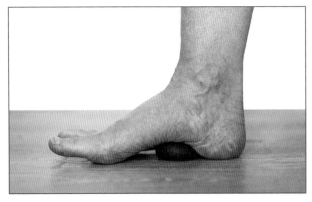

Figure 9.21. *Place the ball under the foot where you feel the intersection of the talar and subtalar joints (see chapter 6, and assessments in chapter 8). The ball should act as a rocker between each axis to provide freedom for dorsiflexion and plantar flexion, and inversion and eversion.*

Change sides and put your left foot forward and the ball directly under the subtalar joint.

- Draw the circle with your left knee moving laterally out to the 9 o'clock position and your foot moving into inversion, around to 12 o'clock and into ankle dorsiflexion, medially to 3 o'clock into eversion and back to 6 o'clock and into ankle plantar flexion.

Repeat 4 times clockwise and 4 times anti-clockwise.

All the above exercises are designed as a beginner's journey for the foot. You will have assessed what your foot is capable of and what your restrictions might be. Armed with this information, you can begin to explore more fully those exercises that will benefit you and your foot type. Regular practice and "foot maintenance" are essential for all feet, and a great way of bringing small global changes to your skeletal structure. Never underestimate the power of your foot to enhance or detract from your overall movement potential.

Below are three short sequences. One for general foot health, and one for each foot type. The exercise number, as it appears in the book, is in brackets at the end of each exercise listed below.

Regular practice with these 10 to 15 minutes sequences will set you on the path to better structural balance in your feet.

Routine for General Foot Health
1. General foot awakening (1)
2. Foot clocks, figure of 8, and tripod of balance (2)
3. Stepping through—toe extension (3)
4. Short foot (doming) (6)
5. Bi-lateral heel raises, knees extended, and ball between heels (7)

6. Single-leg stance—transfer of weight onto one foot—add knee lifts for balance (8)
7. Lengthening off the yoga block (18)

Routine for a Foot That Needs General Strengthening

1. General foot awakening (1)
2. Foot clocks, figure of 8, and tripod of balance (2)
3. Stepping through—toe extension (3)
4. Bi-lateral heel raise—knees flexed (5)
5. Short foot (doming) (6)
6. Bi-lateral heel raises, knees extended, and ball between heels (7)
7. Single heel raises (9)
8. Single heel raises with band and lateral resistance (10a)
9. Abductor hallucis longus—big toe training (12)
10. Small knee bends and small squats with props (11)
11. Kneeling ankle dorsiflexion and plantar flexion with props (17)
12. Lengthening off yoga block knees straight stretch (18)

Routine for a Foot That Needs Releasing
1. General foot awakening and foot release (1)
2. Foot clocks, figure of 8, and tripod of balance (2)
3. Stepping through toe extension (3)
4. Toe extensor and anterior compartment release (16)
5. Knee clock—massaging the subtalar joint (2)
6. Ankle mobilization (14)
7. Foot wringing (15)
8. Bi-lateral heel raises with knees extended (4)
9. Single-leg heel raises with medial resistance (10b)
10. Lengthening off the yoga block (focus on the stretches) (18)
11. Kneeling ankle dorsiflexion and plantar flexion (with prop to drive foot into pronation) (17)

DESIGNED FOR LIFE

A good day starts with the perfect shoes.

—Unknown

▤ INTRODUCTION

It is true that life is better when you are wearing the perfect shoes. But what defines "the perfect shoes"? The correct fit? The perfect style and color? The right height? Comfort?

It can be an emotive question and our answers will vary depending on age, background, gender identification, time of day, culture, religion, the event we are dressing for, the events we hope to be undressing for…

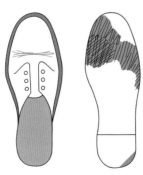

Figure 10.1. A typical, normal wear pattern.

There are few more provocative pieces of clothing than our footwear. As Christian Louboutin, the master of sexualized footwear, reminds us *"Shoes transform your body language and attitude. They lift you physically and emotionally."* But the wrong shoe can bring us down and I am sure most of us have lived through the physical pains of an uncomfortable shoe or the emotional misery of a fashion faux pas.

Shoes have two main functions: they are a fashion statement used to project a variety of social signals, and they provide protection for our feet. Sadly, these two functions have become almost mutually exclusive categories. Fashion-based footwear, it could be argued, alters the form of our feet that they are doing more harm than good. It is hard to find foot-shaped shoes but, due to the pressures of fashion, it is quite easy to find shoe-shaped feet (see fig. 10.2).

There are styles and brands of shoe that can work for our feet, and there are those that pinch and bite—and deform. In this final chapter, we explore the anatomy of the shoe and how it can work with or work against the natural rhythm of our foot. I am sure it is no surprise to learn that ideal mechanics is no longer a major goal for most footwear manufacturers, so knowing a

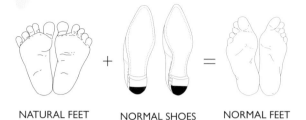

NATURAL FEET   NORMAL SHOES   NORMAL FEET

A LIFETIME IN NORMAL FOOTWEAR CAN CHANGE
THE SHAPE OF YOUR FEET.

VIVOBAREFOOT

Figure 10.2.   Natural feet should be wide across the toes, but most fashion shoes taper toward the toes and change the shape of the feet. Image supplied courtesy of Vivobarefoot.

little about the design features of a shoe can help you make better purchases.

THE IMPORTANCE OF THE RIGHT FIT

He obliged Cinderella to sit down, and, putting the slipper to her little foot, he found it went on very easily, and fitted her as if it had been made of wax.

—Charles Perrault

It is rare to be as lucky as the girl rescued from the downstairs kitchen, as most fashion shoes require some compromise on the part of our feet. More often than not, we are prepared to contort our feet to fit into the shoe, rather than walk away and find a better fit. Although we are not driven to take the drastic flesh-cutting measures of Cinderella's step-sisters, we are often guilty of abusing the adaptability of our feet and compromising foot function in favor of shoe form.

If the shoe doesn't fit, must we change the foot?

—Gloria Steinem

It is the repeated and regular wearing of shoe-shaped shoes that produces shoe-shaped feet. As the Chinese knew, our feet can mold to the form of their encasements. Thankfully, there has been a rise in the number of minimalist footwear companies, and they are rapidly expanding their marketing and technologies to support green, renewable, and vegan-friendly options. Shoes produced by brands such as Vivobarefoot, Lems, and Merrell all have foot-shape and natural function in mind during design and manufacture.

Minimalist shoes are still a small portion of the footwear market and these small brands must compete against global brands that produced 66.3 million pairs of shoes in 2018.[1] That is a lot of shoes, leather, glue, plastic, and moldings, as well as a huge profit and marketing capability.

Like the rest of the fashion industry, the shoe-trade is rife with waste, pollution, and exploitation, and economics should form part of our choice as consumers. We have the power to choose brands that support us—those that do not pollute, use toxic glues, or exploit their workers; those that do pay their taxes and support the welfare of their workers.

Our incomes are like our shoes; if too small, they gall and pinch us; but if too large, they cause us to stumble and to trip.

—John Locke

However, footwear choice is not straightforward. There are the environmental and ethical considerations, there are biomechanical factors, and there are psychosexual and emotional elements. For example, a review by Barnish et al. 2017, found that high heels are still frequently

[1]Data from Hoskins 2020.

worn by many women, despite the known significant biomechanical effects and increased likelihood of musculoskeletal issues. The researchers noted that both "implicit and explicit compulsion" played a part—women are choosing of their own freewill, as well as being encouraged by others, to wear high heels. A major factor in the dynamic was the increased perceived attractiveness of the wearer. The authors were careful to point out that no one should be coerced "into wearing high heels against their will."

Freewill is not straightforward though and we are all open to many factors that influence our choice. A 2016 study of adults in the UK, found that those with "shorter stature and higher BMI were observationally associated with measures of lower socioeconomic status." (Tyrrell et al. 2016). Although the correlation was greater for men in height, and for women in BMI measurements, the message was clear—if you want to get ahead in life, get taller, and get thinner. Wearing high heels can give the illusion of both, and, in a world that clearly values height and appearance over biomechanics, it is important that individual choices are unrestricted and free from judgment.

ANATOMY OF A SHOE

Most shoes are shaped as if feet were made for shoes.

—Mokokoma Mokhonoana

A shoe is the interface between the foot and the ground, and the features of the shoe will affect the reactions that take place. The earliest shoes are estimated to have been designed around 40,000 years ago (Trinkaus and Shang 2008), and are more likely to have been created to protect the foot than with any fashion statement in mind. However, it is interesting to note that the researchers based their assumptions on the fact that there was a reduction of toe length around this time. Is this reduced robusticity of the phalanges an indication of decreased use of the toes, or that they were crammed into elegant toe boxes? Who knows?

There are many temporal markers for the development of "mismatch disorders"—the divergence between the cultural adaptations we have invented and the evolutionary anatomy and physiology developed over millions

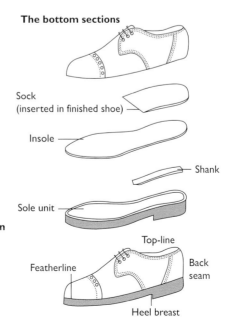

Figure 10.3. General outline of a Gibson/Derby style shoe.

of years. From the invention of agriculture 10,000 years ago, through the industrial revolution 150 years ago, to the ubiquity of personal computing and communication devices in the last 20 years, each change has had an impact on how we use and treat our bodies. We had to adapt our digestive system for new types of food, we had to adapt our cultural and family routines to fit into factory-based life, and we now must fit our bodies around ever-present communication devices. The invention of shoes predates all of those—squeezing our feet into footwear is not a new problem.

Our journey through the anatomy of a shoe will take us from heel strike to toe-off, and a revision of the four rockers we have referenced throughout the text. Although we cannot travel through each style of shoe, the main costs and benefits are similar across shoe types. There is no perfect style—even minimalist shoes have their costs for some feet—so we must keep in mind the abilities of the foot we are placing in the shoe and look for a match. That match should be not just in size but also in capability.

Impact forces at heel strike need to be managed and, as we have seen, the forces will travel in numerous directions. The shoe will affect the management of these forces. The initial impact can be damped by the heel material, and how the heel deflects the shock into the foot depends on the angle and shape of the shoe's heel. The sharp edge of the Gibson shoe, and its distance from the calcaneus will cause the foot to plantar flex more rapidly than normal on heel strike, and give tibialis anterior more work to decelerate the foot on its descent (see fig. 5.2). A sharp-edged heel can be a cause of anterior shin pain and should be considered during clinical examination.

Once the foot is on the ground and weight is being transferred onto it, the calcaneus should tilt. Most shoes have a rounded cup for the calcaneus, and this "heel counter" can vary in fit. If the counter is too tight it stops the calcaneus everting (the trigger for pronation); if it is too loose, uncontrolled tilting of the calcaneus can cause the skin to rub against the stiffened material of the counter, causing irritation. Increased wear around the heel counter also makes the counter a useful indicator of an unstable calcaneus. Although a heel counter can be a useful stabilizer for the calcaneus, there is the Goldilocks struggle of getting just the right amount of support without preventing pronation.

Some pronation is necessary as it contributes to the efficiencies of gait, and the foot needs to absorb some impact forces. To absorb some of the force the bones of the foot need room to spread to allow pronation to happen, which brings us to the next areas of compromise—the quarter, the facing, and the vamp. The quarter and the facing of a shoe hug the mid-foot and these can be adjusted by altering the lacing pattern to match the foot type (fig. 10.4). The vamp forms the upper portion of the toe box and houses the metatarsal heads and the toes—the site of most spreading during pronation, along the MTJ line.

The crease across a well-worn shoe (see fig. 10.1) shows the position of the MTJ joint fold. The crease line should match the widest part of the shoe and the "ball" of the shoe when seen from the side (fig. 10.5). The ball of the shoe should match the position of the forefoot rocker when the foot is inside the shoe. The ball of the foot and the ball of the shoe should both be below a flexible portion of the vamp that can fold and allow extension across the MTJ line.

Fashion normally dictates the shape of the vamp and, often, vanity can dictate its size. There is a difference between what is "normal" and what is "natural", and our natural foot is wider across the toes. But rather than accommodate the full breadth of the foot, it

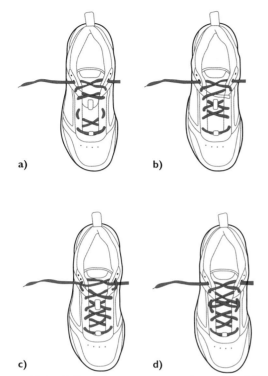

Figure 10.4.   *Different lacing patterns can be used for different foot types. a) A high in-step, supinated-type foot benefits from gapping in the lacing through the middle to reduce pressure on the dorsal aspect of the foot. b) Those with a wide forefoot can create extra space by gapping the lacing at the front of the shoe to provide more space. c) Narrow heels can slip out of the throat of the shoe and therefore require extra support toward the ankle. d) To give extra support to the pronated-type foot, the lacing can be reinforced around the mid-section. (Adapted from Shoe Locker infographic.)*

has become normal for our feet to be cramped into restrictive vamps that, over time, change the shape and therefore function of our feet. Without enough space, the metatarsals cannot spread to tension the transverse tie-bar, the medial longitudinal arch cannot lengthen, and the foot cannot twist to strain the plantar tissues.

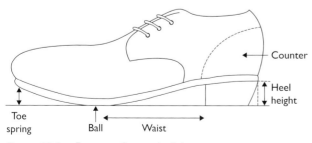

Figure 10.5.   *Features of a standard shoe.*

Some of the work involved in a step can be displaced to the shoe. The shoe can become a stabilizing agent and its materials can be used to dampen GRFs. This is particularly true of performance shoes, where material science has improved significantly to increase efficiency, protection, and effectiveness. This brings new variables surrounding performance into the footwear discussion. Shoes can be chosen to allow natural function or to enhance an individual's performance in terms of speed and efficiency. It is important that we should not fall into the *appeal to nature fallacy*[2] and assume that "natural" is naturally better.

However, in the case of toe boxes and vamps, their unnatural sizing and angulations certainly do not seem to be improving the health of our feet or our performance. The cramping causes the toes, especially the big toe, to adduct, and their joints to misalign. Our ontogenetic plasticity allows our vanity to squeeze us into the latest shoes when we are young, but research is showing that the cost to our health and mobility might not arise until our later years.

A recent study found that walking speeds in 85% of elderly men and 93% of elderly women have reduced so much that they can no longer cross the road at speeds considered safe (Asher et al. 2012). Although this study was only performed in England, the results are in keeping with studies performed in Ireland, South Arica, Spain, and the United States. It is hard not to see how this may relate to other statistics that show that 85% of the population are wearing incorrectly sized shoes (Tyrrell, in Yates 2012), that 87% of older adults have some form of foot dysfunction (Franklin et al. 2015), with up to 74% having a hallux valgus, and one in 40 people over the age of 50 suffer with a hallux rigidus (Rodríguez-Sanz et al. 2018).

_____

[2]The appeal to nature fallacy is the assumption that anything that is natural is better than an invented, unnatural alternative.

In each category of dysfunction, female feet are worse than those of men, and I am sure few people would contest that women's footwear is less foot-shaped than men's. Women's shoes also tend to have higher heels, which places extra stress on the metatarsal heads, realigns the ankle to a plantar flexed position and, over time, can shorten the gastrocnemius and stiffen the Achilles tendon (Franklin et al. 2015).

Each misalignment and every reduced range of motion will affect bone and soft tissue function. As we saw in chapter 5, there are many benefits to tensioning collagenous tissues during natural movement, and joint and soft tissue alignments overlap to ensure the system flows with ease. Changing toe alignment or artificially reducing the range of joint motion robs the system of momentum and the force enhancements from pretensioning.

Shoe design can affect the pretensioning of the plantar tissues in many ways. The most obvious is the toe spring, the upward curve of the sole beyond the ball, which is often used by manufacturers to compensate for the stiffness of the sole. If the material used for the sole of the shoe is difficult to bend, it will stop the MTJs from extending. Shoe manufacturers compensate for this with an in-built toe spring to exaggerate the ball of the shoe.

The effect on the foot is to reduce or remove toe extension and, by doing so, to reduce the amount of work performed by the flexor tissues. It should be no surprise that outsourcing the work of the foot to the shoe causes the foot to weaken, as the muscles are no longer being used for deceleration and control. A study by Sichting et al. (2020) found that toe springs reduce the workload and decrease the stiffness of the medial longitudinal arch, an effect they warn may have long-term consequences for foot health, as the intrinsic muscles become weaker over time due to underuse.

However, we need to be aware to not fall foul of the appeal to nature argument. It is always important to read research with a critical eye as we can learn a clinical lesson from the study. Sichting and colleagues show that toe springs divert work from the plantar tissues and into the form of the shoe, which is not a good thing for a healthy foot. It is a totally different story if the foot is already challenged. In cases of plantar heel pain, plantar fascia pain, or metatarsalgia, toe springs could be a clinically useful device for the temporary unloading of tissues that may be under stress. In cases of plantar heel pain, plantar fascia pain, or metatarsalgia, toe springs could be used to off-load the tissues and give them time to heal without requiring the client to completely rest.

A comprehensive review of related literature by Holowka and Lieberman (2018) showed that habitually shod populations generally had weaker feet and recorded lower height and stiffness of the medial longitudinal arch than habitually unshod populations. In their study, Holowka and Lieberman showed that wearing minimalist shoes could significantly increase the cross-sectional area of abductor hallucis, and, to a lesser extent, the cross-sectional areas of abductor digiti minimi and flexor digitorum brevis. Minimalist shoes allow the foot to spread and the toes to extend, so it should be no surprise that letting the foot follow its natural function makes the associated muscles work a little harder. These intrinsic muscles form part of the "foot core system" proposed by McKeon et al. (2014) that we mentioned in chapter 1 and, like any "core", the muscles benefit from working out. Conveniently, we do not need to go to the gym to exercise the feet, we could be working them with every step—if we are wearing the right shoes!

As part of their construction, minimalist shoes have flexible, thin soles that not only allow the plantar tissues to engage but also enhance sensory stimulation. The foot can feel the surface more clearly and by stiffening the tissues, the mechanoreceptors receive appropriate information regarding the pressure, shear, and stretch that is unavailable to them in a stiff, cramped shoe. Once again though, modern shoes can offer something to the pathological foot. As the major function of shoes is to protect the foot, we must consider those with challenged tissues. Both peripheral vascular and neurological deficits can increase sensitivity or, dangerously, decrease it to the extent that the client is unaware of any tissue damage. All too commonly in cases of diabetes, injury to the foot leads to complications that require amputation. Ensuring properly fitted shoes are worn can reduce injuries and should form part of any quality care package.

In less serious conditions, such as plantar fascia conditions, a shock absorbing sole can temporarily reduce strain on the tissue and speed recovery. In fact, any condition that has challenged the soft tissues can benefit from some rest and recovery time and the support given by a shoe. For example, reduced fat pad coverage can be compensated for with an absorbent heel as the calcaneal fat pads deform up to 60% with minimalist shoes, but only 35% in conventional running shoes.

▨ FINDING THE RIGHT FIT

> **There's one good thing about tight shoes; they make you forget your other troubles.**
>
> —Josh Billings

Getting the right fit matters and there are a number of simple tips that can help.

- The first is to shop in the afternoon as your feet tend to increase in volume by up to 3% during the day. That measurement even increases to 8% during vigorous exercise (Yates 2012) so think about the timing of your shopping trip
- Most of us have one foot a little longer than the other, so buy for the larger foot. It is easy

to add liners or heel pads to decrease the space in the shoe for the smaller foot
- Make sure you are wearing the same type of sock that you will wear with the shoe—do not try your shoes on with thin nylon stockings, only to go home and wear the new shoes with thick woollen socks
- The end of the shoe should be around 10–12 mm from the end of your longest toe—and that could be your second toe, not the big toe
- The line of your MTJs should be at the widest part of the shoe—that line should also be flexible and absent of stitching or design detail that can sometimes alter the vamp when creasing for toe-off
- Be wary of buying longer shoes to compensate for a wider foot. Despite normal human variation, many manufacturers do not make shoes in different width fittings and to find the correct width it can be necessary to buy a longer size. This changes the position of your MTJ line relative to the ball and tread line of the shoe. Commonly, there is also a stiffening rod called a *shank* made of plastic, steel, or wood, embedded within the sole of the shoe (see fig. 10.3—one can often see its outline on the inner sole of a high heel). The shank is there to protect the waist of the shoe but can impinge on your MTJ line if you have bought a longer than usual shoe. It is important that each of the "fold lines" match up—the ball and tread line of the shoe and your MTJ line, which should be beyond the end of the shank (fig. 10.6)

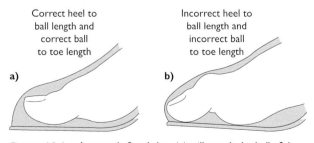

Figure 10.6.   A correctly fitted shoe (a) will match the ball of the foot with the ball and tread line of the shoe. A shoe that is too short (b) creates a mismatch between the foot's MTJ line and the folding line of the shoe to cause cramping of the toes in the toe box.

- The width of the toe box should match or extend beyond the width of your feet. The compliance of the vamp material will affect the importance of the toe box width, as a soft compliant material will still allow your foot to adapt if it is snug. Avoid pairing a stiff material and a narrow toe box

- The heel counter, if there is one, should match the needs of your foot. Does your foot need more support? Is the heel counter too soft or too hard? The height of heel counters also varies, so be aware of those that may be too high for your calcaneus, as they can cause irritation

- A shoe's *pitch* is the change in height from the heel to its tread line (see fig. 10.4). Increasing the pitch puts more pressure onto the metatarsal heads and increases the degree of extension in their resting position. Wearing a higher heel changes the angles at both the ankle and the MTJs, which will alter the foot's ability to stiffen during gait. As the ankle is held in a plantar flexed position by the shoe, the talar joint may have an increased ability to move toward dorsiflexion as it moves from plantar flexion to neutral and then into dorsiflexion. However, the joint is less likely to reach its end of range and naturally stiffen the plantar flexor tendons because of the already extended position of the toes. Altering the pitch interferes with the natural mechanics of the extrinsic and intrinsic tissues of the foot and may cause extra compensation from the hip and back

Shoes can provide necessary support for orthotics, whether they are prescribed or over-the-counter mass-produced options. Shoes should be fitted with the orthotic in place to ensure there is adequate space for the foot to adapt during gait. Finding the right orthotic may require a full professional consultation, but many people find that off-the-shelf devices can provide as much relief as more expensive custom-made options, making the cheaper option a reasonable first resort. However, serious consideration should be given to the effects of choosing orthoses as, like stiff and ill-fitting shoes, they often reduce the stresses and strains on the foot, causing more weakness in the foot and long-term dependency on the device. Like many suggestions above, they can be a useful temporary measure to off-load tissue and provide time for an appropriate exercise and stretching program to take effect.

The shape and angle of the toe box can affect the angle at toe-off. As we saw in the discussion of Morton's foot in chapter 8, misalignment of the joints can change the direction of momentum into the joints further up the limb. Shoes are designed with various degrees of *flaring* (fig. 10.7)—the difference between the measurements of the midline of the last and the outermost parts of the shoe. The bisecting midline is measured along the line from the middle of the heel, and the manufacturer can choose to either increase the distance from that line to the inside or outside of the tread line or keep them balanced. An in-flare will have more shoe to the inside of the midline, an out-flare will have more shoe to the outside of the midline. These deviations can match the

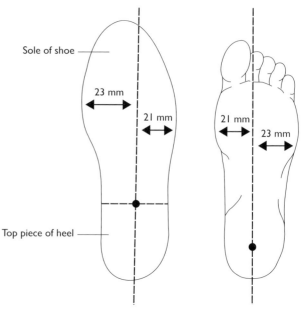

Sole of shoe

23 mm

21 mm

21 mm

23 mm

Top piece of heel

Figure 10.7. The widest points from the midline of the last should be wider than the widest parts of the foot. A shoe with a wider medial portion is referred to as having an in-flare, those with more width laterally are out-flared. If there is equal distance medially and laterally, the shoe is neutral.

needs of a supinated- or pronated-type foot respectively, and prevent irritation of the skin from contact with the inner of the shoe.

▥ THE LAST WORD

Shoes are like friends, they can support you, or take you down.

—Unknown

The overall moral of the story is that our feet and our shoes can be best friends[3] if we take care of our feet and make the best choices in our footwear. We can give them the occasional workout by running barefoot across the sand, or investing in some flexible-soled, minimalist shoes made from a foot-shaped last. We should always make sure our shoes are fit for purpose and, by doing so, help ensure that our feet also remain fit for purpose into our latter years. After all, the alternative is a slower, less satisfying, and sometimes painful gait that reduces our experience and engagement with the world.

In his excellent exploration of gait, neuro-scientist Prof. Shane O'Mara (2019) lists the many benefits to our mental and physical health that we gain from walking. The many paybacks from the simple act of walking range from maintaining muscle strength and tone, defying the weakening effects of sarcopenia, to the emotional and psychological lift. O'Mara reminds us that getting out and about, taking oneself for a daily constitutional, is shown to aid "openness, extraversion and agreeableness" and reduce depression. But the biggest benefits, he says, come from explorations in the natural world and through our *extension*—although O'Mara does not define what he means by extension; I like to think of it as the extended

position just prior to toe-off. In that position, we are literally opened and tensioned along the front of our body.

Retain mobile and adaptable feet, and our feet will give the same gifts back to us.

We need to get out there and extend ourselves. And to do that, well, we need to be able to extend—especially those big toes! Looking after your feet, keeping them strong and mobile, and making good shoe choices will stand you in good stead to stride out—literally striding out to make good use of those ranges of motion—and ensure you can cross roads safely, well into your latter years.

To give Dr. Morton the final word, '*There is nothing of a haphazard nature in the pattern of the human foot.*' (*Human Locomotion and Form*, 1963, pg. 28.)

Each portion of the foot, each tissue, every ligament and tendon passing along bony grooves, has developed for a reason. Balancing many, often opposing demands, the human foot is remarkable, and it is '*a total biotic complex*' that deserves time and attention to understand and appreciate.

Thankfully, as we move ourselves from the tight boundaries of binary thinking, whether it is in society's questioning the concepts of race and gender, or the simplistic approach to muscle action, I hope to have expanded our ability to splash around with the complexity and multi-dimensionality that true anatomy requires of us.

There is much to consider in this short text, and I hope, like any book worth writing, it will also be worth re-reading.

---

[3]Why are your feet your best friends? Because…wait for it…they *understand* you!

RESOURCES

▦ EDUCATION

James Earls & Owen Lewis, Born to Move	borntomove.com
Lucy Wintle	canterburypilates.co.uk
Animatum	animatum.co.uk
Gait Happens	gaithappens.com
Tom Michaud and Human Locomotion	humanlocomotion.com
Dr. Emily Splichal & Barefoot Strong	ebfaglobal.com

▦ PRODUCTS

Correct Toes	correcttoes.com
Mobo Boards	moboboard.com
Sensory Enhancement Soles and Workout Mats	naboso.com

▦ ALTERNATIVE FOOTWEAR

Xero Shoes	xeroshoes.com
Lems	lemsshoes.com
DaVinci Shoes	davincifootwear.com
Feel Grounds	feelgrounds.com
Carets	carets.com
Vivobarefoot	vivobarefoot.com

REFERENCES

Abdalbary, S., E. Elshaarawy, and B. Khalid. 2016. "Tensile Properties of the Deep Transverse Metatarsal Ligament in Hallux Valgus." *Medicine* 95 (8): 2843.

Abitbol, M. 1988. "Effect of Posture and Locomotion on Energy Expenditure." *American Journal of Physical Anthropology* 77 (2): 191–199.

Adstrum, S., G. Hedley, R. Schleip, C. Stecco, and C. Yucesoy. 2017. "Defining the Fascial System." *Journal of Bodywork and Movement Therapies* 21 (1): 173–177.

Aiello, L., C. Dean, and J. Cameron. 2002. *An Introduction to Human Evolutionary Anatomy.* 1st edn. London: Academic Press.

Aiello, L., and J. Wells. 2002. "Energetics and the Evolution of the Genus HOMO." *Annual Review of Anthropology* 31: 323–338.

Asher, L., M. Aresu, E. Falaschetti, and J. Mindell. 2012. "Most Older Pedestrians are Unable to Cross the Road in Time: A Cross-sectional Study." *Age and Ageing* 41 (5): 690–694.

Barak, M., D. Lieberman, and J. Hublin. 2011. "A Wolff in Sheep's Clothing: Trabecular Bone Adaptation in Response to Changes in Joint Loading Orientation." *Bone* 49 (6): 1141–1151.

Barnish, M., H. Morgan, and J. Barnish. 2017. "The 2016 HIGh Heels: Health effects And psychosexual BenefITS (HIGH HABITS) study: Systematic Review of Reviews and Additional Primary Studies." *BMC Public Health* 18: 37.

Batson, E., G. Reilly, J. Currey, and D. Balderson. 2010. "Postexercise and Positional Variation in Mechanical Properties of the Radius in Young Horses." *Equine Veterinary Journal* 32 (2): 95–100.

Benzie, S. 2020. *Lost Art of Running.* London: Bloomsbury Sport.

Biel, A., and R. Dorn. 2015. *Trail Guide to the Body.* 5th edn. Boulder: Books of Discovery.

Bramble, D., and D. Lieberman. 2004. "Endurance Running and the Evolution of *Homo.*" *Nature* 432 (7015): 345–352.

Brockett, C., and G. Chapman. 2016. "Biomechanics of the Ankle." *Orthopaedics and Trauma* 30 (3): 232–238.

Carter, D., and G. Beaupré. 2001. *Skeletal Function and Form.* Cambridge: Cambridge University Press.

Chen, C., and D. Ingber. 1999. "Tensegrity and Mechanoregulation: From Skeleton to Cytoskeleton." *Osteoarthritis and Cartilage* 7 (1): 81–94.

Clarke, R., and P. Tobias. 1995. "Sterkfontein Member 2 Foot Bones of the Oldest South African Hominid." *Science* 269 (5223): 521–524.

Cowgill, L., A. Warrener, H. Pontzer, and C. Ocobock. 2010. "Waddling and Toddling: The

Biomechanical Effects of an Immature Gait." *American Journal of Physical Anthropology* 143 (1): 52–61.

Coyne, J. 2014. *Why Evolution Is True*. New York: Penguin Books.

Crompton, R., E. Vereecke, and S. Thorpe. 2008. "Locomotion and Posture from the Common Hominoid Ancestor to Fully Modern Hominins, with Special Reference to the Last Ccommon Panin/Hominin Ancestor." *Journal of Anatomy* 212 (4): 501–543.

Currey, J. 2013. *Bones*. Princeton: Princeton University Press.

Dalmau-Pastor, M., B. Fargues-Polo, D. Casanova-Martínez, J. Vega, and P. Golanó. 2014. "Anatomy of the Triceps Surae." *Foot and Ankle Clinics* 19 (4): 603–635.

Darwin, C. 1872. *The Origin of Species By Means of Natural Selection*. 6th edn. London: John Murray.

DeSilva, J., E. McNutt, J. Benoit, and B. Zipfel. 2018. "One Small Step: A Review of Plio-Pleistocene Hominin Foot Evolution." *American Journal of Physical Anthropology* 168 (S67): 63–140.

Duda, G., M. Heller, J. Albinger, O. Schulz, E. Schneider, and L. Claes. 1998. "Influence of Muscle Forces on Femoral Strain Distribution." *Journal of Biomechanics* 31 (9): 841–846.

Earls, J. 2020. *Born to Walk*. Nutbourne: Lotus Publishing.

Ellis, T. 1889. *The Human Foot – Its Form and Structure, Functions and Clothing*. 1st edn. London: Churchill.

Farris, D., and B. Raiteri. 2017a. "Elastic Ankle Muscle–Tendon Interactions are Adjusted to Produce Acceleration During Walking in Humans." *The Journal of Experimental Biology* 220 (22): 4252–4260.

Farris, D., and B. Raiteri. 2017b. "Modulation of Leg Joint Function to Produce Emulated Acceleration During Walking and Running in Humans." *Royal Society Open Science* 4 (3): 160901.

Farris, D., J. Birch, and L. Kelly. 2020. "Foot Stiffening During the Push-off Phase of Human Walking is Linked to Active Muscle Contraction, and not the Windlass Mechanism." *Journal of The Royal Society Interface* 17 (168): 20200208.

Fede, C., C. Pirri, C. Fan, G. Albertin, A. Porzionato, V. Macchi, R. De Caro, and C. Stecco. 2019. "Sensitivity of the Fasciae to Sex Hormone Levels: Modulation of Collagen-I, Collagen-III and Fibrillin Production." *PLOS ONE* 14 (9): e0223195.

Fleagle, J. 2013. *Primate Adaptation and Evolution*. 3rd edn. Edinburgh: Elsevier.

Foster, A., D. Raichlen, and H. Pontzer. 2013. "Muscle Force Production During Bent–Knee, Bent–Hip Walking in Humans." *Journal of Human Evolution* 65 (3): 294–302.

Franklin, S., M. Grey, N. Heneghan, L. Bowen, and F-X. Li. 2015. "Barefoot vs Common Footwear: A Systematic Review of the Kinematic, Kinetic and Muscle Activity Differences During Walking." *Gait & Posture* 42 (3): 230–239.

Fukunaga, T., K. Kubo, Y. Kawakami, S. Fukashiro, H. Kanehisa, and C. Maganaris. 2001. "*In Vivo* Behaviour of Human Muscle Tendon During Walking." *Proceedings of the Royal Society of London Series B: Biological Sciences* 268 (1464): 229–233.

Galway–Witham, J., and C. Stringer. 2018. "How did *Homo Sapiens* Evolve?" *Science* 360 (6395): 1296–1298.

Garfin, S., C. Tipton, S. Mubarak, S. Woo, A. Hargens, and W. Akeson. 1981. "Role of Fascia in Maintenance of Muscle Tension and Pressure." *Journal of Applied Physiology* 51 (2): 317–320.

Gosman, J., Z. Hubbell, C. Shaw, and T. Ryan. 2013. "Development of Cortical Bone Geometry in the Human Femoral and Tibial Diaphysis." *The Anatomical Record* 296 (5): 774–787.

Grant, R., and Grant, P. 1993. "Evolution of Darwin's finches caused by a rare climatic event. Proceedings of the Royal Society of London." *Series B: Biological Sciences* 251 (1331): 111–117.

Grant, P., and B. Grant, B. 2008. *How and Why Species Multiply*. 1st edn. Princeton: Princeton University Press.

Hallinan, J., W. Wang, M. Pathria, E. Smitaman, and B. Huang. 2019. "The Peroneus Longus Muscle and Tendon: a Review of its Anatomy and Pathology." *Skeletal Radiology* 48 (9): 1329–1344.

Hanna, T. 2004. *Somatics*. Cambridge, Mass.: Da Capo.

Hicks, J. 1955. "The Foot as a Support." *Cells Tissues Organs* 25 (1): 34–45.

Hicks, J. 1956. "The Mechanics of the Foot, IV." *Cells Tissues Organs* 27 (3): 180–192.

Holowka, N., and D. Lieberman. 2018. "Rethinking the Evolution of the Human Foot: Insights from Experimental Research." *The Journal of Experimental Biology* 221 (17): jeb174425.

Holowka, N., I. Wallace, and D. Lieberman. 2018. "Foot Strength and Stiffness are Related to Footwear Use in a Comparison of Minimally- vs. Conventionally-Shod Populations." *Scientific Reports* 8 (1): 3679.

Holowka, N., Wynands, B., Drechsel, T., Yegian, A., Tobolsky, V., Okutoyi, P., Mang'eni Ojiambo, R., Haile, D., Sigei, T., Zippenfennig, C., Milani, T. and Lieberman, D. 2019. Foot Callus Thickness Does Not Trade Off Protection for Tactile Sensitivity During Walking. *Nature*, 571(7764): 261–264.

Hoskins, T. 2020. *Footwork: What Your Shoes Are Doing to the World*. 1st ed. London: Weidenfield & Nicolson.

Huijing, P., H. Maas, and G. Baan. 2003. "Compartmental Fasciotomy and Isolating a Muscle from Neighboring Muscles Interfere with Myofascial Force Transmission within the Rat Anterior Crural Compartment." *Journal of Morphology* 256 (3): 306–321.

Hutchison, M. 2018. "Can Foot Exercises and Barefoot Weight Bearing Improve Foot Function in Participants with Flat Feet?" *Orthopedic Research Online Journal* 3 (4): 000567.

Ishikawa, M., J. Pakaslahti, and P. Komi. 2007. "Medial Gastrocnemius Muscle Behavior During Human Running and Walking." *Gait & Posture* 25 (3): 380–384.

Jones, F. 1944. *Structure and Function as Seen in the Foot*. 1st edn. Baltimore: Williams & Wilkins.

Kapandji, I., L. Honoré, and R. Tubiana. 2019. *The Physiology of the Joints*. 7th edn. Edinburgh: Handspring.

Kidd, R., P. O'Higgins, and C. Oxnard. 1996. "The OH8 Foot: A Reappraisal of the Functional Morphology of the Hindfoot Utilizing a Multivariate Analysis." *Journal of Human Evolution* 31 (3): 269–291.

Kim, P., Richey, J., Wissman, L. and Steinberg, J. 2010. The Variability of the Achilles Tendon Insertion: A Cadaveric Examination. *The Journal of Foot and Ankle Surgery*, 49(5): 417–420.

Kurihara, T., J. Yamauchi, M. Otsuka, N. Tottori, T. Hashimoto, and T. Isaka. 2014. "Maximum Toe Flexor Muscle Strength and Quantitative Analysis of Human Plantar Intrinsic and Extrinsic Muscles by a Magnetic Resonance Imaging Technique." *Journal of Foot and Ankle Research* 7 (1): 26.

Lai, A., A. Schache, N. Brown, and M. Pandy. 2016. "Human Ankle Plantar Flexor Muscle-Tendon Mechanics and Energetics During Maximum Acceleration Sprinting." *Journal of The Royal Society Interface* 13 (121): 20160391.

Lewis, O. 1989. *Functional Morphology of the Evolving Hand and Foot*. Oxford: Clarendon VIII.

Lidstone, D., H. van Werkhoven, A. Needle, P. Rice, and J. McBride. 2018. "Gastrocnemius Fascicle and Achilles Tendon Length at the End of the Eccentric Phase in a Single and Multiple Countermovement Hop." *Journal of Electromyography and Kinesiology* 38: 175–181.

Lieber, R., and S. Ward. 2011. "Skeletal Muscle Design to Meet Functional Demands." *Philosophical Transactions of the Royal Society B: Biological Sciences* 366 (1570): 1466–1476.

Lieberman, D. 1997. "Making Behavioral and Phylogenetic Inferences from Hominid Fossils: Considering the Developmental Influence of Mechanical Forces." *Annual Review of Anthropology* 26 (1): 185–210.

Lieberman, D. 2014. *The Story of the Human Body*. 1st edn. Vintage.

Lutz, F., R. Mastel, M. Runge, F. Stief, A. Schmidt, A. Meurer, and H. Witte. 2016. "Calculation of Muscle Forces During Normal Gait Under Consideration of Femoral Bending Moments." *Medical Engineering & Physics* 38 (9): 1008–1015.

McDougall, C. 2009. *Born to Run*. New York: Random House.

McKenzie, J. 1955. "The Foot as a Half-Dome." *British Medical Journal* 1 (4921): 1068–1069.

McKeon, P., J. Hertel, D. Bramble, and I. Davis, I. 2014. "The Foot Core System: A New Paradigm for Understanding Intrinsic Foot Muscle Function." *British Journal of Sports Medicine* 49 (5): 290–290.

Medical Massage Therapy. 2020. *Range of Motion*. [online] Available at: <https://www.massagetherapyreference.com/range–of–motion/> [Accessed 3 December 2020].

Michaud, T. 2021. *Injury-Free Running: Your Illustrated Guide to Biomechanics, Gait Analysis, and Injury Prevention*. Chichester: Lotus Publishing.

Mickle, K., C. Nester, G. Crofts, and J. Steele. 2012. "Reliability of Ultrasound to Measure Morphology of the Toe Flexor Muscles." *Journal of Foot and Ankle Research* 5 (S1).

Miller, E., Whitcome, K., Lieberman, D., Norton, H. and Dyer, R. 2014. "The Effect of Minimal Shoes On Arch Structure and Intrinsic Foot Muscle Strength." *Journal of Sport and Health Science* 3(2): 74–85.

Morton, D., and D. Fuller. 1952. *Human Locomotion and Body Form*. Baltimore: Williams & Wilkins.

Morton, D. 1922. "Evolution of the Human Foot." *American Journal of Physical Anthropology* 5 (4): 305–336.

Morton, D. 1935. *The Human Foot*. New York: Columbia University Press.

Nash, L., M. Phillips, H. Nicholson, R. Barnett, and M. Zhang. 2004. "Skin Ligaments: Regional Distribution and Variation in Morphology." *Clinical Anatomy* 17 (4): 287–293.

Navarrete, A., C. van Schaik, and K. Isler. 2011. "Energetics and the Evolution of Human Brain size." *Nature* 480 (7375): 91–93.

Nigg, B. 2010. *Biomechanics of Sport Shoes*. Calgary, Alta: University of Calgary.

Olewnik, Ł. 2019. "A proposal for a new classification for the tendon of insertion of tibialis posterior." *Clinical Anatomy* 32 (4): 557–565.

Olewnik, Ł., M. Podgórski, M. Polguj, and M. Topol. 2019. "A Cadaveric and Sonographic Study of the Morphology of the Tibialis Anterior Tendon – a Proposal for a New Classification." *Journal of Foot and Ankle Research* 12 (9).

Olson, M., T. Lockhart, and A. Lieberman. 2019. "Motor Learning Deficits in Parkinson's Disease (PD) and Their Effect on Training Response in Gait and Balance: A Narrative Review." *Frontiers in Neurology* 10: 62.

O'Mara, S. 2019. *In Praise of Walking*. London: Bodley Head.

Pablos, A. 2015. "The Foot in the Homo Fossil Record." *Mitteilungen derGesellschaft für Urgeschichte* 24 (11): 11–28.

Page, P., C. Frank, and R. Lardner. 2014. *Assessment and Treatment of Muscle Imbalance*. Champaign, IL: Human Kinetics.

Perry, J., and J. Burnfield. 2010. *Gait Analysis*. Canada: Trafford.

Physiopedia. 2020. *Navicular Drop Test*. [online] Available at: <https://www.physio–pedia.com/Navicular_Drop_Test> [Accessed 2 December 2020].

Pontzer, H. 2017. "Economy and Endurance in Human Evolution." *Current Biology* 27 (12): R613–R621.

Pretterklieber, B. 2018. "Morphological Characteristics and Variations of the Human Quadratus Plantae Muscle." *Annals of Anatomy: Anatomischer Anzeiger* 216: 9–22.

Rajakulasingam, R., J. Murphy, H. Panchal, S. James, and R. Botchu. 2019. "Master Knot of Henry Revisited: a Radiologist's Perspective on MRI." *Clinical Radiology* 74 (12): 972.e1–972.e8.

Reach, J., K. Amrami, J. Felmlee, D. Stanley, J. Alcorn, and N. Turner. 2007. "The Compartments of the Foot: A 3–Tesla Magnetic Resonance Imaging Study with Clinical Correlates for Needle Pressure Testing." *Foot & Ankle International* 28 (5): 584–594.

Rios Nascimento, S., R. Watanabe Costa, C. Ruiz, and N. Wafae. 2012. "Analysis on the Incidence of the Fibularis Quartus Muscle Using Magnetic Resonance Imaging." *Anatomy Research International* 2012: 485149.

Robbins, S., E. Waked, and J. McClaran. 1995. "Proprioception and Stability: Foot Position Awareness as a Function of Age and Footware." *Age and Ageing* 24 (1): 67–72.

Roberts, T., and E. Azizi. 2011. "Flexible Mechanisms: The Diverse Roles of Biological Springs in Vertebrate Movement." *Journal of Experimental Biology* 214 (3): 353–361.

Rodríguez-Sanz, D., N. Tovaruela-Carrión, D. López-López, P. Palomo-López, C. Romero-Morales, E. Navarro-Flores, and C. Calvo-Lobo. 2018.

"Foot Disorders in the Elderly: A Mini-Review." *Disease–a–Month* 64 (3): 64–91.

Rolian, C., D. Lieberman, J. Hamill, J. Scott, and W. Werbel. 2009. "Walking, Running and the Evolution of Short Toes in Humans." *Journal of Experimental Biology* 212 (5): 713–721.

Rubenson, J., N. Pires, H. Loi, G. Pinniger, and D. Shannon. 2012. "On the Ascent: The Soleus Operating Length is Conserved to the Ascending Limb of the Force-Length Curve Across Gait Mechanics in Humans." *Journal of Experimental Biology* 215 (20): 3539–3551.

Ruff, C., B. Holt, and E. Trinkaus. 2006. "Who's Afraid of the Big Bad Wolff?: "Wolff's law" and Bone Functional Adaptation." *American Journal of Physical Anthropology* 129 (4): 484–498.

Sawicki, G., C, Lewis, and D. Ferris. 2009. "It Pays to Have a Spring in Your Step." *Exercise and Sport Sciences Reviews* 37 (3): 130–138.

Shubin, N. 2014. *Your Inner Fish*. New York: Vintage Books.

Shubin, N. 2021. *Some Assembly Required*. London: Oneworld Publications.

Shubin, N., E. Daeschler, and F. Jenkins. 2014. "Pelvic Girdle and Fin of Tiktaalik Roseae." *Proceedings of the National Academy of Sciences* 111 (3): 893–899.

Sichting, F., N. Holowka, F. Ebrecht, and D. Lieberman. 2020. "Evolutionary Anatomy of the Plantar Aponeurosis in Primates, Including Humans." *Journal of Anatomy* 237 (1): 85–104.

Silder, A., B. Whittington, B. Heiderscheit, and D. Thelen. 2007. "Identification of Passive Elastic Joint Moment-Angle Relationships in the Lower Extremity." *Journal of Biomechanics* 40 (12): 2628–2635.

Singh, A., Zwirner, J., Templer, F., Kieser, D., Klima, S. and Hammer, N. 2021. On the Morphological Relations of the Achilles Tendon and Plantar Fascia via the Calcaneus: a Cadaveric Study. *Scientific Reports*, 11(1).

Snow, S., Bohne, W., DiCarlo, E. and Chang, V. 1995. Anatomy of the Achilles Tendon and Plantar Fascia in Relation to the Calcaneus in Various Age Groups. *Foot & Ankle International*, 16(7): 418–421.

Solórzano, S. 2020. *Everything Moves*. 1st edn. Edinburgh: Handspring.

Sorrentino, R., K. Carlson, E. Bortolini, C. Minghetti, F. Feletti, L. Fiorenza, S. Frost, T. Jashashvili, W. Parr, C. Shaw, A. Su, K. Turley, S. Wroe, T. Ryan, M. Belcastro, and S. Benazzi, 2020. "Morphometric Analysis of the Hominin Talus: Evolutionary and Functional Implications." *Journal of Human Evolution* 142: 102747.

Stainsby, G. 1997. "Pathological Anatomy and Dynamic Effect of the Displaced Plantar Plate and the Iimportance of the Integrity of the Plantar Plate-Deep Transverse Metatarsal Ligament Tie-Bar." *Annals of The Royal College of Surgeons of England* 79 (1): 58–68.

Standring, S. 2008. *Gray's Anatomy*. Edinburgh: Elsevier Health Sciences UK.

Stecco, C. 2015. *Functional Atlas of the Human Fascial System*. 1st edn. Edinburgh: Elsevier.

Stecco, C., V. Macchi, A. Porzionato, A. Morra, A. Parenti, A. Stecco, V. Delmas, and R. De Caro. 2010. "The Ankle Retinacula: Morphological Evidence of the Proprioceptive Role of the Fascial System." *Cells Tissues Organs* 192 (3): 200–210.

Taleb, N. 2013. *Anti-Fragile*. London: Allen Lane.

Tamer, P., and S. Simpson. 2017. "Evolutionary Medicine: Why do Humans get Bunions?" *Evolution, Medicine, and Public Health* 2017 (1): 48–49.

Thompson, D. 1968. *On Growth and Form*. Cambridge: Cambridge University Press.

Thorpe, S., R. Holder, and R. Crompton. 2007. "Origin of Human Bipedalism as an Adaptation for Locomotion on Flexible Branches." *Science* 316 (5829): 1328–1331.

Trinkaus, E., and H. Shang. 2008. "Anatomical Evidence for the Antiquity of Human Footwear: Tianyuan and Sunghir." *Journal of Archaeological Science* 35 (7): 1928–1933.

Tyrrell, J., S. Jones, R. Beaumont, C. Astley, R. Lovell, H. Yaghootkar, M. Tuke, K. Ruth, R. Freathy, J. Hirschhorn, A. Wood, A. Murray, M. Weedon, and T. Frayling. 2016. "Height, Body Mass Index, and Socioeconomic Status: Mendelian Randomisation Study in UK Biobank." *British Medical Journal* 352: i582.

van der Wal, J. 2009. "The Architecture of the Connective Tissue in the Musculoskeletal System – An Often Overlooked Functional Parameter as to Proprioception in the Locomotor Apparatus." *International Journal of Therapeutic Massage & Bodywork* 2 (4): 9–23.

van Wingerden, J., A. Vleeming, C. Snijders, and R. Stoeckart. 1993. "A Functional-Anatomical Approach to the Spine-Pelvis Mechanism: Interaction Between The Biceps Femoris Muscle and the Sacrotuberous Ligament." *European Spine Journal* 2 (3):140–144.

Venkadesan, M., A. Yawar, C. Eng, M. Dias, D. Singh, S. Tommasini, A. Haims, M. Bandi, and S. Mandre. 2020. "Stiffness of the Human Foot and Evolution of the Transverse Arch." *Nature* 579 (7797): 97–100.

Viseux, F. 2020. "The Sensory Role of the Sole of the Foot: Review and Update on Clinical Perspectives." *Neurophysiologie Clinique* 50 (1): 55–68.

Webber, J., and D, Raichlen. 2016. "The role of Plantigrady and Heel-Strike in the Mechanics and Energetics of Human Walking with Implications for the Evolution of the Human Foot." *The Journal of Experimental Biology* 219 (23): 3729–3737.

Whittington, B., A. Silder, B. Heiderscheit, and D. Thelen. 2008. "The Contribution of Passive-Elastic Mechanisms to Lower Extremity Joint Kinetics During Human Walking." *Gait & Posture* 27 (4): 628–634.

Wilson, A., and G. Lichtwark. 2011. "The Anatomical Arrangement of Muscle and Tendon Enhances Limb Versatility and Locomotor Performance." *Philosophical Transactions of the Royal Society B: Biological Sciences* 366 (1570): 1540–1553.

Wood Jones, F. 1944. *Structure and Function as Seen in the Foot*. 1st edn. Baltimore: Williams and Wilkins.

Yamauchi, J., and K. Koyama. 2019. "Force-Generating Capacity of the Toe Flexor Muscles and Dynamic Function of the Foot Arch in Upright Standing." *Journal of Anatomy* 234 (4): 515–522.

Yates, B., and L. Merriman. 2009. *Merriman's Assessment of the Lower Limb*. Edinburgh: Churchill Livingstone.

Yates, B. 2012. *Merriman's Assessment of the Lower Limb*. Edinburgh: Churchill Livingstone.

Yi, T., G. Lee, I. Seo, W. Huh, T. Yoon, and B. Kim. 2011. "Clinical Characteristics of the Causes of Plantar Heel Pain." *Annals of Rehabilitation Medicine* 35 (4): 507–513.

Young, N., T. Capellini, N. Roach, and Z. Alemseged. 2015. "Fossil Hominin Shoulders Support an African Ape-Like Last Common Ancestor of Humans and Chimpanzees." *Proceedings of the National Academy of Sciences* 112 (38): 11829–11834.

Zelik, K., V. La Scaleia, Y. Ivanenko, and F. Lacquaniti. 2014. "Coordination of Intrinsic and Extrinsic Foot Muscles During Walking." *European Journal of Applied Physiology* 115 (4): 691–701.

Zügel, M., C. Maganaris, J. Wilke, K. Jurkat-Rott, W. Klingler, S. Wearing, T. Findley, M. Barbe, J. Steinacker, A. Vleeming, W. Bloch, R. Schleip, and P. Hodges. 2018. "Fascial Tissue Research in Sports Medicine: From Molecules to Tissue Adaptation, Injury and Diagnostics: Consensus Statement." *British Journal of Sports Medicine* 52 (23): 1497.

Zwirner, J., Zhang, M., Ondruschka, B., Akita, K. and Hammer, N. 2020. An Ossifying Bridge – on the Structural Continuity Between the Achilles Tendon and the Plantar Fascia. *Scientific Reports*, 10(1).

INDEX

CONTRIBUTOR

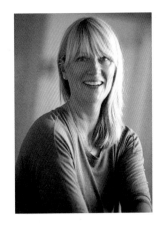

Lucy Wintle has been in the human movement business for over 20 years. She originally trained as a Pilates instructor with Body Control Pilates and owns and runs a busy studio in Canterbury, Kent, UK, where she teaches both mat and equipment-based sessions.

Her desire to deepen her functional anatomy understanding led her to study structural integration, and during this period she met James Earls. She now firmly believes that more attention needs to be paid to giving the skeletal structure the strong foundation that it deserves and often requires, enabling clients to improve their athletic performance, rehabilitation, and slowing down age-related postural tendencies. Foot strengths and weaknesses, general balance issues, and postural alignment are all key components in her teachings. Her loyal customers define her as part educator, part instructor and role model and speak about the lasting changes her classes bring to their bodies.

More recently, Lucy has developed her own brand, Hexology, which encourages clients to look at the broader picture of wellness and to engage in activities in the 'here and now' to promote active aging. The Hexology concept brings together her six essential elements for future health: Pilates, cardiovascular work, muscle mass, bone health, balance training, and general wellness.